Arthritis and You

Also by Naheed Ali

Understanding Alzheimer's: An Introduction for Patients and Caregivers

The Obesity Reality: A Comprehensive Approach to a Growing Problem

Diabetes and You: A Comprehensive, Holistic Approach

Arthritis and You

A Comprehensive Digest for Patients and Caregivers

Naheed Ali, MD

ROWMAN & LITTLEFIELD PUBLISHERS, INC.
Lanham • Boulder • New York • Toronto • Plymouth, UK

Published by Rowman & Littlefield Publishers, Inc.
A wholly owned subsidiary of The Rowman & Littlefield Publishing Group, Inc.
4501 Forbes Boulevard, Suite 200, Lanham, Maryland 20706
www.rowman.com

10 Thornbury Road, Plymouth PL6 7PP, United Kingdom

British Library Cataloguing in Publication Information Available

The hardback edition of this book was previously catalogued by the Library of Congress as follows:

Library of Congress Cataloging-in-Publication Data

Ali, Naheed, 1981–
Arthritis and you : a comprehensive digest for patients and caregivers / Naheed Ali, M.D.
pages cm
Includes bibliographical references and index.
ISBN 978-1-4422-1901-4 (cloth : alk. paper) -- ISBN 978-1-4422-1902-1 (pbk. : alk. paper) -- ISBN
978-1-4422-1903-8 (electronic)
1. Arthritis. I. Title.
RC933.A365 2013
616.7'22—dc23
2012044230

♾   The paper used in this publication meets the minimum requirements of American
National Standard for Information Sciences Permanence of Paper for Printed Library
Materials, ANSI/NISO Z39.48-1992.

Printed in the United States of America

Arthritis and You is dedicated to my students, to arthritis patients, and to all who have provided encouragement and support for my research.

Contents

Disclaimer

This book represents reference material only. It is not intended as a medical manual, and the data presented here are meant to assist the reader in making informed choices regarding wellness. This book is not a replacement for treatment(s) that the reader's personal physician may have suggested. If the reader believes he or she is experiencing a medical issue, professional medical help is recommended. Mention of particular products, companies, or authorities in this book does not entail endorsement by the publisher or author.

Preface

While the importance of being knowledgeable about a disease or condition as a patient or health-care professional is quite obvious,[1] the actual fact is that patients and their caregivers may desire additional information about the condition they deal with. Even in more sophisticated nations, health-care delivery systems find it increasingly difficult to involve their health-care providers in providing sufficient knowledge about a medical condition such as arthritis.

SIGNIFICANCE OF THIS BOOK

Worldwide, arthritis is one of the most prevalent diseases, affecting an estimated 350 million people and 50 percent of people over sixty years of age.[2] Patient education and its place in medical management of a chronic and debilitating or disabling condition such as arthritis are well documented and backed by extensive research.[3] In modern disease prevention and medical management programs, emphasis is placed on a patient-centered approach, also known as the biopsychosocial process of disease management.[4] The educated patient and well-informed caregiver serve as the most important players in this type of disease management.

As the reader will observe in forthcoming chapters, some types of arthritis tend to precipitate more frequently on the obese and physically less active individuals. In rheumatoid arthritis, though the disease cannot be predicted and there is no primary prevention, measurement of c-reactive proteins and rheumatoid factor may signal a future scenario to a certain extent. People who read and become informed about risk factors such as problematic proteins that predispose them to arthritis can take necessary steps to make lifestyle changes.

Arthritis education is to be seen as organized information, and quality, timely, and sufficiently detailed ideas mostly come as reading. Therefore, arthritis patients and their caregivers can have great leverage on the entire system that involves health-care providers, patients, families of patients, and communities they belong to through reading and becoming well informed. The arthritis patient's caregiver is susceptible to injury and other adverse effects due to his or her caregiving activities. Patients receive most of their health care from a family member who is not very knowledgeable about the disease.[5] That can adversely affect the arthritis sufferer's caregiving role as well. A well-informed caregiver will be important in providing optimal care while not getting affected. Relevant and comprehensive information acts as the catalyst of the arthritis patient, caregiver, and health-care provider interaction, making the whole process of patient management more efficient and effective and less stressful for all parties involved.[6]

Proper information and knowledge of a condition in the form of a book may lead to increased patient compliance. Poor patient compliance is a major health issue, especially in chronic and debilitating conditions such as arthritis that require long-term management and care.[7] When it comes to such a condition as arthritis, patient compliance is the patient's willingness and ability to (1) comply with health advice, (2) follow the prescribed medication regimen, (3) visit the physician as scheduled, and (4) go through the required investigations as planned. Patient compliance is also a major determinant of arthritic clinical outcome from a doctor's perspective. That said, learning about arthritis improves patient compliance to a degree that enhances the quality of patient-clinician interaction. The informed arthritis patient is a willing and enthusiastic partner in the doctor-patient relationship. The health-care provider finds it less frictional to engage in a productive and outcome-oriented discussion with well-informed patients and physicians. In the many disorders grouped together as the condition of arthritis, lifelong medication is indicated. Most of the drugs used to treat and maintain a reasonable lifestyle have adverse effects that can easily affect patient compliance. Noncompliance with a specified treatment regimen is a rare occurrence among well-informed patients, and a comprehensive book on arthritis such as *Arthritis and You* provides them with the essential insight that prescription medicine is a balance between the adverse effects of the drugs and the outcome of the natural progress of the disease. Further, an informed caregiver can be a facilitator in the process and an effective agent against patient noncompliance.

Clinical investigations such as those cited throughout this book can reveal many aspects of the condition that a mere clinical examination may lack. Arthritis victims are willing and ready go through the scheduled investigations only if they know their importance and relevance. Patients look to a visit to a doctor with a sense of deep apprehension. Fear of doctors, or iatrophobia, is common among patients who have little knowledge about their conditions.[8] They fear all kinds of interactions with physicians, and most of the time they postpone all doctor visits until the condition becomes worse, needing unpleasant and complicated interventions. An informed arthritis patient knows fully well about the possible outcomes of visits to the doctor, and interacting with the doctor makes the former less anxious.

People with arthritis need to follow a regular schedule of clinical appointments in order to get a proper assessment of the progress of the disease, their response to treatments, and the impact of the disease on the patient's physical and psychological well-being. Only patients who know in detail about their disease will realize the value of keeping to the schedule. They will inform their doctor in a timely fashion of any new significant symptoms and adverse drug reactions. They will negotiate with the doctor before they decide to stop taking a certain medication due to its unpleasant side effects. In many chronic and progressive conditions, including arthritis, the aim is to educate the patient to achieve the best possible quality of life and minimize suffering. In achieving this goal, patients are required to follow a self-management process that involves making decisions. In essence, they are their own problem solvers and need thorough knowledge about how to cope with an ever-changing situation. Self-efficacy is the measure of self-management. It is only with an ongoing and thorough educational program that patients can be properly assisted in self-care and management. Arthritis, as the leading cause of disability in the United States,[9] undoubtedly has a critical impact on the patient's health-related lifestyle. The patient needs a positive perception about living with arthritis and playing his or her role as a member of society. Information will empower the patient, and such a patient can develop a positive attitude toward living with the disease. Pain and stiffness associated with the disease can cause depression, which is prevalent among arthritis patients. Advancing disease causes limited mobility and more "unhealthy days." Well-informed patients are less depressed and feel that they can have a positive impact. Patient satisfaction is an outcome of quality communication with the health-care provider. An arthritis patient who feels that he or she receives the best possible care from his or her providers makes him or her satisfied. In order to know that optimal care is provided, the patient needs to have well-rounded information on the disease itself and the best available treatment and management modalities. The impact of comprehensive health education on reducing health-care costs is well established by research.[10] Arthritis sufferers who are educated demand less of the health-care delivery system. Patients such as those diagnosed with arthritis who are on regular treatment can make necessary lifestyle changes. These changes include a weight-reduction plan and physical exercise. As a long-term result, they may not lose as many workdays.

ARTHRITIS AT A GLANCE

Before moving on to the meat of this book, the reader should know that arthritis affects joints, bones, muscles, and related tissues to varying degrees. There are two major forms of this condition: osteoarthritis and rheumatoid arthritis. Nevertheless, *arthritis* is in fact an umbrella term that covers more than one hundred different disorders involving joints, bones, muscles, and surrounding soft tissues. Osteoarthritis is defined as inflammation of a joint that may lead to changes in the joint's structure. It causes pain and swelling. Rheumatoid arthritis, on the other hand, is a chronic disease that leads to crippling deformities.[11] Rheumatoid arthritis is defined, in more detail, as a chronic autoimmune disease leading to inflammation and deformity of the joints, accompanied by systemic problems affecting blood vessels and blood, lungs, and bones.[12]

There are numerous other disorders classified within the condition of arthritis that cause pain, swelling, stiffness, and limitations of joint movements. They all share certain characteristics. Most of them have no permanent treatment, and the best cause of action is to manage the disorders to optimize the well-being of the patient physically, psychologically, and socially. In many physical conditions, mobility gradually gets impaired. Likewise, in the long term arthritis can cause physical and psychological stress and even depression. Effective pain management, lifestyle changes, and social adaptations are necessary, and reading or writing about such topics certainly helps.

THE LEAD-IN

One common misleading view holds that there is no effective way to manage pain and joint stiffness associated with arthritis. Contrary to the common view, today there are many treatment modalities to ease the pain and stop or slow down joint destruction. Research has proven that surgeries, exercise programs, and other medical treatment options have helped arthritis patients to lead a near-normal, functional, and pain-free life.[13] However, a patient-centered management approach is the most effective of all options. In a patient-centered self-management approach, the arthritis victim is considered the most responsible partner in managing the disease. With the overall care and management of arthritis patients in mind, I hope to provide patients and their caregivers with information organized into a unique regimen. Furthermore, reviewing the ever-expanding problem of the condition in such a way will help to spot the people who are affected so they can be approached by caregivers and treated in a timely manner.

1

Groundwork

Chapter One

Introduction to Rheumatism

Arthritis is very complex because of the many arthritis-related conditions and, consequently, many different treatments for them.[1] Thus, neither the subject matter nor the methodology of the medical subspecialty concerned with these disorders can be defined without effort. This opening chapter attempts to make some clarifications with regard to the origins and evolution of the subspecialty focusing on arthritis and related disorders.

CONSTITUTING A SCIENCE: THE TWENTIETH CENTURY

Roots of Rheumatism

Not until the beginning of the twentieth century was a more systematic approach to arthritis and rheumatic diseases pursued, even though rheumatic diseases have almost certainly been around for ages. The first documented attempt to create a subspecialty concerned exclusively with arthritis-related disorders occurred at a 1925 medical conference in Paris where a Dutch doctor named Jan van Breeman lobbied for the creation of a special branch of the International Society of Medical Hydrology (ISMH) dedicated to the study of arthritis and its nature.[2] The International Committee on Rheumatism—considered the first organized practice of this kind—was founded later, and by the end of 1933, it had generated so much interest that it had to be transformed into a membership association. The American Committee for the Control of Rheumatism was instituted in 1928 and held its first formal meeting in Cleveland in June 1934. After many mergers and alterations, it finally became the American College of Rheumatology in 1988.[3] In the meantime, many different organizations of the same type were created around the world, and rheumatology became one of the fastest-evolving medical specialties of the twentieth century.

HISTORY OF RHEUMATISM AND ARTHROLOGY

Beginnings: From Hippocrates to Islamic Medicine

Interest in theory, even when incomplete and inconsistent, has long precluded systematic practice in the sciences. The informal existence of rheumatology dates back to the fourth century BC, when the Greek physician Hippocrates—widely considered the father of Western medicine—first posited the theory of humorism. It held that through the human body run four bodily fluids, or "humors," whose excess or deficiency influenced both man's temperament and his health. The excess of watery fluid believed to stream down from the brain was named *rheuma* (literally meaning "flowing"), a term widely used in ancient Greece. The terms *rheuma* and *catarrhos* ("flowing down") were used interchangeably to describe many of the illnesses now considered rheumatic.[4] Their clear symptomology, combined with Hippocrates' scrupulous observations and strong deductive powers, resulted in some of the first accurate descriptions of rheumatic diseases in history.[5]

Perhaps the rheumatic condition that he defines the best is gout (also known as podagra when it involves a big toe). Based exclusively on clinical observations, Hippocrates came up with three aphorisms cited in much modern literature covering gout: (1) gout never develops in men before puberty; (2) gout can never be seen in women before menopause; and (3) gout is not common in eunuchs. It is a remarkable accomplishment to have deduced these three axioms without the help of modern medicine, or without being aware of (1) the existence of uric acid and (2) the condition of hyperuricemia (abnormally high levels of uric acid in the blood, detectable after A. B. Garrod invented his renowned "thread test" in 1848).[6] In 1956, an ophthalmologist made a connection between a passage in Hippocrates's *Third Book of Endemic Disease* and what was identified in 1937 as Behçet's disease.[7] The ophthalmologist's only remark on Hippocrates' description concerns the prevalence of the disease, and although thought of as endemic by the latter, Behçet's has since become rare or sporadic.[8] However, it is now known that Behçet's disease (or syndrome) is quite common in Turkey and the Middle East, while being extremely rare in Western Europe and North America.[9] The third rheumatic disease described by Hippocrates was scleroderma, literally meaning "hard skin." Some speculate that his description may even be more accurate than originally thought, illustrating Reynolds syndrome, a rare form of scleroderma.[10] Moreover, different studies have proposed further hypotheses about Hippocrates' familiarity with rheumatic diseases. Rheumatic fever, hip osteoarthritis, sciatica, enteroarthritis, fibromyalgia, lupus erythematosus, and rheumatoid arthritis have all been proposed as possibly originally described by Hippocrates.[11] His description of rheumatic fever can almost certainly be found in his book *On Diseases*,[12] but it is nearly impossible to claim that his description of a form of arthritis manifesting around the age of thirty-five, in which there is an interval between the involvement of the hands versus the feet, is in fact rheumatoid arthritis. Scientists have been attempting for years to understand how a disease whose clinical signs are so evident has been mentioned so rarely in Europe up to the beginning of the nineteenth century. The condition has been frequently observed in skeletal remains of archaic Amerindians. One theory proposes it is a New World disease that achieved worldwide distribution when the Europeans discovered the American continent; another criticizes this assumption, claiming that rheumatoid arthritis also existed in pre-Columbian Europe.[13] Either way, if Hippocrates's description refers to rheumatoid arthritis, his version is possibly the only mention of this condition in Western medical literature for two millennia.

Hippocrates of Cos died around 370 BC, and in a sense, classical ancient Greece did as well, shortly after the civilization was ravaged by Philip II of Macedon and Alexander the Great. The decline of the Greek civilization meant also that the epicenter of medicine addressing the treatment of joint disease, among other types of maladies, transferred to Western Europe, where the Romans had started a new empire largely influenced by Greek culture. It is more than mere coincidence that Aelius Galenus—better known as Galen of Pergamon, an ethnic Greek—was Rome's most prominent physician and surgeon. Galen contributed significantly to the understanding of many scientific disciplines, and his authority remained almost unquestioned until Andreas Vesalius's *De Humani Corporis Fabrica*[14] of 1543 and William Harvey's *De Motu Cordis*,[15] published less than a hundred years later. The demise of the Western Roman Empire in the fifth century meant also a discontinuation of the evolution of medical sciences related to arthritis, though they persisted uninterrupted in the Eastern Roman Empire (Byzantium), albeit without any breakthroughs worth mentioning. Somewhere around the second half of the eighth century, books by Hippocrates and Galen, as well as the ancient Indian surgeon Suśruta's *Samhitā*,[16] were translated into Arabic. Islamic physicians were basically given an opportunity to advance further with medical research. Completed in 1025, *The Cannon of Medicine*,[17] a medical encyclopedia in five books collected by Ibn Sina (better known by his Latinized name, Avicenna), offered a categorized summary of all the available medical knowledge on what is now known as rheumatology and arthrology. The first part of Sina's *Book One* refers to Hippocrates' (as well as Galen's) theory of the four temperaments, which involved all of the following:[18]

- Moral positions
- Intellectual capacities
- Emotional features
- Movement
- Self-awareness
- Dreams

A polymath of Avicenna's rank, as well as one of the foremost physicians of his time, Muhammad ibn Zakariya Razi (known as Razi or Rhazes by way of the Latinists of the Middle Ages) was among the first to use the theory of humorism to distinguish contagious diseases from each other. At least one anecdote of dubious verifiability links him to a notable insight into the nature of arthritis. After being called upon to treat a famous caliph who had a severe form of arthritis, Razi advised him to take a hot bath. While the caliph was bathing, Razi, producing a knife, threatened to kill him. This purposeful provocation allegedly increased a natural caloric, then believed to dissolve the humors causing rheumatic pain. The caliph stood up and started running after Razi,[19] thus illustrating once again the theory of humorism in medical praxis.

From the Middle Ages to Scientific Breakthroughs

Any joint ailment was referred to as *gout* in thirteenth-century Europe; the term—in combination with *gouty diathesis*—was used almost as broadly as the word *arthritis* is used today. Gout derives from the Latin word *gutta*, and its meaning—"a drop" of liquid—ought to have conveyed the idea of a morbid material or noxious humor's "dropping" (falling drop by drop) from the blood into the joints.[20] It is a further testimony to the all-pervasive Hippocratic-Galenic medical legacy in Europe, another indicator of the extent to which the theory of humorism dominated medicine during the Middle Ages.

Holy Circumstances

A Dominican monk named Randolphus of Bocking was the first person to use the word *gout* to describe what had before been called *podagra* (from *pous* meaning "foot" and *agra* meaning "prey"). The term refers to a foot trap, a disorder of the feet. Podagra is used interchangeably with *gonagra*, a disorder of the knees. Both are associated with more general arthritis[21] in a phrase that, interestingly enough, originally reads, "gutta quam podagram velartiticam vocant," or, roughly translated, "the gout called podagra or arthritis."[22] Both a clergyman and a keen observer, Randolphus did not have a particular sympathy for those suffering from gout, which was, in his time, misperceived as a more or less self-inflicted ailment that chiefly affected the upper classes. It was believed, and is now known to be a fact, [23] that diet is strongly related to gout, and overindulgence in food and wine is the primary cause. Only members of the aristocracy could afford such overindulgence. Thus, gout became famous as *morbus dominorum et dominus morborum*, meaning "the disease of kings and the king of diseases." [24] In addition to members of high society, ironically, many priests were frequent gout sufferers. In an age when sciences were censored and controlled by the church, huge advances in the field of what is now known as rheumatology were almost impossible. St. Gregory the Great, also remembered as Pope Gregory I, for example, attributed his own gout to God. He thought of it as a form of humiliation vested upon him due to his apparently unworthy and spiritually ungainly life. [25]

Owing first to this connection between rheumatic diseases and the upper classes and, second, to the apparently low mortality among gout sufferers, the disease gained prominence both in the Middle Ages and the periods that followed. For the latter reason, people were not unhappy to have gout in the thirteenth-century years of plague, famine, and war. For the former reason, people endured gout's exhaustive pains with a smile in the eighteenth and nineteenth centuries. Indeed, for a large part of history, gout was thought of as a welcomed prophylactic visitor among the diseased. Rheumatism patient and author of *Gulliver's Travels* Jonathan Swift, afflicted with gout, expressed it best in his satirical poem *Bec's Birthday*, in which he claims that if doctors were able to confine gout only to the distal parts of the body such as the feet, joy should be present, and life would be prolonged. [26]

Gilbert Sheldon, an archbishop of Canterbury under Charles II, was said to have offered £1,000 to any person who would infest him with gout, apparently to protect his health. A mere hundred years later, in a letter sent to Sir Horace Mann, Horace Walpole, the English eccentric, art historian, and writer, would further testify to the belief in gout's being a prophylactic. Walpole wrote that gout prevented other illnesses and was a better option than apoplexy, palsy, and even fever. [27] This conviction may be best illustrated by the fact that in eighteenth-century Georgian England, patients suffering from melancholy or consumption were frequently sent by their own physicians to the spas at Bath, Somerset. Then a popular spa town, Bath gave people hopes of acquiring gout and, in that way, expelling their other sicknesses. [28]

Drunken Roots

Due to its prevalence among politicians and socially powerful individuals at that time, gout became famous as a socially desirable disease. A comment in the *London Times* in 1900 satirically illuminates the social background of two prominent illnesses. While the common cold has more than deserved its name, the comment says that gout seems instantaneously to elevate the patient's social status.[29] A popular fable dating well back to the ninth century[30] shows that this attitude toward gout and its sufferers is much more ancient than one might be inclined to believe. It was first recorded in English in 1644 in Richard Hawes's medical handbook, perhaps in reference to Petrarch's short story "Aranea et Podagra."[31] The tale is about Monsieur Gout and a spider, his traveling companion. At one point during their adventures, Monsieur Gout is forced to lodge with a poor man while the spider weaves a web in a rich man's house. As they continue their journey, the two start a discussion about their respective accommodations from the day before. Monsieur Gout exclaims that his was the worst he's ever had. Shortly afterwards, the poor man started banging and thrashing his feet, and Monsieur Gout was unable to relax throughout the night. The spider complains of a different problem: no matter how many times he started building his house (the web), a maid would come with a broom and tear down his work, forcing him to start all over again. Upon agreeing about the hardships of their destinies, they decide to exchange places. They are so pleased with their respective new homes that they agree to take up permanent residence: the spider in poor men's houses and Monsieur Gout in rich men's chambers. The webs are left undisturbed in maidless homes, and Monsieur Gout is continuously entertained with warm pillows, soft cushions, hot broths, and a regular dose of sweet caudle.

Sweet caudle, a sugared alcoholic drink, was supposed to have medicinal properties, and its mention in the tale of Monsieur Gout and the spider as part of gout's treatment illustrates the double standard physicians held regarding alcohol. While immoderate consumption of alcoholic beverages was believed to be a main cause of rheumatic ailments, for centuries alcohol was most often prescribed as a cure, or at least a pain reliever, for gout.

Depending on the time and the place, it was falsely believed that while some types of alcohol would provoke gout, others could soothe it. Fortified wines such as port were usually among the former, especially during the epidemic of saturnine gout in eighteenth-century England. The dramatic rise in the number of gout sufferers coincided with the War of the Spanish Succession at the beginning of the eighteenth century, or more precisely, after 1703 when King Pedro II of Portugal decided to switch sides and ally with the British in light of the Methuen Treaty. More of a commercial than a military contract, as it is still known as the Port Wine Treaty, the agreement permitted Portugal to export its wines to Britain at only a third the tariff placed on French wines in exchange for a tax-free admittance of English woolen cloth to Europe's westernmost country. Port and other exquisite Portuguese wines were soon imported in Britain in unprecedented volumes. The problem was that port wine was subject to spoilage, and since ethanol is a well-known natural antiseptic, the shippers started adding brandy to it, thereby "fortifying" the wine, which was at the time stored in lead casks. Lead is soluble in alcohol, and the resultant poisoning causes a predisposition for rheumatic problems such as gout.[32]

Couch Solution

The breakout of the disease in Britain was probably intensified by physicians who regularly prescribed moderate doses of punch, whiskey, and beer to gout sufferers. It is highly unlikely that this had any beneficial therapeutic effect,[33] but it is indicative of the way preliminary, informal rheumatologists treated rheumatic diseases for long periods of history. Instead of grappling with the internal causes of the respective diseases (humorism did not present convincing methods of inhibiting the flow, or *rheuma*, of watery fluid), physicians sought reduction of the most obvious symptoms, such as redness, swelling, outward inflammation, and joint pain. This usually meant providing additional comfort, and the tale of Monsieur Gout and the spider belonged only to the realm of the fictional. To ameliorate the severe attacks of gout he suffered, King Philip II of Spain lived many days of his life either on a sort of movable couch with a horsehair mattress or on a sedan chair carried by several of his servants. He invented the "gout chairs" and approved them for commercial use. They were still in use more than a century after his death, and it is known that Benjamin Franklin, another famous rheumatism sufferer, came across one in Paris in the 1700s.[34]

Gerhardus Feltmann, a legal scholar from the Netherlands, suggested that gout sufferers were sexually more capable than those who did not have the disease, mainly because of the nurturing effect of bed rest on the reproductive organs. This was just another explanation of a well-known fact—an additional reason as to why gout was considered a blessing in disguise was its supposed aphrodisiac power. It was probably a misinterpretation caused by recurrent tales linking rheumatic disease with love goddesses. A famous Greco-Roman myth personified rheumatism, specifically gout, as the deity Podagra, son of Dionysus (Bacchus) and Aphrodite (Venus).[35] Hieronymus Cardanus's *Podagra Encomium* of 1562 implicitly refers to this myth to show that those restrained by gout are protected by the goddess of love and have increased prowess. In a further clarification of the believed phenomenon twenty years later, Michel de Montaigne's essay *Of Cripples* [36] attributes the gout sufferers' sexual energy to the misplacement of food, which, being unable to reach the damaged limbs, nourishes primarily the genital parts.[37] This is a paradigmatic example of the layman's approach taken for thousands of years by accomplished intellectuals in understanding rheumatism. Even the medical breakthroughs of the eighteenth and nineteenth centuries would be marred for many years by the anecdotal prehistory of rheumatism.

UNCOVERING OF A SCIENCE

Thomas Sydenham

Excluding ancient Egypt's polymath Imhotep and his supposed identification of gout as a distinct disorder three millennia before the advent of Christianity, Hippocrates of Cos may rightly be considered the father of rheumatism. However, a more recent pioneer of rheumatism is said to be Thomas Sydenham (1624–1689),[38] a London physician hailed in his time as the English Hippocrates.[39] Sydenham himself suffered from rheumatic disease and is credited with one of the best descriptions of gout pain. In a classical piece of medical writing, Sydenham repeats the old conviction that gouty patients are either old men or youths who have brought upon themselves a premature old age by overindulgence. He then goes on to describe a gout sufferer's after-midnight awakening. The pain is compared to that of dislocation, although—Sydenham adds—at times it feels as if cold water is poured over the painful region. The sleepless night is passed in torture as the pain is followed by chills, shivers, a little fever, and continuous turnings of the affected part, which, he says, is usually the great toe and very rarely the heel or the ankle. Sydenham has indebted medicine with a few lasting discoveries and is credited with first distinguishing acute from chronic, crippling arthritis, the former probably being rheumatic fever and the latter almost certainly what is now called rheumatoid arthritis.[40] Sydenham's *A Treatise on Gout and Dropsy*,[41] published in 1683 as *Tractatus de Podagra et Hydrope*, is a landmark of Hippocratic medicine, but it also proved the seminal text of modern rheumatism that would revive clinical interest and inspire further advancements in the field.

Leeuwenhoek and Others

In the 1670s, the inventor of the modern-day microscope, Antonie van Leeuwenhoek, became the first person to observe urate crystals,[42] the chemical composition of which was unknown at the time. Although unaware of the connection between these crystals and rheumatic pain, Leeuwenhoek gave an accurate description of their appearance when he likened them to chalk particles. However, his discovery did not contribute much to the progress of the study of rheumatism.[43] Noted physician, antiquarian, and rheumatism sufferer William Stuckeley would soon follow through to where Leeuwenhoek could not, and in 1734, he described the uric chemicals causing gout's pain.[44] The chemical identity of uric acid as a constituent of renal calculi (kidney stones) was first established by German-Swedish pharmaceutical chemist Carl Wilhelm Scheele in 1776, and twenty-one years later English chemist

William Hyde Wollaston found urate substances in a tophus from his own ear.[45]

Another Englishman finally identified the abnormal increase of uric acid in the blood as the cause of gout. In 1848, Sir Alfred Barring Garrod, who is also credited with coining the term *rheumatoid arthritis*,[46] described his celebrated thread test, a semiquantitive method used to measure the amount of uric acid in the serum of urine,[47] and eleven years later, in his remarkable *The Nature and Treatment of Gout and Rheumatic Gout*, he stated that deposited urate of soda is not the effect but the cause of gouty inflammation.[48] Researcher Max Freudweiler's demonstrations of (1) the manifestation of gouty arthritis precipitated by an intra-articular injection of tiny crystals of sodium urate, and (2) the formation of tophi as a result of a hypodermic injection of urate crystals experimentally proved Garrod's hypothesis.

D. J. McCarty and J. L. Hollander

The above experiments were pushed aside for more than fifty years until a seminal paper by D. J. McCarty and J. L. Hollander showed that the crystals from gout patients' synovial fluid are composed of monosodium urate.[49] McCarty and Hollander recommended synovial fluid analysis, a laboratory test exclusively used for the diagnosis of musculoskeletal diseases, in the early 1960s, when they introduced polarized light microscopy of synovial fluid as a way to identify urate and pyrophosphate crystals seen in rheumatism. Such a technique would soon be established as a definitive method for diagnosing rheumatism, and pseudogout. Since then, rheumatism papers have recommended the use of synovial fluid analysis in the diagnosis of any form of acute arthritis, as well as when there is doubt as to the real cause of chronic arthritis.[50]

WHAT A NAME CONTAINS

After a long period of the interchangeable use of *rheuma* and *catarrhos* as a way to describe many joint problems, French physician Guillaume de Baillou in the 1640s coined the term *rheumatism* and distinguished rheumatic diseases that affected the joints from those that caused *catarrh* (head colds, hay fever, sinusitis).[51] Today, the word *rheumatism* is sometimes characterized as an old-fashioned lay term used to describe aches and pains in and around the joints.[52] Nevertheless, it is still widely used, and the science that deals with arthritis and arthritis-related problems is simply called *rheumatology* Rheumatism is in fact almost an obsolete term since it means "state of the rheuma"—that is to say, state of the watery humor that causes joint-related problems. No alternative names for this science have been proposed thus far. *Arthrology* (from *arthron* , meaning "joint," and *logy* , meaning "study of") is a newer term referring to the science concerned with the anatomy, function, and dysfunction, as well as the treatment, of joints. Since rheumatic diseases are also diseases of the joints, there is a clear overlap between the subspecialties, which may lead at times to certain ambiguities. For example, arthrology is not the science dealing with arthritis but rather the much broader science dealing with joints in general.

Chapter Two

Understanding Bone and Joint Health

The medical science behind the understanding of bone and joint health, unlike philosophy and religion, cannot afford the luxury of speculation. Causality of bone and joint disease is the basic foundation of the scientific method. For instance, if an effect such as bone and joint pain cannot be presented experimentally as a regular consequence of a familiar cause, the phenomenon cannot be considered a scientifically studied event. This distinguishes medical facts from other facets of knowledge. When speaking of bone and joint health, the scientific method requires systematic observation, testing, and modification of original hypotheses in order to be objective and let reality speak for itself. Even if contested by reality, philosophical and religious concepts may still stand. Medical confirmation must not claim that something is true unless it has taken into account all the possible causes while repeatedly proving that some (or all) of them contribute to the occurrence of the studied phenomenon. The detailed causes of arthritis are discussed in a later chapter, but it is important now to look at how causality plays a crucial role in understanding the health of bones and joints.

MEDICAL AND PUBLIC HEALTH CARE

Unveiling the Differences

There are basically two types of care for bone and joint patients: medical and public health care.[1] Medicine has been concerned first and foremost with palliative and curative treatments for conditions such as arthritis. Public health, on the other hand, is almost exclusively concerned with the prevention and control of such diseases and disorders. To simplify, medicine is oriented toward either finding a cure for an existing medical condition (curative care) or relieving the suffering of patients (palliative care). Public health really encompasses preventive care and refers to the procedures taken to avert injuries or diseases rather than to ameliorate their symptoms or cure them. Medicine belongs to the postcausal, and public health to the precausal, state of a disease. Medicine is engaged in treating conditions such as those of the bones and joints. Public health involves educating and instructing the healthy. There is another important difference between medicine and public health: while the former focuses on the treatment of individuals, public health focuses on the evaluation and reduction of health problems in the population. A bone and joint physician needs to diagnose the problem using an individual's medical history and an array of diagnostic tests, such as blood screens or tissue samplings. The entire approach includes prescribing medicines, surgery, or rehabilitation. A public health professional needs surveys and disease registries in order to "diagnose" a growing health problem. Informal treatment includes developing programs and advocating for medical reforms, while educating the community on discovered bone and joint health problems to reduce their prevalence. Public health research programs emphasize epidemiology and social sciences in their efforts to determine risk factors pertaining to a large percentage of the population.[2]

Primary Prevention

Primary prevention (neither bone and joint illness nor disease is present) is the prevention readers might be most familiar with: it includes methods for preventing the disease itself. As far as infectious diseases of the bones and joints, such as reactive arthritis, are concerned, primary prevention means identifying the microorganisms causing the disease and then developing a vaccine that will help keep hosts from being infected, even when exposed to the microorganisms in the future. A famous example is the discovery and development of the first polio vaccine by Jonas Salk in 1955.[3]

Primary prevention of a chronic bone or joint condition is again related primarily to etiology, although in this case risk factors (not microorganisms) are to be identified. The intervention includes either pharmacologic treatment or a suggested lifestyle change, and in some cases both. Weight reduction, for example, shows success in the primary prevention of diabetes, whereas a regular treatment with antihypertensive drugs reduces the risk of coronary heart disease in men suffering from high blood pressure.[4] Prevention of Type 2 diabetes can be achieved through prophylactic use of metformin, even though lifestyle changes have proven more effective,[5] while hypertension can also be primarily prevented without the use of medications if effective lifestyle modifications, such as the following, are practiced regularly:[6]

- Consuming a diet rich in fruits and vegetables
- Reducing dietary sodium intake
- Lowering dietary saturated fat
- Limiting alcohol consumption
- Engaging in regular physical activity

Secondary Prevention

Secondary prevention of bone and joint conditions (illness is absent; disease is present) refers to the methods used to diagnose and treat a disease in its early stages. Detecting a disease in its preclinical, or silent, phase, when no visible symptoms can be observed, usually yields a great chance of preventing the unwanted consequences of the bone or joint disease, such as disability or death. An example that will further illustrate the definition is the use of mammography to detect breast cancer at a stage when early treatment can be initiated, thereby reducing breast-cancer-related deaths.[7]

Tertiary Prevention

Tertiary prevention (both illness and disease are present) may be safely considered in the realm of bone and joint health because it refers to the treatment of an already-clinical disease (a disease at a symptomatic stage) with the main objective being, again, the prevention of important consequences such as disability and death.[8] Tertiary prevention of a bone and joint problem covers measures aimed at maximizing the life quality of a patient after he or she has been diagnosed with a long-term disease or injury. A good example would be the elimination of offending allergens from the nearby surroundings of patients diagnosed with asthma.

Quaternary Prevention

Quaternary prevention (illness is present; disease is absent), a newer concept that is more ethical than medical in nature, refers to overdiagnosis and overtreatment of bone and joint diseases. The idea is to evade excessive interference by the health system to prevent unnecessary medical activity where possible. In accordance with this attitude, theorists and practitioners of quaternary prevention consider it foremost among all prevention levels since it enacts the principal precept of medical ethics: *primum non nocere*, or "first, do no harm."[9]

PUBLIC AWARENESS AND CONTRIBUTIONS
OF PUBLIC HEALTH

Importance

Understanding the importance of bone and joint health goes hand in hand with understanding any other form of health. An ounce of prevention is worth a pound of cure, regardless of the problem in question, and many diseases, including those of the bones and joints, have been carefully studied and shown to be consequences of recognizable causes and risk factors. Public health promotion programs that raise awareness of medical issues such as bone and joint conditions and stimulate regular examinations among the population have been a massive factor in reducing the overall prevalence of many ailments. More specifically, it is important for the field of medicine to discover a cure for bone and joint conditions.

Contributions of Public Health Initiatives

Perhaps people tend to forget public health's contributions to improvement in the general quality of life, but recent public opinion polls have shown that, at least in the United States, public health is highly valued. [10] Even when pertaining to bone and joint health, public health initiatives are not without cause. Specific health initiatives may have contributed to the increase in the lifespan of the population almost five times more than medical care has. Medical advances account for around five years of a thirty-year improvement in life expectancy, [11] which means that public health's prevention facets are responsible for almost twenty-five years. [12] Acknowledging public health and preventive medicine as factors affecting bone and joint health, the following sections highlight great public health achievements of the twentieth century. [13]

Vaccination

Population-wide vaccination programs have completely eradicated smallpox, a feat described as the greatest achievement in twentieth-century medicine. [14] Elimination of polio and control of diphtheria, measles, tetanus, rubella, and *Haemophilus influenzae* type B are also direct consequences of vaccination.

Motor Vehicle Safety

By advocating decreased drinking and increased use of safety belts, motorcycle helmets, and child-safety seats, public health promotion programs have largely curbed motor-vehicle-related deaths and, by extension, reduced injuries to bones and joints.

Control of Infectious Diseases

Infections such as cholera and typhoid have been diminished due to improved sanitation. Control of tuberculosis and sexually transmitted diseases has resulted from public health efforts to promote the development of antimicrobial therapies.

Decline in Deaths from Heart Disease

In a study conducted in Britain from 1981 to 2000, 79 percent of the increase in lifespan for people afflicted with coronary heart disease was ascribed to risk factor modifications such as blood pressure control and smoking cessation.[15] Death rates for coronary heart disease have decreased by more than half since 1972.

Safer and Healthier Foods

Nutrition-deficiency diseases such as pellagra, goiter, and the bone disorder rickets have been almost eliminated in the United States due to the identification of essential micronutrients and the establishment of food-fortification programs.

Recognition of Tobacco Use as a Health Hazard

A major report[16] had a lasting effect on worldwide awareness of the consequences of smoking, including the effects on bones and joints. Since then, health-promotion activists are working ceaselessly to prevent millions of smoking-related deaths around the world.

More Reasons for Public Health Initiatives

Even in ideal conditions, learning about any disorder, then eliminating all factors that can cause or worsen it, does not imply immunity from that disorder. Even the fittest athletes can die of cardiac arrest, and even the most adamant nonsmokers may develop lung cancer. However, choosing a suggested risk-free lifestyle drastically reduces the probability of developing problems related to bone and joint health. Despite public perception to the contrary, it has been estimated that only one athlete in three hundred thousand will die suddenly, with the majority of deaths related to a previously undiagnosed underlying cardiac condition.[17] Scarcely 10 to 15 percent of lung cancer sufferers are nonsmokers, with most cases easily attributed to exposure to substances including radon and asbestos, or to air pollution or secondhand smoke.[18] A healthy way of life may not only diminish the risks of developing a bone or joint disease but also increase the chances of curing it or accelerate the process of recovery, even in some cases if behavior modifications are pursued only after diagnosis. There is also a point of no return after which preventive medicine will be unable to help. Understanding certain bone and joint disorders and their risk factors, and complying with the suggestions provided by health organizations around the world, is the simplest way for any person to ensure a better future.

SOCIETY'S CHALLENGES

Bone and Joint Dilemma

As with many things in life, people undervalue the most valuable things they own, until one day they lose them irreversibly. Bones and joints are no exception. Patients and caregivers take them for granted until the pain starts. As a result, almost half of Americans over the age of eighteen, more than 48 percent, are afflicted with bone and joint conditions.[19] This makes bone and joint problems the most widespread cause of severe, enduring pain and physical disability around the world.[20] In fact, ailments of the musculoskeletal system are the second most common reason why patients visit doctors in most countries, accounting for up to 20 percent of primary care consultations.[21] These ailments include anything from broken bones, to bone and joint trauma caused by accidents, to back, hip, knee, or foot pain, to arthritis and osteoporosis.

From Words to Action

The Bone and Joint Decade, a global multidisciplinary initiative that aims to help people with bone and joint disorders, has been formally launched. In a statement, then secretary-general of the United Nations claimed that medicine has discovered effective ways to prevent and treat musculoskeletal diseases, providing reason enough to act as soon as possible. The program envisaged four long-term goals when initiated:[22]

- To raise awareness of musculoskeletal disorders as a growing burden on individuals and society
- To empower patients to participate in their own care
- To promote cost-effective prevention and treatment
- To advance the medical knowledge of musculoskeletal disorders through research in an attempt to improve prevention and treatment

The initiative's proposal, titled *Decade of the Bone and Joint*, was the culmination of the worldwide recognition of bone and joint disorders' impact on individuals and society.[23] It was also a warning statement about the public's increasing neglect of musculoskeletal health. Bone and joint health enables an active and healthy way of life. It is imperative for people of all ages to be aware of the existence of the most prevalent musculoskeletal diseases because lack of knowledge may result not only in painful and progressive illness but also in disability and death. After all, there are many musculoskeletal and rheumatic symptoms, disorders, and diseases. Musculoskeletal diseases alone account for more disabilities and more costs to the US healthcare system than any other medical problem.[24] Simple preventive procedures such as dietary modifications or lifestyle changes may reduce the risk and prevalence of many of these conditions significantly.

ON THE MATTER OF GOUT AND BACK PAIN

Dietary Origins

Gout, widely known today as a joint disorder, was virtually unknown for a long period of history in Asia. Traditional Asian diets are based on rice and vegetables and are low in dietary purines, which are directly related to gout and can be found in high concentrations in foods such as the following:

- Herring
- Sardines
- Mackerel
- Anchovies
- Scallops
- Red meat

European and American diets are usually high in both seafood and meat, with beer being the most widely consumed alcoholic beverage among Europeans.[25] Consequently, gout was much more widespread in the Western Hemisphere. During the last twenty years, however, the economic growth of China and other Asian countries has resulted in an expansion of the number of people pursuing a westernized diet, and this has caused an increase in the prevalence of gout around the world.[26] The Western diet pattern often leads to obesity and is implicitly responsible for the worsening of many bone- and joint-related diseases, especially osteoarthritis.[27] Obesity is the most significant risk factor for the development of osteoarthritis of the knee, the hand, and the hip and for osteoarthritis progression in the knee and the hip. For development of osteoarthritis of the knee and the hip, certain jobs and physically demanding activities are also well-known risk factors. Among them, farming really stands out.[28] It is highly unlikely, however, that farmers will consider lifestyle changes based on statistical information. Most of the population, in fact, avoids health advice and risks over- or underusing the bones and the joints. Diet in relation to arthritis will be discussed in further detail later.

Attribution

A lack of understanding of bone and joint disorders can lead sufferers to ignore pain endured at the onset of a disease. Lower-back pain, for instance, is a serious health and socioeconomic problem in Western countries, mainly because people tend to disregard the risk factors and even the pain itself when it first appears. Depending on the description, lower-back pain is defined as pain below the line of the twelfth rib and above the gluteal folds. More than 90 percent of low-back-pain cases are nonspecific, meaning the pain is not due to any suspected pathological cause.[29] Most of these cases are attributable either to strain or sprain of the muscles of the back or to an injured or torn ligament in the back due to hyperactivity of the muscles. An injury to one of the intervertebral discs (e.g., disc herniation or tear) is also a possibility. In all these cases, the one to blame is not the one suffering, despite the fact that low-back pain is associated with lack of physical fitness, excess body weight, smoking, and the strength level of abdominal and back muscles. Moreover, the expected occupational factors, such as heavy work, bending, twisting, lifting, pushing, and pulling, as well as psychological factors such as emotional instability, depression, or anxiety, have been suspected as possible causes. Though it is still a matter of debate, back pain may be directly related to job dissatisfaction.[30]

Understanding Back Pain as a Major Bone Issue

Lower-back pain is the main reason why Americans miss work and one of the most significant contributors to the worsening of the quality of life for a large, but hardly estimable, part of the population.[31] This is due to the lack of verified treatments and the fact that preventative activities are seemingly ineffectual once the pain (re)appears. The idea that exercise, for example, prevents recurrence of long-term pain has shown mixed results if the pain is prolonged for more than two weeks.[32] Bed rest and inactivity are considered counterproductive, and sufferers who prefer passivity usually aggravate their condition.[33] Of the patients suffering from low-back pain, 10 percent are absent from work for more than two months, and if that absence goes on for more than six months, more than half are likely never to return to work again.[34] This is just the beginning of a long series of socioeconomic problems associated with musculoskeletal diseases; thus, development of cost-effective treatments is a primary goal of the Bone and Joint Decade. Musculoskeletal conditions indeed account for more disability and for more costs to the US health-care system than any other disease.[35] They are also the most expensive disease category in the cost-of-illness study in Sweden, representing nearly a quarter of the total cost of illness, mainly due to indirect costs related to disability and morbidity. The direct cost for the use of health services as a result of musculoskeletal conditions totals 0.7 percent of the gross national product in the Netherlands, 1 percent in Canada, and 1.2 percent in the United States. The indirect costs (lost wages and productivity), as expected, were much greater, corresponding, for example, to over 2 percent of Canada's gross national product.[36]

GOALS AND ACCOMPLISHMENTS

As far as bone and joint diseases are concerned, especially during the last decade, preventive medicine is continually making advances, whether in the diagnosis or treatment of a disorder. For example, one primary arthritis prevention trial proved that a vaccine for the spirochetes (twisted bacteria) related to Lyme disease, which cause joint swelling, reduced the risk of getting the disease in endemic areas. Many musculoskeletal diseases are directly related to obesity and lack of exercise—most notably osteoarthritis—but although these have frequently been identified as serious risk factors, there is still no global primary prevention program that includes experimentally checked data. Musculoskeletal diseases are usually observed after the first symptoms appear, but secondary prevention has so far found many ways to detect arthritis-related problems during the asymptomatic phase. Screening for osteoporosis with dual-energy X-ray absorptiometry (DEXA) has been shown to reduce fracture rates and consequent disability by detecting the disease in its early stages and allowing for early treatment. The sooner the treatment ensues, the less severe the ultimate disability. This is true with many diseases, and musculoskeletal disorders are no exception. In fact, there is near certainty in the medical community that secondary prevention of rheumatoid arthritis will be very successful because of the effective medical treatments that limit joint destruction. The challenge is to develop a suitable screening test that will diagnose rheumatoid arthritis during its asymptomatic stage.[37]

Call to Action

Through leadership and involvement in the National Arthritis Action Plan, the National Committee on Quality Assurance and the Arthritis Foundation have tried to meet the everlasting challenge of promoting the health of people with and at risk for bone and joint problems such as arthritis. Depending on the program, long-term aims range from increasing public awareness of arthritis as a leading cause of disability and a public health problem of utmost importance, to preventing arthritis with early diagnosis and maximizing the number of healthy years, to increasing health-care-provider counseling about weight loss and exercise and reducing the impact of arthritis on employment. Major types of activities used to achieve these aims include epidemiology, surveillance and prevention research, education and communication, and policy development.

BASIC STRUCTURE OF HUMAN BONES AND JOINTS

The adult human skeleton consists of 206 bones. Newborns have up to 270,[38] because many of their bones harden or fuse as they grow. In infants there are four or five bones in the sacral region, which eventually form one sacrum, while the pubis, ischium, and ilium fuse into the pelvic girdle. Similarly, an adult human coccyx is formed through a gradual fusing of three to five bones in that same region.[39]

AGE- AND GENDER-RELATED SKELETAL DIFFERENCES

The pelvis and coccyx are significant for another reason: the differences in these two bones are the most prominent among the many differences that can be observed when male and female skeletons are compared. This is because of the process of childbirth. The female pelvis is more rounded and flatter. It is also proportionally larger in order to allow the passing of a fetus's head. Whereas a female's pelvis is about one hundred degrees in angle, a male's is about ninety degrees or less. The orientation of the coccyx differs as well. While the male's coccyx is typically oriented anteriorly (more or less), the coccyx of a female's pelvis—again, in order to leave more room for childbirth—is oriented differently.

Makeup Not Needed

The bone structures of the face and head also have distinctive female or male features. The earlier onset of puberty in women and subsequent shorter periods of growth produce size and shape differences most perceptible in the skull. Women's faces stop growing a few years earlier than men's, which results in differences that allow for gender identification of an adult human with great precision even in the absence of hair, other facial features, or enhancements, such as facial makeup.[40] Throughout history, however, these differences have been either understudied or radicalized, for the most part in favor of men. The female skeleton was considered either unfinished or deformed, either as a sign of natural female inferiority or as an indicator of women's childishness.[41] Although this latter view is almost a staple in the history of human ideas, it was not always perceived as derogatory. While the ancient world's figurative idols described in chapter 1 used the comparison as a disparaging comment on women's immaturity, nineteenth-century thinkers used the similarities in order to exemplify females' freshness, innocence, and youth in comparison with men's apparently distinct, corruptive nature.[42]

In any case, the differences between men's and women's adult skeletons enable gender identification even when remains are so fragmentary that complete bone dimensions are not preserved.[43] The gender of children, however, cannot be distinguished solely on the basis of observation and measurements of skeletons,[44] despite a few attempts to devise a methodology for accurately determining the gender of juvenile bones.[45] Interestingly, it is possible for archaeologists and forensic experts to determine not only the sex (the biological, genetically controlled category) but also the gender (the performance category, the cultural construct) of a human skeleton based on an analysis of the patterns of arthritis and bone health.[46]

SKELETAL STRUCTURE AND PURPOSE

Axial Skeleton

This area consists of eighty axial bones: twenty-nine in the head region and fifty-one in the trunk, or torso. The axial bones usually remain in place, with the important exception of the spinal column, so they are less susceptible to repetitive-motion disorders or overuse injuries. They are, however, apt to attain secondary infections as a result of viruses, bacteria, or allergens affecting the facial or sinus cavities.

- Head: The skull contains twenty-two bones (eight flat cranial bones and fourteen irregular facial bones) with the small, *U*-shaped hyoid bone at the base of the tongue and the six tiny middle ear bones, called ossicles, all comprising the twenty-nine bones of the head.
- Torso: There are fifty-one centrally located bones, mainly consisting of the vertebral column (twenty-six irregularly shaped bones of the spine) and the rib cage (twenty-four curved bones, divided into fourteen true, six false, and four floating ribs). The long, flat breastbone, called the sternum, is the fifty-first bone of the torso.

Appendicular Skeleton

This area consists of 126 bones (64 in the upper extremities and 62 in the lower). Due to this part of the skeleton's mobility, overuse syndromes and torn ligaments are common, as are bone breaks and sports injuries. Osteoporosis, osteoarthritis, and other degenerative bone and joint conditions usually affect the more mobile regions of the appendicular skeleton. The upper extremities include ten bones in the shoulder and arm, sixteen bones in the wrist, and thirty-eight bones in the hand. The lower extremities include ten hip and leg bones, fourteen anklebones, and thirty-eight foot bones.

Purpose of the Skeleton

In addition to being part of a highly complex musculoskeletal system that provides stability, form, and support for the body, the human skeleton also serves five major functions:

- Movement: Movement is coordinated by the nervous system and powered by the skeletal muscles. The bones and joints of the body provide the most important mechanics for movement.
- Protection: Almost all the vital organs are protected by the skeleton, with the skull protecting the brain, the eyes, and the inner ears. The rib cage, spine, and sternum protect the heart, the major blood vessels, and the lungs.
- Storage: Calcium can be stored in the bone matrix, while iron can be stored in the bone marrow. Thus, the skeleton is involved in both calcium and iron metabolism.
- Blood cell production: When fully developed, the bone marrow takes over the task of producing most of the blood cells for the organism. Hematopoiesis, or the formation of blood cellular components, takes place in the red marrow.
- Endocrine regulation: Osteocalcin, a hormone that bone cells release, contributes to the regulation of glucose (blood sugar) and fat deposition. It increases insulin secretion while boosting the number of insulin-producing cells and reduces the amount of stored fat. [47]

The next chapter examines these functions more closely; this chapter looks at the basic structure of the human bones and joints, as well as at the evolutionary changes that shaped them into the forms known today.

PHYSICAL AND INTELLECTUAL EVOLUTION OF THE HUMAN SKELETON

Bipedalism and Human Skeletal Changes

Humans are the only routinely bipedal mammals, although scientifically it would be also safe to say "animals" instead of "mammals." The beginnings of bipedalism can be traced back as far as 4 million years, [48] with bipedal specialization already found in *Australopithecus* fossils from around that period. [49] There are many different hypotheses for why and how bipedalism evolved in humans, with reasons ranging from Charles Darwin's original idea of men needing their hands for carrying and tool usage,[50] to adaptation for locomotion on flexible branches[51] and changes in habitat requiring a more elevated eye position (from jungle to savanna), to reduction of the amount of skin exposed to the sun.[52] More importantly, many alterations in the morphology of the human skeleton are direct consequences of the evolution of human bipedalism, including changes in the size, shape, and arrangement of some of the bones of the foot, hip, knee, skull, and vertebral column. Most of these alterations are due to the adaptive methods of weight transference, which are very much different in bipedal versus quadrupedal animals. The human foot evolved to be a platform supporting the entire weight of the body and stopped being a grasping structure, as it was in the early hominids. This is why humans have relatively small toes as well as a foot arch rather than flat feet.[53]

In order to support the greater amount of weight passing through them, modern humans' hip joints are larger than those of their quadrupedal ancestors. This has resulted in a closer connection between the vertebral column and the hip joint, which means a more stable base for trunk support during an upright walk.[54] The vertebral column itself has changed. In humans, it takes a backward bend in the upper region (also called the thoracic, consisting of twelve vertebrae) and a forward bend in the lower region (the lumbar area, consisting of five vertebrae). The bending helps people use less muscular effort to walk upright,[55] since without the curve, the body's gravitational center would not be located directly over the feet.[56] Resting on the vertebral column is the human skull. The foramen magnum (the "great hole," or the opening in the occipital bone, to which the spinal cord is attached) is located inferiorly under it which means that most of the head weight is put behind the spine. As a result, forehead muscles in humans are relieved of head-balancing tasks and are used only for facial expressions.[57] Human knee joints are enlarged in order to better support body weight, while the elongation of legs since the evolution of bipedalism changed how leg muscles function. A longer leg allowed the use of the typical swing of the limb, meaning humans had less need to use muscles again when advancing the other leg for the next step.[58] Moreover, humans have adapted their femurs, the bones of the thighs, to bipedalism. Not only are femurs perhaps the strongest bone in the human body, but—unlike apes' vertical femurs—they are also slightly angled, starting from the hip and ending with the knee. This brings humans' knees closer to each other and locates them directly under the body's center of gravity, resulting in minimum effort from the muscles to stand up straight.[59]

It is important to know that even though these modifications of the bones and joints have helped people dominate the animal kingdom, some features of the human skeleton are, more or less, faulty and badly adapted to bipedalism. Lower-back pain and pain in the knee joints are almost unavoidable consequences of these maladaptations, and arthritis became a problem only after hominids became bipedal. Some suppose that arthritis was even more prominent in prehistory, frequently referring to it as the most widespread ailment of prehistoric peoples.[60] Recent reports suggest that other bipedal animals, such as dinosaurs, may have suffered from arthritis similar to that found in humans.[61]

MEDICAL SCIENCE OF BONES

Classification

Bones are usually classified by size and shape. The shape of every bone provides information about its function and creation. For example, the previously mentioned femur ensures maximum strength with minimum mass due to its hollow cylindrical build, another skeletal change due to human bipedalism. Nevertheless, there are four different types of bones in the human body, although some consider the sesamoid bones to be part of a separate group. Here they are presented as a subtype of short bones.

Short Bones

Short bones are generally cube shaped and located in the wrist and ankle. They consist of a thin layer of compact bone that surrounds a spongy interior. Sesamoid bones, whose name is associated with their shape resembling a sesame seed, are an unusual type of short bone embedded in tendons. The kneecap and patella are examples of this type of bone. Sesamoid bones differ in size and number for different people.

Long Bones

Long bones are noticeably longer than they are wide. The majority of the bones in the limbs are made of compact bone with lesser amounts of marrow and spongy bone. The bones of the fingers and toes, contrary to those in the wrists and ankles, are categorized as long bones. This is mainly due to their internal structure since these bones are shorter than other long bones in the body.

Flat Bones

These bones are flattened, thin, and usually slightly curved. The cranial bones of the skull belong to this group, as do the ribs, the breastbone, and the shoulder blades. Flat bones consist of a layer of spongy bone pressed between two layers of compact bone.

Irregular Bones

These bones have a variety of shapes and thus cannot be included in any of the previous categories. Like short ones, irregular bones consist of a thin layer of compact bone surrounding a spongy interior. The vertebrae and hip bones are examples of irregular bones.

OSSEOUS BONE TISSUE

Osseous tissue is the major structural connective tissue of the body. This category of tissue forms the rigid part of the bone organs and consequently gives them a three-dimensional coral-like internal structure. There are two types of biologically identical osseous tissue, although both are microstructured differently. The first is compact osseous tissue, synonymous with cortical bone, which is strong, solid, and resistant to twisting. The second is spongy osseous tissue, synonymous with cancellous or trabecular bone, which is responsible for the bone's elastic strength. The term *cancellous* relates to the lattice-shaped spicules, which are needlelike structures, shaped like honeycomb, that compose the tissue. When compared to the compact bone, the spongy bone has a larger surface area, but it is also weaker, softer, less rigid, and less solid. First accurately illustrated by Crisóstomo Martinez,[62] the spongy bone is generally found at the ends of long bones, near joints, and inside the vertebral column. Where hematopoiesis occurs, spongy bone is intensely vascular and regularly contains red bone marrow.

The cortical bone eases the main functions of the bone, which are essentially (1) to support the whole body, (2) to provide protection for all vital organs except the intestines, (3) to give levers for movement, and (4) to accumulate and release chemical elements, primarily calcium. As the name indicates, cortical bone forms the cortex, or the external case, of most bones. The term is also linked to the second most important aspect of compact bones: their denseness. About 80 percent of the weight of a human skeleton may be attributed to the overall weight of the compact bone. The main anatomical and functional component of this type of bone is the osteon. Osteons are cylindrical formations that in cross-section resemble a cut tree trunk, with its concentric rings. They are normally quite a few millimeters long and have diameters of around one millimeter. Osteons are present in most mammals; they can be observed in several bird species as well.

OTHER BONE TISSUES

Marrow

Bone marrow is the spongy, soft, flexible tissue found inside the bone. It composes nearly 4 percent of humans' entire body mass, meaning that for an average adult body mass of sixty-five kilograms, bone marrow occupies almost three kilograms. The bone marrow in the large bones contains cells that generate new blood cells. The hematopoietic compartment, which is responsible for the formation of blood components, generates nearly 500 billion blood cells each day. [63]

There are two different types of bone marrow: red marrow (medulla ossiumrubra) and yellow marrow (medulla ossiumflava). The first consists mostly of hematopoietic tissue, and the second is mainly made up of adipose, or fat, tissue. The red marrow is where thrombocytes (or platelets), red blood cells, and the majority of white blood cells are produced. Both types of bone marrow include numerous blood vessels and capillaries. All bone marrow is red at birth but gradually changes to yellow until the amounts of yellow and red marrow are balanced. Red marrow is mostly found in the flat bones, such as the pelvis, cranium, sternum, scapulae, ribs, and vertebrae. It can also be found in the spongy substance at the epiphyseal ends of some long bones, such as the humerus and the femur. Yellow marrow is located within the medullary cavity, the empty interior in the middle fraction of a long bone. The yellow marrow works as an emergency reserve in case of severe blood loss. In such a case, the body converts yellow marrow into red to increase the production of the blood cells. The tissue of the bone marrow that is not directly involved in the primary function of hematopoiesis is called stroma. The largest part of the bone marrow, stroma is generated from the yellow bone marrow. Only small concentrations of stromal cells can be found in the red bone marrow. Bone marrow stroma is constituted by the following cells:

- Fibroblasts (reticular connective tissue)
- Osteoclasts
- Osteoblasts
- Adipocytes
- Macrophages
- Endothelial cells forming the sinusoids [64]

Macrophages contribute significantly to the production of red blood cells because they deliver iron for the production of hemoglobin.

Cartilage

Cartilage is a partially rigid connective tissue, more flexible and elastic but weaker when compared to bones. It plays a crucial role in the protection and amortization of the joints. Cartilage can be found in many areas throughout the body, such as the following:

- Joints between the bones
- Tip of the nose
- Outer part of the ear
- Rib cage
- Intervertebral discs
- Elbow
- Knee
- Ankle
- Bronchial tubes

Cartilage is composed of numerous specialized cells, scattered throughout a matrix of protein fibers surrounded with a gel-like ground substance rich in elastin fibers and protoglycan. The collagen fibers inside the matrix provide cartilage with its elastic strength. Cartilage flexibility is attributed to distensible fibers and variations in the type and quantity of ground substance elements, as well as water. The cells that produce the matrix of the cartilage are called chondroblasts. Chondrocytes, also known as mature chondroblasts, occupy small chambers in the matrix that are known as lacunae and ensure that the matrix remains healthy. Mature cartilage is avascular, meaning it is not penetrated by blood vessels; because of that, nutritive elements must circulate through the matrix. Cartilage has at least the following two vital functions in the body:[65]

- It provides support to the soft tissues. C-shaped hyaline cartilage rings in the trachea, for example, give support to the connective tissue and musculature of the tracheal wall. Fibrocartilage provides both flexibility and toughness to the pubic symphysis and intervertebral discs, while elastic cartilage supports the fleshy, outer part of the ear known as the auricle.
- It provides a model for the creation of nearly all of the bones in the body. Beginning in the embryonic period, cartilage serves as a gliding surface and a rough schematic form that is afterward replaced by bone tissue.

There are three types of cartilage: hyaline cartilage, elastic cartilage, and fibrocartilage.

Hyaline Cartilage

Hyaline cartilage looks similar to frosted glass and is the most common type of cartilage. Its primary function is to support the soft tissue. It has, however, other important functions, one of which is to create most of the fetal skeleton and serve as a model for most future bone growth. Hyaline cartilage is found in numerous areas of the body, such as the nose, the trachea, most of the larynx, and the articular ends of long bones.

Elastic Cartilage

Elastic cartilage has many elastic fibers in its matrix. It appears yellow when placed under a microscope lens and gets its color from the higher concentration of elastic fibers in its fresh sections. The chondrocytes of the elastic cartilage are almost identical to those of the hyaline cartilage. They are usually closely packed and surrounded by a small amount of extracellular matrix. The elastic fibers are denser and more highly branched in the central region of the extracellular matrix, where they form a kind of a network lattice around the chondrocytes. The epiglottis bends down to cover the opening of the larynx during swallowing and is made of elastic cartilage. The highly flexible cartilage in the external ear is also composed of elastic cartilage.

Fibrocartilage

Fibrocartilage is an unusual tissue resisting not only strong compression but also strong tension forces.[66] Its extracellular matrix has abundant coarse, visible fibers, which are organized as irregular bundles between large chondrocytes. There is a small amount of ground substance, and the chondrocytes are usually arranged in parallel rows. Fibrocartilage is a structural intermediate between dense regular connective tissue and hyaline cartilage. This form of cartilage is found in the pubic symphysis, the intervertebral discs, and the menisci, the C-shaped cartilage pads of the knee joint.

BASIC STRUCTURE AND FUNCTION OF JOINTS

Joints are fundamental components of the human body. It is safe to say that they make human movement possible. Without joints, the arthritis patient's body would just be a rigid structure of bones and would never be able to move. Joints hold the skeleton together and are responsible for its agility and flexibility. Joints, also called articulations, are usually defined as functional junctions between bones. Support and movement are the two most important functions of joints. Even though joints are the weakest parts of any skeleton, their structure allows them to resist tearing, crushing, and many other outward pressures that would force them out of alignment. Joints can be classified by either function or structure. The functional classification is based on the degree of movement that joints make possible. According to this classification, there are three types of joints in the human body:

- Synarthroses are immovable joints.
- Amphiarthroses are slightly movable joints. Together with synarthroses, amphiarthroses make the sturdiness of the axial skeleton possible.
- Diarthroses are freely movable joints that predominate in the limbs.

The most commonly used classification of joints is the structural,[67] focusing on the type of tissue that binds the bones at each junction and on the absence or presence of a joint cavity.[68] The structural classification will be used here for a better understanding of the nature of joints, divided structurally into three main groups: fibrous, cartilaginous, and synovial.

Fibrous Joints

The bones in the fibrous joints are connected by fibrous tissue, specifically dense regular connective tissue. A joint cavity is absent in this type of joint. Most fibrous joints are either immobile or only slightly mobile. There are three types of fibrous joints: sutures, syndesmoses, and gomphoses.

Sutures

The bones of suture joints (literally meaning "seams") are closely bound by a small amount of fibrous tissue. Sutures are found only between the skull bones, and their fibrous tissue is connected with the periosteum around these flat bones. The edges of the articulating bones at sutures are wavy and interlocking. Sutures' function is to weave the bones together and to allow growth so that the skull can develop with the brain during childhood. Infant skulls are incompletely developed, and several of the bones are connected by fontanels, the membranous areas that allow the skull to change shape slightly during childbirth. As the bones continue to grow, the fontanels close and are replaced by sutures. The fibrous tissue ossifies during middle age, and the skull bones fuse into each other. At this juncture, the joined sutures are called synostoses, or "bony junctions." The immobile nature of sutures works as a protective mechanism since the brain would be easily injured if movement of the cranial bones were a possibility.

Syndesmoses

The bones in syndesmoses are entirely connected by ligaments, the bands of fibrous tissue longer than those that can be found in sutures. The name *syndesmosis* itself is derived from the Greek word for "ligament." The syndesmosis is a flexible junction and may be twisted, so partial movement is possible. Unlike sutures and gomphoses, which are synarthrotic, syndesmoses are amphiarthrotic joints.[69] The amount of movement depends on the length of the connecting fibers. If the fibers are short, only minimal movement is possible. Such is the case with the distal tibiofibular articulation. If the fibers are long, as is the case with interosseous membrane between the radius and the ulna, then numerous movements can occur.

Gomphoses

Gomphoses (from the Greek word for "bolt") are almost immovable, although considerable movement can occur over a long period. These are fibrous joints where a conic bony process is placed into a socket-like segment. Because of this, the gomphosis is sometimes referred to as the peg-in-socket joint.[70] The only example of this type of joint is the articulation of a tooth with its bony socket (dental alveolus). The connecting ligament is a short one named the periodontal ligament.

Cartilaginous Joints

Either hyaline cartilage or fibrocartilage unites the articulating bones in cartilaginous joints. Cartilaginous joints do not have a joint cavity and are almost immobile. There are two types of cartilaginous joints: synchondroses and symphyses.

Synchondroses

These are cartilaginous joints in which hyaline cartilage is the fusing mechanism. Most are temporary since they disappear during growth. In immature long bones, synchondroses participate in bone lengthening, but by the time ossification completes (usually before the age of twenty-five), the joints turn into synostoses, or bony synarthrotic joints. The epiphyseal plates are synchondroses, as are the immobile joints between the first rib's costal cartilage and the manubrium of the sternum.

Symphyses

In these joints, fibrocartilage unites the bones. The intervertebral discs and the pubic symphysis of the pelvis are examples of this kind of joint. Hyaline cartilage is present in symphyses, with the main function of reducing friction between bones during movement. Fibrocartilage, on the other hand, withstands both tension and pressure and works as a flexible cushion or shock absorber. Symphyses are slightly movable joints—amphiarthroses—that give the skeleton strength and flexibility.

Synovial Joints

Synovial joints are the most common and most movable joints in the human body. They are all classified as diarthroses, the easily movable joints. The basic difference between this type of joint and the fibrous or cartilaginous types is the existence of a fluid-filled joint capsule surrounding the articulating surfaces. The following sections outline the general anatomy of synovial joints.

Joint Cavity (Synovial Cavity)

This is a feature unique to the synovial joints. All-important for the movement of humans, the joint cavity is nothing but a latent space that retains a small amount of synovial fluid.

Articular Capsule

This double-layered capsule surrounds the joint cavity. The external layer is a fibrous capsule of dense connective tissue that strengthens the joints and prevents the pulling apart of bones. The inner layer of the capsule is a synovial membrane, composed primarily of areolar connective tissue. This membrane covers all the internal joint surfaces that are not covered by cartilage and lines the articular cartilage. The synovial membrane secretes the synovial fluid.

Synovial Fluid

This viscous, oily fluid inside the joint cavity resembles raw egg white. Thus, the name derives in part from *ovum*, meaning "egg." Synovial fluid is composed of secretions from the synovial membrane cells and a filtrate from blood plasma.[71] Synovial fluid has three main functions: (1) lubricating the articular cartilage on the articulating bones, (2) nourishing the chondrocytes in this cartilage (cartilage, as mentioned above, is avascular), and (3) distributing stresses evenly across the joint surfaces when pressure suddenly increases. Synovial fluid not only occupies the joint cavity but also appears within the articular cartilages.

Articular Cartilage

This is composed of hyaline cartilage covering the ends of the opposing bones. These spongy cushions absorb the forces placed on the joints and in this manner prevent the crushing of the bone ends. The repetitious process of compressing then relaxing during exercise is essential to the health of the articular cartilage since the pumping action that accompanies it enhances its nutrition and waste removal.[72]

Reinforcing Ligaments

These bandlike ligaments give additional force and strength to the synovial joints. Usually the ligaments are intracapsular, meaning they are thickened parts of the fibrous capsule. If they are not, they can be either extracapsular or situated just outside the capsule. The fibular and tibial collateral ligaments of the knee are well-known examples of the intracapsular variety, such as the anterior and posterior cruciate ligaments in the knee. Intracapsular ligaments are covered with a synovial membrane that separates them from the articular cavity through which they run.

Nerves and Vessels

Sensory nerve fibers are abundant in the synovial joints and innervate the joint capsule. Some of these fibers detect pain, but most merely evaluate the amount of physical extension the capsule is subjected to. This monitoring of the extending and stretching of the joints is one of the many ways by which the nervous system recognizes posture and adjusts body movements. The blood supply of a synovial joint is obtained through the arteries sharing in the anastomosis around the joint. In addition to these six main anatomical elements, synovial joints are usually accompanied by at least four accessory structures: articular discs, bursae, tendons, and articular fat pads.

Articular Discs

The disc of fibrocartilage that can be found in some synovial joints is called a meniscus (meaning "crescent") or an articular disc. Articular discs occur in the knee joint, the temporomandibular (jaw) joint, the sternoclavicular joint, and a few others. The meniscus extends internally from the capsule and usually divides the articular cavity in two. Articular discs typically occur in joints with articulating bone ends of rather different shapes. The bone ends touch each other only at small points, meaning that the pressure there is highly concentrated. This can damage the articular cartilage and lead to osteoarthritis. The meniscus fills the gap and, like a missing puzzle piece, improves the fit between the articulating bones.

Bursae

Bursae are fibrous, saclike structures containing synovial fluid and lined by a synovial membrane; their very name, *bursa*, derives from the Latin word for "purse." Bursae may be either connected to or separated from the articular cavity. As with most additional joint components, bursae are designed to alleviate the friction within the joint. That is why they usually occur where tendons, muscles, bones, skin, or ligaments are in contact and rub together.

PHYSIOLOGY OF HUMAN BONES AND JOINTS

Physiology is a branch of biology that deals with the normal functions of organs and organ systems in living creatures.[73] This includes all the physical and chemical processes that go on inside living things and that are necessary for proper functioning of the body. Physiology is closely related to anatomy, the study of different organs in a body and their relative positioning. This is because an understanding of the functions of body parts requires a prior understanding of how the body is built. Human physiology is the specific study of the workings of the human body.

Organ Systems

The following sections outline the body's organ systems.[74]

Musculoskeletal System

This system consists of the bones of the skeleton, joints, muscles, connective tissues, ligaments, tendons, and cartilage. The musculoskeletal system provides a framework for the body, protects many critical organs, and facilitates the movement of movable body parts.[75]

Nervous System

This system transmits signals between different parts of the body in order to coordinate body movement and other vital functions. The nervous system comprises the brain, the spinal cord, sensory cells called sensory neurons, or sensory nerve cells, and the nerves that connect these sensory cells.

Cardiovascular System

This system includes the heart, blood, and blood vessels. It supplies nutrients to all parts of the body through the blood. The system works in close conjunction with the respiratory system.

Respiratory System

This system consists of the lungs, air passages, and respiratory muscles. It arranges for oxygenation of the blood and release of carbon dioxide from blood.

Endocrine System

This system is made up of numerous glands, each secreting some hormone. These hormones are released directly into the bloodstream for regulation of the body's metabolism. This organ system includes glands such as the pituitary, adrenal, thyroid, and pineal glands and the pancreas and thymus. The pancreas is also a part of the digestive system and functions as an endocrine as well as an exocrine gland.

Digestive System

This system absorbs nutrients from consumed food and disposes of waste. It consists of the mouth, esophagus, stomach, small intestine, large intestine, rectum, and anus. The liver and pancreas, which secrete digestive juices, are also part of this system. This system works in active collaboration with the nervous and cardiovascular systems.

Urinary System

This system produces, stores, and disposes of urine. It is made up of two kidneys, two ureters, one bladder, and a urethra.

Reproductive System

The reproductive system is involved with the production of reproductive cells. It also provides a mechanism through which these cells are combined. This system consists of external genitalia as well as the organs that produce the reproductive cells.

Immune System

The immune system protects the body against disease. It includes the bone marrow, white blood cells, lymph system, antibodies, spleen, and thymus.

Integumentary System

This system safeguards the body from damage and comprises the skin and appendages of the skin, such as nails and hair.

The study of human physiology includes an exhaustive focus on all these systems. This study has to be combined with a fundamental understanding of the molecular-, cellular-, and tissue-level principles that form the basis of the functions of these systems. Proper functioning of the human body requires all these systems to work smoothly. The overall health of the human body is determined by the efficiency of the collective or integrated working of all these systems.[76] An important concept in physiology is homeostasis. This refers to the maintenance of certain physiological parameters within a narrow range despite frequent changes in the external environment. Such a control is essential for proper functioning of all the organ systems. The physiological parameters that need to remain within limits include body temperature and the concentrations of electrolytes and glucose within cells.[77]

PHYSIOLOGY EXPLAINED

Origins of the Term *Physio*

The term *physio* is derived from the Greek word *phusis*, meaning "nature," and was used by the people of ancient Greece around 1000 BC. The word *phusis* is also said to refer to the Greek goddesses of nature, who maintained the balance of nature. The term also implied normality, as opposed to monstrousness or perversity.[78]

Differences

Considerable physiological differences exist between humans, other animals, and microorganisms. These differences can usually be ascribed to the process of evolution. Darwin's theory of evolution proposes that all life on earth started from a single-celled organism that slowly diversified into numerous species. In order to adapt to surroundings, the physiologies of organisms changed slowly. Different climatic conditions triggered different types of changes and over the millennia led to the development of varied life forms. Humans have an average brain-to-body mass ratio of 1:40, which is exceeded only by that of small birds (1:12).[79] This highly developed brain is said to be the reason why humans are more intelligent than other animals. Such a brain is also the reason why people have a longer memory than most other animals. Usually, animals outside the human species live in the moment and are therefore free of emotions such as spite, guilt, and self-consciousness.

Differences in Fingers and Legs

The thumb is most developed in people. During early evolutionary stages, mankind had greater need of a thumb; hence this body part developed better than in other species. The thumb added a whole new dimension to the activities that humans were able to perform. They could make and use tools and advance scientifically. While a superbly developed brain provides the arthritis patient with ideas, the thumb helps in the realization of some of those ideas in practice.

Humans walk on two hind legs while most other animals walk on four legs.[80] Certain types of monkeys do walk on two legs, but that is not their normal mode of mobility. This feature provides arthritis sufferers with an erect posture and frees their hands for other, more important activities. This is also why humans have a running speed that is slower than most other animals of comparable size.

Cardiovascular, Communication, and Sensual Differences

The number of chambers in the heart varies among animals. Humans have four chambers, reptiles usually three (except crocodiles, which have four), fishes two, and so on. Moreover, communication skills are very highly developed in humans as compared to other animals. Man is the only animal capable of articulate and coherent speech, as opposed to the sounds and gestures made by animals, which can convey their emotions only in a broad sense. As compared to many other animals, humans have an inferior sense of smell, as well as worse eyesight and hearing. During the course of evolution, humans made steady progress and started to tailor their environment to their needs. In a partly customized environment, the need for these senses declined as compared to when humans lived in open and often unprotected environments.

Microbiological Differences

Humans and animals have numerous organs, which are collections of many cells and tissues. Each organ has one or more functions. This specialization is either absent or limited in microorganisms, as the number of cells is limited. Organ systems such as the musculoskeletal, nervous, and cardiovascular systems are usually absent in the bodies of microorganisms. Many microorganisms are capable of rapid reproduction when the temperatures are moderately high. This rate is very high compared to that of humans and most other animals. Reproduction slows in cold environments. Microbes such as bacteria can freely exchange genes with other similar species, leading to quick mutation and evolution. This process of horizontal gene transfer poses great challenges for medical science as the variant species can resist even targeted medication. Reproduction in microbes can be asexual, sexual, or both.[81] Fungi reproduce asexually, while bacteria can reproduce in both ways. Barring a few exceptions, most animals reproduce sexually. Sexual reproduction in bacteria can lead to mutation and associated problems for medical science. This process is called conjugation and involves transfer of DNA from one bacterium to another via a thread-type structure known as a pilus. Such a transfer enables bacteria to pass characteristics and leads to the formation of a varied species capable of survival in newer, more hostile environments.

NORMAL FUNCTIONS OF BONES AND JOINTS

Purpose of Bones

All the bones and joints in the body form the skeletal system, which is inherently linked with muscles to form the musculoskeletal organ system. The skeletal system serves three fundamental functions.[82] By now, the arthritis patient should know that the skeletal system supports all the other organ systems of the body by providing a framework of bones and joints on or inside which other organ systems rest. This structure also gives shape to the body. Bones provide protection to internal organs such as the brain, lungs, uterus, and others. This is a notable function and therefore merits a somewhat detailed treatment.

- The skull encases the brain and protects the eyes and the middle and inner ears.
- The sternum, rib cage, and spine shield the heart, lungs, and critical blood vessels.
- The vertebral column forms a covering around the spinal cord.
- The spine and ilium safeguard the hips and the digestive and urogenital systems.

Movement

Movement is provided by bones in combination with attached muscles. Skeletal muscles operate in pairs; when one relaxes, the other simply contracts. An example is the bicep-triceps combination. When the arm is stretched, the bicep relaxes with contraction of the triceps, and vice versa. Many times, bones provide leverage by amplifying the magnitude and changing the direction of force generated by the muscles.[83]

IMPAIRED BONE HEALTH

Overview of Consequences

Unhealthy bones are unable to perform all or some of their functions related to support, movement, protection, blood cell production, and serving as a reservoir and dumping location, respectively, for useful and toxic minerals. Bone disease is a generic term for disorders that make bones weak and brittle and, therefore, more likely to break. Sources for bone disorders include heredity, nutritional deficiencies, injuries, and infections. The general effects include a pronounced decrease in quality of life due to the inability to move efficiently, as well as to frequent bone injuries and possibly fractures. Premature death can result in extreme cases.

Infectious Arthritis

This can happen in people with weak joints. The source is a fungal, viral, or bacterial infection in such joints, and the symptoms include swelling and redness around the joint, joint pain, and fever. The infection is transferred through the blood or can be the result of injury, surgery, or injection. Infectious arthritis is discussed further in chapter 12.[84]

Rickets

Found in children, rickets is due to a vitamin D deficiency. It makes the bones weak and soft. The effects include restricted movements, with bone and muscle pain. Low bone density is due to insufficient development of bone mass during childhood. This can turn into osteoporosis later in life.[85]

Bone Cancer

This affects the normal functioning of bone cells and tissues. Usually, cancer in the bone results from the spread of cancerous cells to bones from another part of the body. Very rarely does bone cancer originate in bone cells. Different types of bone cancers affect bone cells, cartilage cells, and the bone marrow. Symptoms include swelling, pain, weak bones, fatigue, unexplained weight loss, night sweats, and chills. This disorder can assume serious proportions if it affects a load-bearing bone, such as the femur, forcing the patient to use a wheelchair for a considerable portion of the treatment.

Paget's Disease

This bone disease interrupts the cycle of continuous breakdown and rebuilding of bones. Symptoms of this disorder, which can enlarge and weaken the bones, include severe pain and swelling in the joints. This can intensify into other disorders, such as deafness and arthritis.

Osteogenesis Imperfecta

Osteogenesis imperfecta (OI) is a genetic disease that causes bones to break easily, as well as other conditions, such as curved spine, weak muscles, brittle teeth, and hearing loss. The disease-causing gene is inherited and affects the development of collagen, a protein that in turn affects bone development.

Fibrous Dysplasia

This results in replacement of bones with fibrous tissue, thereby causing excessive growth and swelling of bones. Weak bones affect the ability to walk, and the disorder can also cause endocrine problems. This disorder inspires a certain degree of awe because its cause is unknown, it cannot be prevented, and treatment only aims to mitigate its adverse effects.

Osgood-Schlatter Disease

This malady affects the area where the kneecap and tibia (shinbone) connect. It is more likely to afflict adolescents and causes swelling, tenderness, and pain in the affected area. The pain can range from mild to severe and from occasional to constant. [86]

PHYSIOLOGY OF JOINTS

Purpose of Joints

Joints are those locations where two or more bones are attached; they provide connectivity between different bones of the body. The fact that almost all bones are connected to form the skeletal system and that the muscles are connected to the skeleton ensures coordination of movement between different parts of the body. This connectivity integrates all the body parts into one whole entity. Joints facilitate movement through contraction and relaxation of muscles. Purposeful movement is fundamental to animals' behavior and enables them to execute all activities necessary for survival, leisure, and reproduction. Joints, which also serve as shock absorbers, lend the skeletal structure a certain amount of flexibility.

Although evolution has yielded different structures for different types of joints in different animals, their essential functions remain unchanged. An example is the joints in the hind legs of land-based carnivores, which are designed for pouncing on prey. This is why these animals can jump high using their hind legs. At the other end of the spectrum are the herbivores with hind-leg bones and joints geared for high speed. The joints of monkeys are designed for quick climbing and rapid movement in trees. Reptiles' joints enable them to crawl and pounce at high speeds.

Joints in the human body can be classified on the basis of the type of movement they provide physiologically:

- Hinge joints facilitate movement similar to that of a hinged door—along one axis only. They allow movement up and down but not from side to side, and vice verse. Examples of such joints are the elbow, knee, and upper and lower jaw.
- Ball-and-socket joints allow movement in all directions—upwards, downwards, and sideways. The shoulder is an example of such a joint. Another example is the acetabulam, or the hip joint, where the thighbone is connected to the pelvis.
- Pivot joints permit pivotal movement of one part around the other. For example, the skull rotates around the topmost bone of the backbone.

- Gliding joints are characterized by the gliding movement of one bone or bone part over the other. The wrist joint is an example of such a joint.

Joints can also be classified according to the mechanism that holds the bones together at the joint. Application of this criterion renders the following types of joints.[87]

- Fibrous or immovable joints are held together by ligaments only. Examples of such joints are the radioulnar and tibiofibular joints, the joints of bones inside the forearm and shin, respectively.
- In cartilaginous joints, cartilage provides the connection between bones. An example is the joints between the vertebrae.
- Synovial joints are held together by a synovial capsule made from the protein collagen. The inner layer of this capsule, known as the synovial membrane, secretes a lubricant called synovial fluid. Furthermore, hyaline cartilage pads the ends of the bones in these joints. Synovial joints can be hinge, ball-and-socket, pivot, or gliding joints. They can also be saddle or condyloid joints. Different finger bones of the same finger are joined by saddle joints, while condyloid joints join the metacarpal bones to the first phalanges.

DEVELOPMENTAL ASPECTS OF MALE AND FEMALE BONES

Overall Bone Similarities

The skeletons of all primates exhibit certain generic features, such as a large brain, highly developed fingers and thumbs, generalized dental patterns, forward-facing eyes, and bony eye sockets. Considerable similarities also exist between the human male and female skeletons in terms of bones and joints. Both have exactly the same number of bones: 206. The same number of bones also means the same number of joints, although the precise number of joints in the human body is a matter of debate in view of differences of opinion about what constitutes a joint. The shape of most bones in the male and female skeletons is similar, although some bones are differently shaped in view of the different roles of males and females. The femur, or thighbone, is the longest and strongest bone in both human males and human females. The stirrup bone, or stapes, is the smallest bone in the human skeleton irrespective of gender. The average human bone density is approximately 1,062 kg/m^3 for a normal, healthy adult, although males have slightly higher bone density than women.[88] Here again, different researchers[89] have obtained varying results, ranging from 1,000 kg/m^3 to 1,900 kg/m^3. Nevertheless the human skeleton comprises a significant percentage of the total body weight.

Exceptions

Certain peculiarities or exceptions are common to male and female skeletons. The presence of fused bones in the cranium and pelvis serves as an example.[90] These bones are not connected through joints but fit into each other like the pieces of a jigsaw puzzle. The three bones in the middle ear, collectively referred to as ossicles, connect only with each other. The hyoid bone located in the neck serves as a connection point for the tongue; it is not connected to any bone in the skeleton and is held in position only by muscles and ligaments.

Overall Bone Differences

Different hormones affect the development of bones in males and females, and this is the primary reason for bone differences. Testosterone is the main hormone that affects bone development in males, while estrogen does the same for females.[91] The differences between male and female skeletons can be better understood when seen in the context of differences in race, lifestyle, and physical activity. When comparisons are made between males and females of the same race with similar lifestyles, the following points of difference can be observed.

In Relation to Childbirth

There are two differences in relation to the process of childbirth. Females have a more movable coccyx, or tailbone, and a wider and flatter sacrum connected to the pelvis. The coccyx is the last bone of the backbone, and the sacrum is similarly located near the end of the spinal column. Such a structure allows the head and shoulders of the fetus to pass through the cavity during childbirth. Bones that make up the arms and legs are thicker, longer, and therefore stronger in males. Bones in the arm include the humerus, which supports the bicep, and the radius and ulna, which support the forearm. Males possess relatively larger phalanges, or finger bones.

Size

Male skeletons are usually larger and heavier than female skeletons. Traditionally, men have assumed responsibility for hunting, gathering, and working outdoors, while women have borne children and taken on domestic responsibilities. Men therefore have traditionally needed more strength, which explains the strength-related differences in the male and female skeletons.

Face

The facial bone structure in males and females is different on account of differences in the structure of the skull. Men have a more developed bulge at the back of the head and more noticeable brow ridges. Men's chins are more angular and square as compared to female chins, which are more pointed.

Spine Length and Other Differences

Women's spines are shorter than men's. The shorter spine creates the illusion that females' legs are longer than those of males. Other differences include a narrower rib cage, more rounded shoulder blades, and smaller teeth in the female skeleton.

DEVELOPMENTAL ASPECTS OF MALE AND FEMALE JOINTS

Overall Similarities

Human male and female joints have certain common features. The first similarity is the number of joints. Since the number of bones in the bodies of males and females is same, the number of joints is also same. The number of joints is between 250 and 350.[92] There is no exact number due to lack of unanimity about what precisely constitutes a joint. Another prominent similarity is the types of joints. Both males and females have the same types of joints according to the mechanism for holding joints together. The functions of most of the joints in males and females are similar. This point of similarity is a natural corollary to there being an equal number and the same types of joints.

Differences

Men have broader shoulders and hip girths, while women have wider hips and narrower shoulders. This makes the angles of muscle alignment and tendon attachment different in the joints of males and females.[93] Female joints are, on average, more flexible and have a greater range of movement than male joints.[94] On account of this significant point, the following dissimilarities are observed:

1. It is easier for women to perform mobility exercises and exhibit actions such as hurdling and the fosbury flop during high jump.
2. Men are better at events such as the long jump, shot put, and hammer throw.
3. The unique center of gravity also makes women less susceptible to injuries during the execution of jumps over hurdles; on the downside,

this feature lowers the efficiency of the muscle pull and makes women more prone to muscle injuries

4. Elbows and ankles in the male skeleton are smaller and have a smaller carrying angle as compared to female skeletons, which makes male elbows and ankles stronger. [95]

The above are due to women having a lower center of gravity owing to their wider hips and greater distribution of weight around the hips and thighs.

Chapter Three

The Real Meaning and History of Arthritis

The word *arthritis* derives from two Greek terms: *arthron*, meaning "joint," and *itis*, meaning "inflammation." Taken literally, the whole term means "inflammation in joints."[1] As discussed to this point, a joint is a location where two bones in the body are held together by different mechanisms. Arthritis is a generic term that encompasses a whole range of disorders related to joints. In the simplest of terms, this disorder causes bones at a joint to rub against each other. This friction can be due to (1) the wearing down of cartilage, (2) a shortage of synovial fluid in the joint cavity, (3) infection in the joints, (4) an autoimmune reaction, or (5) a combination of these factors. This increase in friction results in inflammation, stiffness, and pain.[2]

ROOTS OF THE DEFINITION

Arthritis as a medical condition is very old; in fact, it is one of the oldest to affect humans and others in the animal kingdom. The condition can be traced back in time to as early as 4500 BC. Skeletal remains of Native Americans dating back to that period testify to the existence of this disorder. Documented descriptions that closely match the symptoms of arthritis have been found in ancient Indian texts of around AD 123. Another piece of the documentary record is *De Arthritide Symptomatica*, composed by William Musgrave in 1715.[3] Genuine progress for describing this condition started in the nineteenth century when great strides were made in medical science and, for that matter, in the entire scientific field. Augustin Jacob Landre-Beauvais, a French physician, was the first to provide a comprehensive and scientific description. Then, in 1859, an English physician named Sir Alfred Barring

Garrod coined the term *rheumatoid arthritis*.[4] Considerable trial and error has gone into the diagnosis of this condition and finding possible remedies. Pinpointing one cause or one definitive symptom of arthritis is almost impossible. It cannot be said with absolute certainty that a particular symptom indicates arthritis. Symptoms of many other abnormal conditions are similar to those of this disorder. Finding the meanings and definitions of the condition is therefore a very tricky business. William Röntgen's discovery of X-rays in 1895 greatly augmented the capacity to define arthritis accurately.[5]

Ambiguity

Since a number of abnormal conditions are included under the rubric of arthritis, there is a certain ambiguity as to the cause of the disorder. Arthritis can result from multiple causes related to overloading and overusing joints, the endocrine or autoimmune systems, or conditions during and after infection. Another dilemma is that despite numerous experiments and concerted efforts, genuine treatment is still not available. Physicians' efforts are directed toward reduction in the severity of inflammation, pain, and stiffness in joints. Therefore, the disorder cannot be precisely defined. This is why arthritis, classified broadly as a disorder, is medically categorized as a condition and not a disease. The term *arthritis* is confused with numerous joint-related disorders, and its vagueness delayed developments related to diagnosis and treatment. The late 1930s and early 1940s marked the beginning of a fresh approach in dealing with this problem. H. L. Tidy came up with *A Synopsis of Medicine*,[6] which is widely believed to have introduced the therapeutic outlook employed at present to deal with arthritis.[7] The disorder and its treatment have received their fair share of recognition only after the outbreak of World War II in 1939. In 1951, Guillaume de Baillou produced the first authoritative text on arthritis.[8] In mitigating the intensity of this disorder, Philip Hench, a physician during the mid-twentieth century, demonstrated the effectiveness of moderate doses of corticosteroids discussed in chapter 16.[9]

THE DEFINING MOMENT

Numerous definitions of arthritis are available today. Arthritis can be defined as:

1. joint inflammation with pain, stiffness, and swelling that can be a result of infection, degeneration, trauma, metabolic disturbances, or other causes and can assume many forms, such as rheumatoid arthritis, bacterial arthritis, or osteoarthritis;[10]

2. joint inflammation that is a result of infection, constitutional changes, or metabolic changes;[11]
3. acute or chronic joint inflammation that usually occurs with structural changes and pain and is a result of multiple causes, such as injury, infection, or crystal deposition;[12]
4. a condition or disorder that causes joint inflammation due to trauma or wear and tear.

These definitions really include more than a hundred abnormalities, many of which can last a lifetime. Many forms of arthritis in such a context are a result of the body's immune system attacking its own tissues.[13]

On Common Ground

The points common to almost all definitions are inflammation and joint ache. Joint ache is included here because bones rub directly against each other due to the wearing down of cartilage, lack of synovial fluid in the joint cavity, infection, autoimmunity, or some combination of these causes. Not every incidence of joint ache and inflammation can be said to be arthritis. Many other disorders manifest themselves similarly through joint ache and inflammation. This is the precise problem that makes it virtually impossible to adopt a definition that encompasses all such conditions—hence the variation in meaning.

A CONDITION BUT NOT A DISEASE

In general parlance, the terms *disease* and *medical condition* are often used interchangeably. However, there is a slight difference between them that is not immediately apparent. The definitions of these terms have to be examined minutely in order to pinpoint the differences. Furthermore, there is a considerable overlap in the definitions as both terms refer to deviation of the state of the body or mind from what is considered normal.

Definition of a Condition

A medical condition such as arthritis can be defined as a defective state of physical or psychological health. It can also be described as a medical problem that has to be treated or managed.[14] This is fairly similar to certain aspects of a disease. The difference lies in the degree of subjectivity and vagueness associated with the diagnosis, causes, and treatment of the disease. The term *condition* is largely used to refer to psychological abnormalities that, inherently, are not very easy to define. The perception of the patient and of the physician plays a capital role in the diagnosis and treatment of the condition. The patient has to be able to express his or her problem correctly, and the doctor has to understand it the right way. The role of tests in the diagnosis of a condition is fairly limited.

Other Information on Diseases versus Conditions

The crux of the difference between a disease and a condition is the element of intangibility. The presence of a disease can be definitely verified or diagnosed. Such verification is done on the basis of specific tests, signs, and symptoms. A disease is therefore an objective condition whose existence can be proved on the application of definite criteria. There can be very little debate between two physicians about whether a patient is affected by a disease when certain tests confirm its existence. A medical condition, on the other hand, is vague and subjective. The confirmation of the existence of a condition is not as straightforward as it is for a disease. What might be diagnosed as a certain condition by one physician can be diagnosed as some other condition by another physician, and both physicians will put forth equally convincing arguments. The overlap in the symptoms of arthritis and many other conditions has already been noted in detail. The term *condition* is used more in the context of mental disorders that are more difficult to define and diagnose and therefore treat.

If an abnormal condition such as arthritis is difficult to define, it will naturally be difficult to trace the cause, for the physician can only guess what the disorder is. The disorder will also be difficult to treat, for the physician will not know exactly what he or she is dealing with. This also means that there will be more than one course of treatment available for a similar set of symptoms, and the efficacy of all of these will be a matter of debate. A treatment that has been effective for certain persons may not be so for another set of people because the diagnosis and treatment have been largely correct for the first group and not for the second. This is precisely the greater element of intangibility referred to in the earlier part of this chapter. Intangibility adds a vague dimension to the condition that in turn lends an aura of incurability to the deviant condition. The aura is reinforced by the fact that the treatment of numerous conditions focuses only on mitigation of the symptoms and discomfort. Genuine cure is not usually available. This is true for arthritis and for many psychological conditions. All the same, such conditions can be managed.

Most diseases can be prevented and cured because the cause is known. This also makes it possible to develop vaccines against diseases. No such vaccines are available against mental conditions or arthritis. Trauma is known to cause certain mental illnesses, but not everyone under stress will be mentally disturbed. A specific type of traumatic situation cannot be said to produce a certain psychological condition. Similar situations can produce different conditions in different individuals and might even fail to produce any response in those who are mentally tough. The degree of vagueness and subjectivity is more for conditions as compared to diseases.

Where the Meaning of Arthritis Stands

If one accepts the degree of vagueness regarding symptoms, causes, and treatment as the criteria for differentiating between a disease and a condition, arthritis has to be classified as a condition and not as a disease. A number of disorders have symptoms similar to those of arthritis, and these have already been discussed at length. The causes for arthritis are also a bit vague. Destruction of the cartilage and synovial membrane leads to arthritis. This breakdown can be caused by infection, lifting of weights that exceed the capacity of joints, stress due to excessively repetitive joint movements, or an autoimmune response. These very causes can result in other joint-related disorders with similar symptoms. Treatment of the "disease" is another important criterion that makes arthritis a condition. All types of treatments for arthritis are aimed toward (1) reduction of pain, swelling, and inflammation; (2) prevention of further joint damage; and (3) improving the mobility of joints. The underlying cause is not usually cured.[15] Arthritis can be mitigated through lifestyle changes, medication, and surgery. Changes in lifestyle include the following:

- Ceasing to stay in one position for too long, elimination or reduction of movements that put excessive stress on joints, and stress-reduction activities such as meditation and yoga.
- Tailored exercise routines that include motion exercises, aerobic activity, and strength building for muscles around the joint to reduce the load on the joint.
- Physical therapy such as massage, external support for joints, water therapy, and heat or ice treatment.
- Reduction in weight, which will automatically reduce the load on joints.
- Getting an ample amount of sleep, including brief naps during the day.
- Consumption of a diet rich in vitamins, minerals, and omega-3 fatty acids. These elements are contained in fresh fruits and vegetables, soybeans, cold-water fish, walnuts, soybean and canola oil, and pumpkin seeds.
- Simple changes around the house, such as installation of grab bars near the toilet and bathtub to distribute the load on various joints while standing up.

The preceding list of measures applies to many other joint-related disorders, but none of these can be described as specific to the approach of arthritis alone. Medication includes acetaminophen, aspirin, naproxen, ibuprofen, immunosuppressants, corticosteroids, biologics, and disorder-modifying anti-rheumatic drugs. When these treatments do not work, joint-replacement surgery, or arthroplasty, can be performed to replace joints.

KNOWING THE REAL MEANING OF ANY DISEASE

Consequences of Not Knowing

Prevention is always much better than a cure. Attempting to narrow down true definitions of diseases can help patients and caregivers avoid them and lead healthy lives. Apart from negatively affecting the personal lives of people, diseases produce other deleterious social, economic, and political consequences. At the personal level, diseases and conditions reduce the quality of health by restricting the normal movements and mobility of the patient. A certain amount of dread is also inspired by highly infectious diseases with a lethal track record, and this can introduce psychological insecurity. Those with limited incomes are burdened with the cost of disease treatment. Diseases also reduce human productivity and can lead to loss of employment for workers. Epidemics come with a huge social and economic cost that can also generate political fallout. The onset of an epidemic can lead to mass migrations away from the affected areas with disruption of the economy in the source region and straining of the infrastructure in the destination area. Trade, tourism, and commerce get disturbed, causing heavy losses. Examples include the 1991 cholera epidemic in Peru, which resulted in estimated losses of $775 million to the country's fishing industry, trade, and tourism.[16] Disruption of trade and commerce and imposition of restrictions on imports from areas where an epidemic breaks out usually lead to political tensions on both sides. Similar straining of relations results from mass migrations that are more common in developing countries and least-developed countries.

More Power to Fight

Knowledge of the real meaning of a condition such as arthritis and how it is spread can go a long way in devising methods to prevent it. It was the knowledge of etiologic agents obtained through years of painstaking research that enabled the development of vaccines and medicines, respectively, for the prevention and cure of diseases. The success in preventing the onset and spread of diseases has been so great that the incidence of most infectious disorders has been eliminated from the developed world. Such disorders are, however, still a major concern in a great part of the developing world. Health concerns in present-day developed countries are focused on the control of those disorders that result from sedentary lifestyles. These disorders[17] include the following:

- Cardiovascular disorders
- Diabetes
- Obesity
- High blood pressure
- Lipid disorder
- Depression
- Anxiety

As the cause for the above disorders is known, steps can be taken to improve physical fitness, which will automatically prevent them. Some mental disorders are a result of loneliness; therefore, these can be prevented by keeping in touch with family, friends, relations, and acquaintances. Forewarned, after all, is forearmed.

Letting Others Know the Real Meaning of Arthritis

Medical conditions such as arthritis are vaguer as their causes, symptoms, and treatments can only be generalized. The moment there is uncertainty about how a condition can be addressed, quacks step in. Myths and legends get associated with the disorder, and the field is left open for dubious physicians to make a quick buck, many times at the cost of the patient's health. The fact that arthritis cannot be completely cured makes it more prone to hijacking by quacks. This is precisely why it is so important to let others know the true meaning of conditions such as arthritis. A realistic presentation of the nature of the condition, especially the extent to which it can be cured and the long duration involved in decreasing its intensity, will provide patients with a clear outlook to deal with it. Patients will be less prone to getting cheated by unqualified "health coaches" if they can compare the proposed treatment with the basic facts of their condition. This also means that arthritis patients will be less likely to choose an incorrect course of treatment suggested to them during informal discussions with friends and acquaintances. Disseminating the correct meaning of arthritis will help patients improve the health of their joints. At the very least, it will prevent them from doing more damage to their joints in the quest for quick and unrealistic solutions.

HISTORY OF ARTHRITIS

Arthritis has been a cause of pain and discomfort in human and animal joints since time immemorial. Evidence of this disorder has also been found in the joints of the Neanderthal, a distant relative of modern humans. The discovery of such fossils has been a fairly recent phenomenon, and the modern therapeutic approach to deal with arthritis was defined only in 1939.[18] Proper understanding and documentation of the multiple conditions that can be classified as arthritic started thereafter. Although arthritis is ancient, scientific attempts to understand and deal with it are relatively recent.

DISCOVERIES

Early Findings of Arthritis in Animals

Fossilized remains of a pack of Iguanodons, a kind of dinosaur dating as far back as 85 million years ago, indicate arthritic joints.[19] These remains were discovered in Belgium, and the creatures, when alive, were troubled by a form of arthritis called ankle osteoarthritis. Most dinosaur fossils exhibit incidence of secondary arthritis resulting from injury and congenital conditions, which makes the above discovery a very rare one indeed. A recent discovery has taken the arthritis clock further back in time to 150 million years ago, when another type of dinosaur called a pliosaur suffered from degeneration of the jaw joint. This is very similar to arthritis.[20] The pliosaur was an apex sea-based predator with an eight-meter-long, whale-type body, short neck, and crocodile-like mouth. The animal had huge twenty-centimeter-long teeth and massive jaws. The enormity of its teeth and jaws, and the fact that its jaws had to deal with struggling prey, may have been the reason for the weakening of the jaw joint. The fossil was discovered in Westbury, Wiltshire, and indicates an arthritis-like condition in the jaw joint. Crocodiles and sperm whales suffer similar jaw-related disorders during their lifetimes. Arthritic conditions are common in a wide variety of animals, both wild and domestic. This diversity suggests that diet and lifestyle do not cause this disorder. The gradual rupture of joints with age is believed to be the main reason as deterioration of joints has not been observed in younger animals. Small mammals do not develop arthritic joints, but medium- and large-sized mammals do, with the large ones being the most vulnerable.

Early Findings of Arthritis in Humans

Arthritic joints were a cause of concern even for the Neanderthals, a distant evolutionary relative of modern man. Neanderthals developed secondary osteoarthritis due to a strenuous lifestyle and a tendency toward continuous injuries. Neanderthals inhabited the planet around 30,000 BC, and such discoveries of arthritis further strengthen the conclusion that this disorder is ancient from a human standpoint. Arthritic joints have also been detected in the skeletal remains of Native Americans. These remains have been discovered in Tennessee and Kansas in the United States and date as far back as 4500 BC. This is the earliest date to which arthritis in humans can be traced. Another famous piece of evidence that indicates arthritic joints is the Ötzi mummy, popularly referred to as "the Iceman."[21] These remains were discovered in the European Alps and can be traced back to 3000 BC. The Iceman is believed to have made a failed attempt to cross the Alps near the present-day Italy-Austria border. These remains, along with a pouch of medicinal herbs discovered with them, provide valuable links in tracing the history of arthritis in human beings.

Related Texts

In addition to fossils, descriptions can be found in numerous ancient texts of a number of civilizations. These descriptions seem to enumerate the symptoms of arthritic conditions. The Ebers Papyrus, composed around 1500 BC by the Egyptians, is believed to be the earliest documented evidence of rheumatic and arthritic conditions. Around 400 BC, Hippocrates described similar symptoms, as mentioned in chapter 1. The *Charak Samhita*, an Indian masterpiece in medicine composed sometime in the third century BC, describes the pain, swelling, and loss of joint function that is now known as arthritis. A disorder described by Aretaeus sometime in the first or second century AD is fairly similar to polyarticular gout. Another ancient description of an arthritis-type condition can be found in the treatise of Soranus of Ephesus (AD 98–138). These descriptions are, however, of a general nature and may have depicted arthritis or other nonarthritic conditions exhibiting similar symptoms.[22]

Learned from This

Certain arthritis-related deductions can be made from a minute examination of the disorder among humans and animals. One is the relation between size and the onset of arthritis. Humans are comparable to a medium-sized animal, and arthritis has been observed in the skeletal remains of most medium- and large-sized animals. Age is another point of concurrence. The skeletal remains of older, but not younger, animals were found to be affected with arthritis. Presently, arthritis is found to affect older humans and animals more than younger ones. Arthritis, therefore, is most likely to affect the joints of older humans and medium- to large-sized animals, irrespective of the historical era.

COINING OF THE TERM

The First to Label Arthritis

The term *arthritis* entered the English vocabulary through Latin and has a certain relation to the Greek language. Alfred Barring Garrod coined the term *rheumatoid arthritis* in 1859 when he argued that it was a separate disorder.

Hitherto, the term has been confused with other disorders such as chronic rheumatism, scorbutic rheumatism, rheumatic gout, and rheumalgia. To put things in a better context, it will be important to note that even today, in view of a certain degree of vagueness associated with its diagnosis, symptoms, and treatment, arthritis is classified as a condition and not a disease. The diagnosis, symptoms, and treatment of the disorder are common to numerous other joint-related conditions. This apparent similarity has introduced some amount of confusion into the nomenclature of this disorder, which, at least in general parlance, persists to the present day. Garrod discussed at length the differences in diagnosis of these related disorders and argued for a separate term. He chose *rheumatoid arthritis* after providing detailed illustrations. In doing so, he rejected the terms *rheumatic gout* and *chronic rheumatism*, respectively coined by Henry Fuller and William Heberden.[23] The fact that the term is still used speaks volumes about the accuracy of Garrod's diagnosis and analysis.

ARTHRITIC FAME

Arthritis has troubled athletes, politicians, artists, surgeons, and film stars alike. Unfortunately, the hit list is as inclusive as it gets. Famous people who have suffered from this disorder include the following:

- James J. Braddock, former heavyweight boxing champion of the world[24]
- Pierre Auguste Renoir, a French painter who developed the impressionist style of painting
- Kay Kyser, a famous radio personality and bandleader of the 1930s and 1940s
- Dr. Christian Barnard, the surgeon who performed the first heart transplant
- Gerald Durrell, a famous author and naturalist
- Rosalind Russell, a Hollywood actress who is perhaps the most glamorous sufferer of rheumatoid arthritis

As one can see, arthritis has been an irritant for famous people across the barriers of time, gender, and profession.

Chapter Four

Anatomy and Pathology of Arthritis

The study of human anatomy can be broadly divided into two levels: macroscopic, or gross, anatomy and microscopic anatomy,[1] also known as histology. As the term *macro* suggests, in gross anatomy the body is studied from an overall perspective, seen as a whole from the outside. The study from this perspective is further divided into two approaches: the regional and systemic approaches. In the former, for the purpose of study, the body is divided into different regions, such as upper limb and back, head and neck, chest, abdomen, pelvis, and lower limb. In the systemic approach, the functioning of the organs, muscles, skeleton, nerves, and other structures lying within these systems is examined. The study through a microscope of the inner structures of the body, such as organs or the tissues and fluids of a joint, defines histology. A third method of study is basic anatomy, which actually introduces the subject of anatomy and how it is to be studied.

NOTABLE ANATOMISTS FROM AROUND THE WORLD

Greece and Italy

History provides us with names of pioneers in the field of anatomy, the earliest and most prominent among them being Hippocrates and Herophilus, both Greek physicians around 400 BC. Hippocrates' works describe the initial understanding of the musculoskeletal system—the system that provides form, support, stability, and movement to the body. While Hippocrates was regarded as the father of medicine, Herophilus had the distinction of being known as the father of anatomy, as he was one of the first to dissect human bodies to understand how they work.

Aristotle, an eminent anatomist among other contemporaries in the fourth century BC, based his findings on animal dissection before the use of human cadavers was an option. Even artists such as Leonardo da Vinci (1452–1519) and Michelangelo (1475–1564) were anatomists in their own right.[2] Through drawings and illustrations, they provided medical students with the visuals necessary to understand their subject and carry out dissections more confidently.

France

France's Jean Cruveilhier (1791–1874) was yet another renowned anatomist. During his long and distinguished career, he served as president of the Académie Nationale de Médecine (National Academy of Medicine) and the Société Anatomique de Paris (Anatomical Society of Paris) for over forty years. His contributions included studies on the nervous system and inflammation of the blood vessels. Cruveilhier's contributions in the field of forensic science and the study of vascular disorders were the precursors to further extensive development in these areas.[3]

England and Scotland

Author of the anatomical book titled *Gray's Anatomy*, Henry Gray (1827–1861) was also one of the greats in the field of anatomy. Recipient of the Triennial Prize from the Royal College of Surgeons for his essay *The Origin, Connexions and Distribution of Nerves to the Human Eye and Its Appendages, Illustrated by Comparative Dissections of the Eye in Other Vertebrate Animals*, he also won accolades for his work on the human spleen. Gray's book on anatomy was tremendously successful, mainly due to the excellent illustrations it contained. The book is, even today, hugely popular with medical students.[4]

On the subject of famous anatomists, two Scottish brothers, William Hunter (1718–1783) and John Hunter (1728–1793), deserve mention. While William Hunter was recognized as one of the best-known teachers of anatomy of the time,[5] his brother John, who was taught by William, outshone his mentor and was acknowledged as the more famous of the two. A fellow of the Royal College, William Hunter acquired his anatomical skills at St. George's Hospital in London, where he specialized in obstetrics. Although acknowledged as London's leading obstetric consultant, he acquired fame in the field of orthopedics for his account on bone and cartilage. His achievements included becoming physician to the wife of King George III, Queen Charlotte, in 1764, then being elected as fellow of the Royal Society in 1767, and a year later being appointed professor of anatomy at the Royal Academy of Arts in London. He founded the famous anatomy theater in 1768, which became the alma mater of some of the best-known anatomists and surgeons of that time. John Hunter, who started out as an assistant to his famed brother, turned out to be a prodigy in his own right. His achievements, which made him more renowned than William, included becoming surgeon at St. George's Hospital (1768), then a member of the Company of Surgeons a little later, and in 1776 being elevated to the position of surgeon to King George III. Ten years later, in 1786, John Hunter was with the British army as a deputy surgeon and rose to become the surgeon general in the army's Defence Medical Services in 1790.[6]

BONE AND JOINT ANATOMY AND AGE

Overview

The human skeleton is made up of 206 bones,[7] which together support the body and give it its rigid form. Minus the skeleton, the body (flesh and soft tissue organs) would simply collapse, as would a tent with no poles to keep it erect. Bones are strong and rigid, yet lightweight. In addition to holding the body upright, they allow mobility and provide protection to the delicate organs of the body by encompassing them within its frame. Although bones are strong, their tissues change constantly. Old bone tissues are replaced by new ones, with the entire skeletal system having been renewed every seven to ten years.[8]

Changes in Composition

Although bones appear dry, hard, and lifeless in skeletons on display in museums and laboratories, bones in all living creatures are actually quite alive, inasmuch as they are constantly growing and changing, just like the various other parts of the body do.[9]

Two elements that provide bones the structure and strength to carry the weight of the body—and, more importantly, the ability to regrow and repair themselves during the arthritis patient's lifespan—are calcium and phosphorus. The body's absorption of calcium is at its peak during its optimum growth period, which begins at the age of ten and starts to decline when a person is around twenty years old. Phosphorus carries the calcium to the bones. Without these two elements, broken and worn-out bones would not heal, and individuals would have to live with deformities. Bone health is all the more vital inasmuch as it is responsible for the production of the red and white blood corpuscles that keep the body alive.[10] In addition to their role in the formation of bones and teeth, these elements (phosphorus and calcium) have other functions. Phosphorus filters waste matter from the kidneys and assists the body in the storage and use of energy. Calcium, stored in the body, contributes to the health of the cardiovascular and nervous systems.

All bones are made up of four distinct materials:

- A thin, dense membrane of nerves and blood vessels that formed on the outer surface of the bone, called the periosteum
- A hard and even surface referred to as the compact bone
- Bone marrow, a thick, semisolid substance in the innermost part of the bone, which produces the blood cells
- The cancellous layer, a spongy yet strong substance inside the compact bone, which protects the innermost part of the bone

Men's bones are denser than females'. Women are born with smaller bones, which absorb less calcium than the bones of men. Because estrogen, a hormone that protects bones from calcium loss, starts depleting after menopause, women may become vulnerable to calcium deficiency after this stage. This is why the bone-density loss, a problem associated with age in both sexes, speeds up in postmenopausal women. [11]

Bone density lessens with age primarily because the body's ability to absorb calcium from foods dwindles. Another contributing factor is diminishing levels of vitamin D, the vitamin that absorbs calcium and phosphorus. Increased consumption of calcium to build healthy bones and teeth is of no consequence if there is a deficiency of vitamin D. As the body's natural function of generating hormones reduces and the intake and absorption of vitamins and minerals decreases, the bones become weak and susceptible to fractures. Cartilage and connective tissues in joints become thinner, and the structure of the cartilage begins to undergo change. This causes the joints to become less flexible and more prone to damage. [12] Age, combined with wear and tear, contributes to damage to the ligaments and tendons in the joints, which become stiffer and more fragile. With time, bones become brittle and break more easily. The shortening of the spine and trunk causes an overall reduction in height. Common ailments that afflict the elderly are aches and pains, acute stiffness, and in some cases varying degrees of deformity. For instance, the posture becomes bent and the knees and hips rickety; the neck begins to tilt, and shoulders gradually narrow. [13] Due to these changes, stamina takes a beating, the gait of the arthritis patient becomes wobbly, energy levels drop, and tiredness sinks in. A reduced level of physical activity, as one ages, is equally to blame for the early arrival of the above symptoms. While the body can be reinforced with essential vitamins and minerals, the bones require a certain level of mechanical stress for rejuvenation. Traditional beliefs that physical exertion should be reduced with age, as well as over-cautiousness about falling or straining some part of the body for fear of pain, are limiting factors in the repair and longevity of the skeletal system of the elderly.

ARTHRITIS-AFFECTED JOINTS OF THE UPPER BODY

Hands

Arthritis affecting the hands and wrists, besides being very painful, can be a functionally restricting condition. The distal interphalangeal joints, which separate the bones in the fingers, are frequently affected by degenerative arthritis. In this condition fingers may become twisted and distorted—in extreme cases to the extent that even holding simple daily-use items such as newspapers and toothbrushes becomes a challenge. [14]

In addition to infection and gout, psoriasis, a condition in which the skin becomes inflamed, can also trigger arthritis of the hand. Osteoarthritis of the hand usually occurs in the wrist; at the starting point of the thumb, where it connects with the wrist; at the middle joint of the finger; and at the last joint, nearest to the fingertip. Along with the severe pain, this condition creates discomfort in carrying out routine activities, such as opening cans, holding utensils, and turning keys, to name a few. [15]

Neck

Arthritis begins to affect the cervical vertebrae when the cartilage that fits between them degrades and the foramen (space) that lies in between narrows remarkably. This region becomes inflamed, resulting in neck pain, which may even radiate to the arms. As the situation deteriorates, the vertebrae develop spurs, which subject the spinal nerves to pressure. The result is acute pain and restricted movement of the neck. This condition usually affects the aged. [16]

Shoulders

Arthritis may affect both the joints of the shoulder. This is typified by the gradual wearing away of the cartilages, resulting in the bone becoming exposed. The resulting friction can be immensely painful. [17] Almost all daily activities become tedious with shoulder arthritis. With the loss of flexibility of the shoulder, driving, domestic chores, and even simple actions such as shaking hands or hugging become restricted.

Vertebral Column

The vertebral column can be broadly divided into four areas.

Cervical Vertebrae

This part of the vertebrae, referred to as the upper back consists, of the first seven vertebrae, which start at the bottom of the skull and connect at the lower end to the thoracic area of the spine. Age-related degeneration of the joints in the cervical portion results in a condition called cervical spondylosis, a form of arthritis that leads to intense pain and restricted movement.

Thoracic Vertebrae

The thoracic, or middle, part of the vertebral column consists of twelve vertebrae. Lying between the neck and the diaphragm, the thoracic area, due to its structure and the support it provides to the rib cage, has limited spinal movement. Despite its limited mobility, this section also undergoes wear and tear. The ensuing chronic inflammation of the spine causes severe back pain, an arthritic condition referred to as ankylosing spondylitis. [18]

Lumbar Vertebrae

Five vertebrae form this section of the spinal column, simply referred to as the lower back. The lumbar region connects the thoracic region to the sacrum, which is a fusion of several bones that connect the spine to the pelvis. With the spread of lumbar arthritis, the exposed bones rub against the nerves, causing pain and loss of sensation in the legs—a condition referred to as spinal stenosis. Although an age-related ailment, spinal stenosis also afflicts individuals who have suffered spine injuries, the obese, and persons engaged in heavy labor. [19]

Sacrum or Sacral Region

The sacrum is at the lowermost portion of the spine and lies between the fifth vertebra of the lumbar region and the coccyx, or tailbone. Arthritis affects this region too. While intense activity aggravates this condition, long periods spent sitting or standing also take their toll. Patients suffering from this condition experience loss of sensation or piercing pain in the lower back, buttocks, and legs. [20]

ARTHRITIS-AFFECTED JOINTS OF THE LOWER BODY

Hips

Compared to other weight-bearing joints, such as the ankle and knee, the hip is considered the largest. It is a ball-and-socket joint wherein the rounded head of the femur oscillates in the curved cavity (acetabulum) of the pelvic bone. Strong ligaments and muscles hold these two bones firmly together.

Hip arthritis tends to affect people over fifty, especially if they are over-weight. This condition seems to be genetic in nature, and it is not uncommon to find it being passed from one generation to the next. Hip arthritis can also occur due to trauma or injury. While several conditions produce disability and pain of the hip joint, entailing surgery, the majority of hip-replacement procedures are necessitated by arthritis.[21]

Knees

Each knee joint is actually a configuration of three bones: the femur, the tibia, and the patella. The knees are actually the largest joints in the body and carry its entire weight when the body is in motion. Activities such as running, walking, climbing, and jumping are possible because of the intricate arrange-ment of the knee joint. This makes it the most important joint in the human body. Pain in the knee is a common malady that afflicts the aged. Although it can be caused by trauma or misalignment, the most common factor is degen-eration due to wear and tear.[22]

Ankles

The foot and the leg meet at the ankle, or talocrural joint. Arthritis affects the ankle joint much less often than other joints. Wearing out of the joint be-tween the shinbone (tibia) and anklebone (talus) is the most common factor leading to ankle arthritis. However, ankle arthritis can also be a result of previous injury and not necessarily old age.[23]

Feet

Arthritis of the foot can be mild to disabling, depending on the severity of the condition and the part of the foot affected. Osteoarthritis is the most common type of arthritis and usually results from injury or many years of activity. Its symptoms include pain and swelling (usually noticed in the ankle) and a decline in joint flexibility. Another form of arthritis that affects the feet is rheumatoid arthritis. In this condition the feet are prone to deformity due to the wearing away of the connective tissues, making walking extremely diffi-cult. While the ball of the foot is the part most affected by rheumatoid arthritis, ankylosing spondylitis can also impact the feet. The symptoms[24] are the same: pain, swelling, and disability. In fact, the symptoms in most forms of arthritis are similar—pain, swelling, and disability—with slight variations in each. For instance, the big toe is the part of the foot affected by arthritis brought on by gout. The toe appears red and is sensitive to the touch. Reac-tive arthritis, usually caused by infection, makes the feet break out in rashes. Psoriatic arthritis affects the joints of the phalanxes (the digital bones of the feet), and the discomfort it causes can be disabling, making normal day-today activities very burdensome. Patients with psoriatic arthritis develop a severe skin condition called psoriasis.[25] In psoriasis, new skin is formed faster than old skin dies. Normally, the skin cells of the outer layer die and are replaced at regular intervals by new skin cells that grow below. In this form of arthritis, the accumulated dead skin cells become dry and scaly, appear red, and are prone to blistering. While these symptoms are visible in toes and fingernails, psoriatic arthritis affects skin in other regions of the body as well.

PATHOLOGY OF ARTHRITIS

Pathology is the branch of medical science that deals with the examination and detection of abnormalities, such as changes in the structure and function of the body, with a view to understanding their causes, progression, and effects. The term *pathology* derives from the ancient Greek word *pathos*, meaning "feeling" or "suffering," and *logia*, meaning "study." A pathology can also be referred to simply as a disease.[26] The term *physiology* derives from the Greek word *physio*, meaning "physical" or "natural," and *logia*. Physiology, therefore, refers to the branch of science concerned with the functioning of all living organisms and their parts. It deals with the mechanical, physical, and biochemical processes within animals and plants. While physiology is concerned with the study of "normal" biological functions in humans and animals, pathology is the study of "abnormal" functions, or diseases.

PATHOLOGY OF ARTHRITIS AT THE MOLECULAR LEVEL

To understand the causes and symptoms of arthritis at the molecular level, it may be useful to know what atoms and molecules are and how they differ from each other.

Atoms and Molecules

Atoms are the basic building blocks of almost all matter present in the universe. All elements are made up of atoms, which ares the smallest units into which an element can be divided. Combinations of atoms form molecules. Molecules are made up of two or more atoms held together in specific proportions by chemical bonds.

Molecules Involved in the Pathology of Arthritis

Pathologists have yet to gain a clear understanding of what causes arthritis besides natural occurrences such as ageing and trauma. Interestingly, a team of scientists from California and Japan has thrown fresh light on this debilitating condition. These scientists have discovered that naturally occurring molecules within the body can counteract the advance of arthritis.

Human Leukocyte Antigens

One such important molecule within the human body is the human leukocyte antigen (HLA), which was identified when organ transplants were, more often than not, being rejected by recipients' bodies. These molecules are actually genes present on human chromosomes and are closely associated with the human immune system. Some of these genes encode proteins known as antigens. An antigen is essentially any substance that causes the immune system to produce antibodies. This came to light only as a result of studies done during organ transplants. An important role, attributed to this group of antigens, is encouraging the growth and rapid reproduction of helper T cells, about which the following paragraphs provide more detail.[27] HLAs have several other important functions within the human immune system:

- They play an important role in disease defense.
- They may be responsible for rejection of organ transplants.
- They may defend—or, conversely, fail to defend (if they are down-regulated by infection of any kind)—the individual against cancers.
- They may intervene in autoimmune diseases, such as those affecting the digestive and endocrine systems.

The types of HLA present within each person are inherited. Thus, people with certain HLA antigens are more susceptible to developing certain diseases than others.

CD4+

CD4+, also called T4, is a large glycoprotein molecule found on the surface of lymphocytes that serve as a receptor for HIV. Glycoproteins play a crucial role in the body. These molecules contain carbohydrates as well as proteins, and in the immune system almost all the main molecules are glycoproteins. With advances in medicine, scientists have recognized the vital role CD4+ plays in immune responses in human autoimmune diseases, including rheumatoid arthritis. As knowledge of CD4+ continues to expand, it will help scientists understand and explore effective steps to arrest and cure this debilitating disease.[28]

Tumor Necrosis Factor

Cytokines, small protein molecules secreted by numerous cells, seem to be useful for signaling between one cell and another. One such cytokine, TNF-M, plays a crucial role in the advance of arthritis in humans and animals. Scientists hypothesize that removing the TNF-M molecule from an inflamed joint might have an effect on the progression of arthritis.[29]

Kinases

Another group of enzyme molecules found in the human body are kinases. Over five hundred different kinases have been identified in the human body, and of these, the largest group is protein kinases. Their main function is to act on or alter the activity of specific proteins within the body. The activity of the kinases is actually believed to modify around 30 percent of all human proteins.[30]

GTPases

Scientists have identified Rho GTPases in the human body, the main function of which is to regulate cytoskeletal activities as well as several kinds of signaling pathways within the system. They may be described as a very small but significant family of G proteins known to regulate many aspects of intracellular dynamics. Scientist have been conducting experiments, particularly with three members of the Rho family: Cdc 42, Rac 1, and Rho A.[31]

Rho GTPases (specialized enzymes) were actually first identified back in the mid-1980s, but investigation into them continues even today. Rho A proteins are known as "molecular switches" and play an important part in cell multiplication, as well as several other common cellular features. They are recognized as pivotal coordinators of immune responses. A more complete understanding of the role played by Rho GTPases will show scientists the way forward in the treatment of arthritis.

Interleukins

Interleukins form another group of cytokines that were first seen to be associated with the white blood cells. They are protein-secreting, signaling molecules. The term *interleukin* is derived from *inter*, meaning "between" but in this case referring to intercellular communication, and *leukin*, due to the fact that many of the proteins secreted by the interleukins are either produced by or act on leukocytes. The name, however, has proved to be a misnomer because subsequent studies have revealed that several other cell types actually produce interleukins as well.[32]

It has been established that the functioning of the immune system depends heavily on interleukins. An interleukin deficiency seems to result in autoimmune diseases or immune deficiencies. There are several forms of interleukin, each with its own significant role to play in the human immune system. For instance, interleukin-1 accelerates production of interferon and stimulates the growth of disease-fighting cells. Interleukin-3 regulates the production of blood cells, and interleukin-35 is believed to play a role in skin inflammation.

PATHOLOGY OF ARTHRITIS AT THE CELL AND TISSUE LEVELS

All living beings, both plants and animals, are made up of cells. A cell can be described as the structural, functional, and biological unit of all organisms. Cells are usually microscopic in structure and contain nuclear and cytoplasmic materials that are bound within a semipermeable membrane. In plants, the cells are surrounded by an outer cell wall. Cells may exist alone or function together with other cells. Tissues are a collection of similar cells that group together to perform a specialized function. *Tissue* derives from the Middle English word *tyssew*, a rich fabric. Organs are structures made up of at least two or more tissues that function together for a common purpose. The body is made up of several different organs (e.g., heart, liver, and kidneys), as well as the skin, which covers every part of the body and is actually the largest organ. The skin is made up of three tissues: (1) the outer epidermis, which protects the body; (2) the connective tissue, which contains the blood vessels that nourish the skin and the nerves that give the skin its ability to feel and make it pressure sensitive to the touch; and (3) fat layers, which provide cushioning to the skin.

Introduction to Cells Affected by Arthritis

The parts mainly affected by rheumatoid arthritis are the joints, tendons, and bone and muscle cells. In some cases, rheumatoid arthritis is also known to affect the internal organs. Fresh insights into the possible causes of arthritis have been uncovered only in the last decade or so, with over one hundred different kinds of arthritis being identified. Scientists have yet to identify a single cause that could set off the cellular symptoms of rheumatoid arthritis and, consequently, a single type of cell responsible for that disease—let alone for arthritis in general. While they continue to look for the cellular root cause of arthritis, valuable information is continuously being uncovered that helps medicine and science understand how to diagnose and treat this disease. Rheumatoid arthritis is now recognized as an autoimmune disease, which arguably relates to the fact that autoimmune conditions involve cells. [33] When a person develops symptoms of rheumatoid arthritis, the body begins to produce antibodies against its own tissues. To understand what causes the production of these antibodies, it is essential to understand the workings of the immune system.

Macrophages

These are leukocytes, or white blood cells, that are part of the human body's defense mechanism. The term *macrophage* originates from *makros*, meaning "large," and *phagein*, meaning "to eat." Macrophages are created in the bone marrow. When foreign bodies, such as bacteria, enter the bloodstream and encounter macrophages, the macrophages engulf and thereby destroy them. [34]

Researchers believe that macrophages play a significant role in rheumatoid arthritis because they appear abundantly at the site of inflamed, arthritis-affected membranes and cartilage. Studies indicate that while macrophages do not seem to be the root cause of rheumatoid arthritis, they do seem to possess an inflammatory and destructive capacity and to be active during all stages of arthritis. There is also ample evidence that the abundance of macrophages at the site of an inflamed, rheumatoid-affected area directly correlates with the severity of the disease.

Red Blood Cells

Studies have shown conclusively that a common complication of rheumatoid arthritis is the abnormally low number of red blood cells in the bloodstream. This leads to a condition called anemia. Contrary to popular belief, all the problems associated with arthritis are not necessarily related to the bones and joints. Between 30 to 60 percent of people with rheumatoid arthritis suffer from anemia. [35] Anemia seems to become more acute in people who have contracted severe forms of arthritis involving a higher number of bones and joints and a greater degree of pain and disability. Arthritis, by way of cellular pathology, is by no means the only cause for anemia; in fact, several other conditions can lead to the latter. However, it is important to note that in people suffering from rheumatoid arthritis, this condition can lead to acute fatigue and shortness of breath and an overall feeling of malaise.

Two types of anemia are associated with arthritis: (1) Iron-deficiency anemia is primarily caused by loss of blood, which contains red blood cells. This may include gastrointestinal bleeding in severe cases. (2) In anemia of chronic diseases, the patient has both rheumatoid arthritis and anemia. The abnormal chemicals and proteins that inflame the joints also affect the cells that produce red blood cells in the bone marrow. Studies show that this form of anemia inhibits or reduces the production of new red blood cells despite the fact that the body may have sufficient iron to produce new blood cells. [36]

B Cells and T Cells

Two types of lymphocytes (white blood cells) are present in the immune system: B cells and T cells. Scientists believe lymphocytes play a major role in ensuring that the activities of the immune system continue. B cells (also called B-lymphocytes) develop from stem cells in the bone marrow and supply antibodies to the human system. Studies have revealed that any change in the development and function of B cells may significantly affect rheumatic disorders. B cell depletion therapy is being investigated actively by researchers today as a treatment for arthritis and many other immune system–related diseases.[37]

Studies have revealed that the B and T cells distinguish between "self molecules" and "nonself molecules," such as bacteria and viruses, which may have invaded the body. Interestingly, B cells produce antibodies that get attached only to nonself molecules. Each B cell seems to produce antibodies for only one type of nonself molecule, and this production of antibodies takes place only with the assistance of T cells, which first need to recognize parts of the same nonself molecule. It is believed that T cells actually direct antibody production.[38]

Since T cells actually direct normal immune reactions, scientists theorize that sometimes T cells confuse self molecules with nonself molecules and begin directing the production of autoantibodies. This marks the beginning of autoimmunity, such as that related to arthritis, which, once started, continues for the rest of the lifespan. This type of autoimmunity seems to be typical only of humans. A clear explanation of what causes most forms of autoimmunity simply does not exist. There is no evidence to support the idea that factors outside the body are "fooling" the T cells into mistaking self for nonself molecules within the body. It seems clear, however, that hereditary factors make some people more susceptible to developing autoimmune disease than others. It appears that even within families with autoimmune disorders, it is impossible to predict who will develop them and when. It is therefore reasonable to conclude that arthritic autoimmunity gets initiated by a chance incident within the immune system. This progresses into a nonending, self-perpetuating vicious cycle. This chance event is the manufacture of an autoantibody with the abnormal ability to reproduce itself prolifically, which causes damage to body tissues.

RARE AND SPECIAL CELLS RELATED TO ARTHRITIS

Synovial Fibroblasts

The synovial membrane is the soft tissue found between the joint and the joint cavity. The term *synovium* comes from *synovia*, which means "synovial fluid," a clear fluid secreted by the synovial membranes. The term may have originally derived from the Latin words *syn*, meaning "with," and *ovum*, meaning "egg," because the liquid secreted is very much like egg white. Synovial fibroblasts are mesenchymal cells known to be abundant in arthritis. Mesenchymal cells are rare cells found in the bone marrow that are capable of developing into connective tissues, lymphatic and blood vessels, and blood. They are considered vital in the diagnosis and treatment of rheumatoid arthritis due to their ability to self-replicate and produce inflammatory cytokines as well as enzymes that destroy the cellular matrix of the cells. However, since rheumatoid arthritis is considered an immunity-related disease, scientists were not able to make a clear connection between the disease and immunity-related symptoms. One characteristic feature of arthritis is the inflammation of the synovial joints. All kinds of cells, such as macrophages, T cells, and neutrophils, migrate to the synovial tissues, become activated, and produce the substances that cause inflammation and degradation of joints and cartilages.[39]

Th-17 Cells

Scientists have been on an elusive quest for years to identify some key factor that triggers the onset and progression of rheumatoid arthritis. So far, all studies have proved futile inasmuch as there does not seem to be a single organism or condition that can exclusively be held responsible for this debilitating disease. A fairly recent study has shown that interleukin-17 (IL-17)–producing helper T cells (Th-17 cells) have a significant influence on the initiation of immune response in arthritis. However, the connection between local chronic inflammation and immune response is still not evident.[40]

Advances in osteoimmunology (the study of the relationship between bones and the immune system) have thrown new light on how bone destruction takes place in rheumatoid arthritis. Osteoclastogenesis and diseases of the bone have been shown to have advanced in the presence of Th-17 and related cytokines, mainly through the conduit of synovial fibroblasts. It is possible to conclude that mesenchymal cells influence the development of rheumatoid arthritis, and there is a clear link between the immune response and localized inflammation and destruction of joints and bones.

BONES AND OTHER TISSUES CONNECTED TO ARTHRITIS

Bones, being specialized tissues composed of cells, play a central role in both the physiology and the pathological status of arthritis patients. Besides giving all vertebrates their shape, they support and protect the body organs, produce red and white blood cells, and store minerals. Bones are multifunctional and are shaped differently according to their position and function. They have a complex internal structure, and osseous, or bone, tissue consists of dense connective tissue. Osseous tissue gives bones their rigidity and three-dimensional, coral-like internal structure. Bones are fairly hard and not too heavy. Other tissues found in the bones include the bone marrow, endosteum, periosteum, nerves, blood vessels, and cartilages.[41]

Bone Pathology and Arthritis

Arthritis affects more than 10 percent of humans between the age of thirty and sixty,[42] and it appears to affect women more than men. A person suffering from arthritis may have inflammation around the joints. This in turn releases enzymes that cause the surrounding bone and cartilage to wear away. If the condition becomes acute, secondary conditions set in that can affect surrounding tissues and organs, lead to bone loss, and give bones a greater tendency to fracture. When the bone tissue becomes damaged, the body automatically replaces it with scar tissue somewhat similar to the scar tissue that forms over an injury on the outer surface of the body. Scar tissue forming on the bone leads to the normal spaces in the joints becoming narrower, and some of the bones actually fuse together, leading to further complications.

Joint Tissue Pathology and Arthritis

Arthritis leads to inflammation of the tissues of the joint lining (synovium), which is the body's automatic response to any kind of infection or foreign invasion. Synovitis, as the disease is called, causes pain and swelling and, if not arrested in time, results in permanent damage to the affected joints and their surrounding blood vessels, nerves, ligaments, tendons, and cartilages.

Cartilage Pathology and Arthritis

Cartilages are flexible connective tissues found in different areas of the bodies of humans and vertebrate animals. Cartilage is less hard and rigid than the bone but not as flexible as the muscles. It is the cushioning agent between bones and ribs and is found in the ears, nose, and bronchial tubes, as well as between the vertebrae of the spinal column. Cartilages do not contain blood vessels like other connective tissues do; as a result, the healing process of the arthritis-affected area is relatively slow. On the whole, in comparison to other connective tissues, cartilage repairs and expands at a considerably slower pace. One pathological manifestation of arthritis is that the cartilage continues to wear away over time. This may lead to a condition in which adjoining bones begin to rub against one another. As an automatic response, the bones start to regenerate at this point, causing the joint to become rough and uneven. As the condition worsens, ridges of bone are formed on the surface of the affected area, making movement difficult and excruciating. Arthritis is the broad term applied when concerning any part of the bone, joint, or synovial membrane, or even the ends of the bone. One consequence of arthritis is the deterioration or atrophying of muscles attached to and in the vicinity of the joint.

When the cartilage in a joint is affected by arthritis, this leads to other negative occurrences, such as the following:

- Wear and tear: Cartilage attached to a joint can be compared to the rubber soles on shoes or the treads on a tire. With constant or heavy use, the soles of the shoe or treads of the tire become worn down and lose their original elasticity. Similarly, the cartilage becomes thinner with continuous use. Importantly, studies have shown that joint cartilage wears out much faster in heavy-built people.
- Dryness: Cartilage covering the joints, also called articular cartilage, is soft and smooth, as well as strong and long-lasting. The water content in the cartilage is very high, almost 60 percent.[43] One consequence of arthritis is that the persistent inflammation, which is one of its manifestations, can lead to reduction or loss of the ability to absorb and store water. If the problem persists, the cartilage becomes brittle and more likely to crack, flake, and crumble.
- Loss of cells: One of the greatest issues with cartilage is its inability to self-reproduce. Once pathologically damaged, there's no way it can be repaired or regenerated. This is extremely worrying, because as more cartilage in the joint becomes worn-out, the bones below become visible and get stressed due to pressure from carrying weight. This can lead to acute strain and pain.
- Traumatic rupture or detachment: The cartilage in the knee gets damaged, sometimes permanently.
- Costochondritis: Inflammation of cartilage in the ribs results in chest pain.
- Spinal disc herniation: An intervertebral disc becomes compressed unevenly, causing rupture of the sac-like disc, which in turn leads to herniation of its soft content. This often compresses the neighboring nerves and creates back pain.
- Relapsing polychondritis: This is probably an autoimmune condition of the cartilage, especially of the nose and ears, causing disfiguration. In extreme cases, death occurs due to suffocation as the larynx loses its rigidity and collapses.

Cartilage is normally smooth and unblemished. When this is altered in anyway and its original appearance and characteristics change or become flawed, cartilage is said to be arthritic.

2

Clinical Picture

Chapter Five

Causes and Symptoms of Arthritis

It is not uncommon to hear people describe age as a state of mind. Old age is therefore a time when one feels old, worn-out, incapacitated, or less capable. Old age is often considered one of the root causes of arthritis, and indeed it is. However, one can quite easily delay the onset of this condition if one accepts that an unhealthy or unkempt body ages faster than one that is less used or abused. This is where the subject of a healthy lifestyle comes into play.

OVERACTIVITY VERSUS INACTIVITY

Overactivity and Its Impact On Bones

Until recent times, body pains were associated with old age and a normal process of regression of the bony structure of the body. This perception is now changing, with people in the younger age bracket showing more and more signs of fatigue and pain brought on by the rigors of today's socioeconomic and lifestyle changes, the root cause being long hours of work confined at workstations, excessive television viewing with restricted movement, and, more importantly, the absence of adequate rest for the body. Though manual workers have always been affected by lumbar disc herniation, today this condition is visible among vehicle drivers and even white-collar workers who spend long hours sitting behind desks, working on computers, and carrying heavy laptop bags. This phenomenon is a clear indication that some kinds of overactivity can lead to bone diseases.[1]

That said, it is necessary to put this matter in its correct perspective. Most doctors would not discourage any form of physical exercise or perceive that overactivity could affect bones adversely. Importantly, all the conditions mentioned above can be remedied by keeping a well-toned body, which is only possible with a good deal of exercise combined with a healthy lifestyle.

Overactivity and Its Impact on Joints

The ever-increasing number of complaints about body dysfunction among younger people, who are subjected to excessive physical stress in their workplaces, serve as enough evidence that overactivity is a major contributor to joint diseases such as arthritis. For instance, cervical spondylosis, or abnormal wear and tear of the cartilage and bones of the neck (cervical vertebrae), is most often the upshot of excessive trauma to the joints of the neck. Patients engaged in long-term computer use may suffer from this due to long hours of craning to look at the computer monitor.[2] While some forms of overactivity have a negative impact on the joints, there is enough evidence that more good is derived from activity than from its absence. Overactivity can mean different things to different people. It is important to know one's endurance limit and to find an exercise pattern suitable for one's body type, age, and state of health. It is not only "all work and no play" that is responsible for joint disorders. Although cartilages are nourished by activity, and playing games can help maintain healthy cartilage, overactivity due to aggressive and intense sports such as boxing, wrestling, mountaineering, tennis, and cycling can cause irreparable joint disorders. Joint injuries, sustained by athletes, can affect cartilages, which can lead to the development of arthritis.[3]

Inactivity and Its Effects on Bones

It is a fact that patients prone to bone diseases[4] include the obese,[5] and while obesity has more causes than just excessive calorie intake, more often than not, it is just that. The key to weight loss is simply a combination of physical activity and a proper nutritional regime. However, expecting overweight people to be agile is, more often than not, an exercise in futility. A recent study shows that obese patients find relief from knee pain after they shed weight following bariatric surgery,[6] which serves as evidence that a heavy body can cause irreparable damage to the knees and weight-bearing bones of the body. The bones of individuals engaged in physical activity get thicker, increase in weight, and become stronger when subjected to stress. This in turn increases the bones' ability to endure more strain. Conversely, individuals who lead a sedentary life are less flexible, have lower pain thresholds, and suffer more injuries than those who are active. Poor balance and flexibility increases the risk of falling and breaking bones already rendered fragile due to mediocre growth and strength as a result of inactivity.[7]

It is important to understand that physical activity is the best way to treat arthritis. It is therefore ideal to deal with the positive impact that activity has on the bones. With exercise, one can actually begin to deal with the pain, gradually improving mobility and thereby one's quality of life. A regular routine of physical activity is good for persons of all ages, whether or not they have symptoms of arthritis. Having understood that, the next step is to find a form of exercise that will get a person started. However, getting someone to accept regular physical activity in the form of exercise, particularly if that person is not the active type, is easier said than done. A bit of counseling is recommended for the not-so-active, be they plain couch potatoes, housewives, or office executives who think they are getting enough exercise doing what they do, whether at home or in the workplace. Cooking, cleaning, or sitting behind a desk for long hours can be stressful and tiring, but that kind of activity may not be what is required to exercise those body parts that need strengthening. Time can be a major factor when one tries to find a slot dedicated to exercise. However, the slot must be found to fit in an exercise regimen that is suitable to one's age, state of health, and available time.[8]

Inactivity and Its Effect on Joints

A healthy body weight is central to the health of the complete body, and that includes the joints. Joints bearing the burden of excess weight suffer extensive wear and tear, inflammation, and stiffness, leading to arthritis. In the past, medication and rest were prescribed for those afflicted by arthritis. Today, it is commonly accepted that arthritis can be kept at bay with regular activity, which strengthens muscles and keeps joints flexible. Inactivity is known to have a severe damaging effect on bone tissue, which in turn hampers bone formation and the regeneration of cartilages. For this reason doctors advise plenty of exercise to prevent osteoporosis, a condition in which bone density declines and the bones become weaker and fracture easily. Uneven weight distribution across the knees or hip joints causes the bone below the cartilage to thicken on the side that is compressed, and the other joint, with less compression, begins to degenerate more rapidly.[9]

PHYSICAL AND MENTAL STRESS LEADING TO ARTHRITIS

How Physical Stress Leads to Arthritis

The body is designed to bend, stretch, jump, climb, carry weight, and absorb numerous other physical stresses during its lifespan. The skeletal structure, equipped with muscles, ligaments, and tendons, provides the body with the dexterity and efficiency to perform all bodily movements. The movements of the body and the amount of weight it has to carry impact the body as a whole. Continuous demands on the arthritis patient due to incessant stress can lead to severe pain in the joints. Sedentary lifestyles and bad posture also add to the stress and make aches in the legs, back, shoulders, and neck quite unbearable. Physical stresses, which are the root cause of distended cartilages, tenderness in the joints, and damage to soft body tissues, can be categorized as follows. [10]

Repetitive Stress Injuries

Repetitive stress injuries (RSIs) are caused by performing the same action repeatedly. Certain games or routine jobs that involve repetitive action—such as tennis, typing, climbing stairs, and any other action that is stressful to a joint—quite frequently cause injuries that fall under this category. While walking is a good form of exercise, climbing up and down stairs requires the knees to bear three to four times the actual body weight. If this is done on a regular basis, the cartilage of the knee joints slowly deteriorates and cracks. Such activities do not allow the area sufficient time to recover, resulting in pain and swelling and ultimately leading to arthritis. [11]

Obesity

Arthritis caused by obesity affects a large number of people, especially now, with the present generation's obsession with junk foods. Needless to say, if the body is to stay healthy, it's important that it not be stressed by carrying cumbersome loads. The burden of carrying excess kilos takes a toll on the joints, which begin to show wear and tear and become swollen and inflexible—symptoms typical of arthritis. [12]

High-Impact Activities

Physical stress caused by running and jumping or unarmed combat training of the sort that soldiers are subjected to may be worse for cartilage health. Persons whose activity level is high and not commensurate with their age or state of health—which may include several hours of walking, sports, or even household chores or yard work—also run the risk of developing arthritis. For instance, middle-aged men and women who engage in excessive levels of bodily activity may be causing damage to the cushioning disks of the joints of their spinal vertebrae or knee joints. [13]

How Mental Stress Leads to Arthritis

While it is easy to correlate physical stress with arthritis, mental disturbances can also trigger it. Sometimes a period of illness or some emotional upheaval, such as a death, divorce, financial worries, or other mentally stressful situation, can lead to a state of turmoil in which essential dietary needs are given a go by. Such situations can be a major contributing factor in the advancement of arthritis. Stressful situations also contribute to the increase of antibodies and inflammatory chemicals within the joints, which in turn aggravates arthritis. Some arthritics may become so overwhelmed by their condition that they become depressed and withdrawn to the point that the need for exercise and to take medication in a timely fashion is ignored. This causes further deterioration of the existing arthritic condition.[14]

CULTURAL FACTORS RELATED TO ARTHRITIS

Introduction to the Role of Culture

Traditions, taboos, and physical activity are contributing factors to the health of various ethnic groups and the treatment of the diseases peculiar to them. Understanding the factors affecting physical activity and occupational patterns is critical in the control of arthritis in these communities. For example, dietary habits, religious beliefs, lifestyles, and awareness (or lack of it) influence a population's susceptibility to arthritis.

Dietary Habits

Obesity is more prevalent in Native Americans than in whites and people of Asian origin. This is also true of Hispanics and blacks, who are more heavily built than whites and Asians.[15] Because obesity is so strongly related to arthritis, it's important to understand the eating habits of different racial groups. For instance, Americans are known to be heavy and large in build and also to be among the least healthy people in the world, primarily due to their diet, which is high in saturated fats, red meat, taste-enhancing add-ons, and fast "junk" food. In contrast, the Asian diet, characterized by vegetarianism, boiled food, and fewer or no preservatives, is now acknowledged to be the model to follow for a healthier lifestyle.

Differences among Cultures

The lifestyles of arthritis sufferers differ from culture to culture. In regions with a more Western-oriented lifestyle, where luxuries are there for the asking, people become more and more dependent on the comforts they have grown used to. Air-conditioning, effortless travel via the best modes of transport, tasty but harmful foods, late nights, a hectic pace of life, high stress levels, and inadequate time for exercise make them more vulnerable to the rigors of life. Sitting before a computer all day, munching oily tidbits and foods rich in carbohydrates while watching television, and other such excesses tend to make people weaker than those in regions that have not yet reached that level of indulgence. Unfortunately, in many parts of the world where inactivity is not the norm, people have become keen to live more like their Western counterparts. [16]

The result of such excessiveness is reduced pain endurance, weaker bodies, fragile bones, inflexible joints, and higher instances of arthritis. In contrast, in regions where lifestyles are more grounded and closer to nature, where the body is put to the test daily, where walking and physical work are a part of life, the people become sturdy, have a higher capacity to endure pain, remain more supple, and are less prone to arthritis. Following an Asian or Eastern lifestyle would be the paradigm shift that could make the difference between living on the edge and living life at its healthiest, with the simple pleasures of biking, walking, and other physical activities that will help one lose weight, raise immunity levels, and prevent diseases such as diabetes, heart problems, and arthritis. [17]

Some societies consider it uncivilized not to wear shoes, whereas others, particularly in the tropics or underdeveloped countries, find barefooted walking acceptable; members of the latter also seem to be less prone to contracting arthritis. It is an acknowledged fact that most shoes increase loads on the joints of the leg. Modern lifestyles requiring the wearing of shoes could do with closer evaluation, particularly with reference to the increasing number of persons suffering from osteoarthritis in urbanized cultures. For instance, in India it is reported that incidences of arthritis and varicose veins are relatively more common among urban Indians as opposed to the people living in rural areas, where wearing of shoes is uncommon. The report [18] indicates that people living in the villages suffer less from stiffness and pain in the joints, a fact attributed to walking barefoot.

Awareness

One reason for the predominance of arthritis in certain communities is the lack of awareness of the symptoms of the condition and its safeguards. Therefore, keeping in mind both the ethnic variance in knowledge about dealing with arthritis and the level of literacy, spreading awareness of the value of physical activity and other arthritis-control measures is the best way forward. This will help people in different communities understand how to deal with pain and what they must do to enhance the level of dexterity among individuals afflicted with arthritis. Information about such strategies, in a comprehensible vernacular and modified to suit every racial or ethnic group, should be made accessible to all societies vulnerable to arthritis, particularly those with a higher degree of pain sensitivity and activity limitations. [19]

ENVIRONMENTAL FACTORS RELATED TO ARTHRITIS

While the most common factor contributing to the increase of arthritis world-wide is lifestyle, environment can also be responsible for an increase in the number of such cases.

Terrain

The knee joint is a composite of three compartments, each with individual functions. The inner and outer compartments, referred to as the medial and lateral compartments, respectively, form the union of the lower end of the femur and the tibia. The third compartment, known as the patella, or knee-cap, joins the front part of the femur, and this joint, called the patellofemoral joint, is prone to arthritis, particularly in hilly terrain. While the medial and lateral compartments are crucial for walking on even surfaces, the patellofemoral joint comes into play for people walking on inclined surfaces, kneeling, crouching, getting up from a sitting position, or climbing stairs. People who live in the hills, whose daily routine involves climbing up and down steep gradients, will either be conditioned with a body suited to that kind of activity or suffer from joint disease in the long run. Similarly, in buildings without elevators, the daily routine of ascending and descending stairs can aggravate the joints and cause the onset of arthritis. Subtalar arthritis is caused when the rear portion of the foot is aggravated by excessive periods of standing or walking on uneven or sandy terrain. Inhabitants of sandy regions, such as denizens of fishing communities, those living in Middle Eastern deserts, people living in coastal areas, and beachgoers or sunbathers who already have a history of arthritis, run the risk of further harm to their lower extremities when walking on sand or any other unstable or undulated surface.[20]

Pollution

The Swedish Epidemiological Investigation of Rheumatoid Arthritis study and the US Nurses' Health Study reveal that prolonged exposure to air pollutants, particularly sulfur dioxide, increases the chance of developing rheumatoid arthritis.[21] Sulfur dioxide is one of the most common pollutants, and city dwellers run the risk of contracting this condition far more than residents of rural or semiurban areas. To understand the relation between pollution and arthritis, it is important to know that people who are prone to this form of autoimmune disease are greatly affected by their environment.[22] Some of the pollutants known to trigger the onset of autoimmune disease are jet fuel fumes, UV radiation, chemicals in food, chemicals in the atmosphere, and even secondhand smoke, just to name a few.[23]

GENETIC FACTORS RELATED TO ARTHRITIS

Overview

Genetics plays an important role in passing characteristics down to successive generations. Many human and animal diseases, including the various forms of arthritis, have genetic influences, but each case of arthritis has a distinct level of severity and hereditary pattern. Different genes work differently to create an impact in terms of vulnerability to and the severity of the disease.

The study of genetics investigates how human characteristics are passed from one generation to another. The process by which these characteristics appear in subsequent generations is attributed to genes. Around twenty-five thousand genes[24] influence human traits such as personality and vulnerability and resistance to different diseases. When mutations take place, the genes undergo changes, some of which are harmful and may cause deformities or diseases in offspring. Unifactorial or multifactorial diseases are the abnormalities passed on due to genetic mutations or variations. Unifactorial diseases occur when a mutated gene or a pair of genes is passed on to a child by one or both parents. A multifactorial disease results from a combination of multiple genes and factors such as environment, nutrition, infection, age, and gender. Osteoarthritis is believed to be a multifactorial and polygenic disease (result of a multigene mutation).

Role of Genes in Arthritis

Understanding the role of genes and genetic factors in the precipitation of arthritis will pave the way for dealing with this serious medical and socioeconomic challenge that affects people all over the globe. As it is prevalent worldwide, arthritis will have characteristics unique to different ethnic groups, each of which will have its own distinctive set of genetic factors. Some genetic factors will be common to all humans, and others will be more population specific.

The significance of identifying the genes for arthritis is that the genes provide an insight into the molecular route to the disease and will pave the way for developing suitable therapies. This will facilitate identifying groups or individuals at risk of developing arthritis and considerably improve the possibility of going straight to the root (genetic) cause of the problem.

Studying the influence of genes on twins reveals more facets of the genetic transfer of traits and diseases. Identical twins, referred to as monozygotic pairs, possess the same genetic structure, while nonidentical twins, or dizygotic pairs, share only half their genes. It has long puzzled scientists that a disease such as rheumatoid arthritis can strike one identical twin and not the other, despite their having identical genes. A relatively recent discovery[25] has shed light on this conundrum: scientists have discovered three or more new genes that seemed to be overactive in the case of the twins suffering from rheumatoid arthritis. This breakthrough will obviously show the way for researchers to get an even deeper understanding of the disease and all its variations and guide them toward finding new line of prevention and treatment. Therefore, arthritis caregivers can conjecture, from the study of twins subject to similar environmental and other exposures, that genetics plays an important role in disseminating traits and diseases.[26] Once the ethnic and genetic background of the different symptoms of arthritis is established, based on studies of different groups, identifying the genes responsible will be the next step in understanding the biological progression of the condition.

SIGNS AND SYMPTOMS OF ARTHRITIS

Medical Difference between a Sign and a Symptom

Although there is plenty of literature regarding the signs and symptoms of arthritis, this chapter aims to dispel some common misconceptions. Moreover, the ability to recognize these signs and symptoms can lead to early diagnosis, dramatically increasing the chances of therapeutic success. Medical symptoms are often mistaken as medical signs, and vice versa, while some practitioners prefer to use the term *symptom* to encompass both signs and symptoms of conditions such as arthritis.

Even though the terms *sign* and *symptom* might appear synonymous to most, they have quite different connotations in the clinical context. Symptoms are sensations felt by the patient, whereas signs are visible to anyone, including the doctors. A sign usually manifests itself externally in a manner that is observable to everyone, including medical professionals. A symptom is characterized by a feeling within the patient himself; it has meaning for and is limited to the patient only. Signs are objective assessments; symptoms are subjective feelings.[27] Patients often feel symptoms but fail to understand their medical meaning. Patients might observe signs which they fail to understand, but the same signs might be full of meaning for the medical professional.

The basic difference between a sign and a symptom lies in perspective. In other words, the identity of the observer determines whether a particular indicator is a sign or a symptom. If a patient notices it, then it is a merely a symptom; when a doctor observes it, it becomes a sign. Headache, pain, anxiety, and fatigue are symptoms. These can be considered sensations or feelings that only a patient can perceive or feel. No one can observe whether someone is having pain apart from the sufferer. A sign, on the other hand, is objective evidence of the presence of a disorder. A patient is the only person who can accurately define the symptoms, but a pale face is a characteristic easily detectable by anyone.

Examples

Examples are presented here to further clarify the difference between medical signs and symptoms. Breathlessness is a symptom (a feeling) associated with the sign of a fast pulse rate (measurable externally). Fatigue or tiredness can be considered a symptom, whereas bodily weakness is a sign. Nervousness is a feeling, which is a symptom, while trembling of the hands is a sign. Symptoms are feelings restricted to the domain of the patient, whereas signs are measurable.

Signs of Arthritis

There are many different signs of arthritis, some of which are discussed here. The particular signs depend on the type of arthritis the patient is suffering from, but there are some telltale, universal signs of arthritis in any form. The most common universal sign of arthritis is joint swelling. The onset of swelling can follow either prolonged use of the joints or simply casual use. The swelling is usually painful, often accompanied by inflammation, and sometimes warm to the touch. The joints that most frequently swell are the wrists, knuckles of the fingers and toes, elbows, shoulders, hips, knees, and ankles. [28] If, after performing any normal activity, one experiences a chill or fever, this also points to the existence of arthritis. These signs are often noticeable after one awakes from a night's sleep, but they can be experienced at other times as well. One noticeable sign of arthritis also includes a crunching feeling or the sound of bone rubbing on bone (known as crepitus) when the joint is used. A lot of people are unable to understand the signs of arthritis and mistake them for something else. For instance, if one has an injury that is hard to heal, the reason might be arthritis rather than something else. A sprained ankle that is not healing as fast as it should could be a sign of arthritis rather than a sprained ankle. Locked joints are another sign. Sometimes the swelling around the joints can be so great that they become locked and cannot bend. Another sign, often exhibited only in advanced stages of arthritis, is the presence of firm lumps, known as nodules, that grow underneath the skin near the affected joints.

Symptoms of Arthritis

Symptoms are defined as the sensations noticeable by the patient only. There are no visible manifestations of symptoms, which are specifically limited to the patient's own body. [29] Symptoms play a crucial role in the diagnosis and treatment of arthritis. The symptoms of arthritis are very common and are generally experienced by everyone at some level. However common these symptoms may be, they should not be taken lightly as ignoring them will only worsen the disease.

Joint pain and progressive stiffness are the most common symptoms of the condition. The pain is experienced by the patient to varying degrees and can be accompanied by swelling or fever. Joint pain experienced during normal daily activities points to the onset of arthritis. The reason behind the pain is quite simple. Whatever the particular type of arthritis, it eventually results in two opposing bones eroding each other. This erosion naturally causes pain, which can be persistent. Pain associated with osteoarthritis can arise from other parts of the body too. The areas around the joint are especially susceptible to this sort of pain. The areas most affected include the bone, ligament, and muscle, and the pain is especially acute after periods of physical activity. People with osteoarthritis react to the pain by completely stopping the use of the affected joints, but this can lead to further loss of permanent motion and other side effects. Osteoarthritis patients suffer from pain and stiffness coming on quickly, whether from an injury or from an unknown cause. As already mentioned, the pain can be accompanied by fever, which points to the presence of infectious arthritis. The pain and stiffness are noticeable in the arms, legs, or back after sitting for short periods or after a night's sleep.[30] Joint pain experienced by the infectious arthritis sufferer is often persistent in nature. Extreme fatigue, lack of energy, and a general feeling of malaise are also symptoms of infectious arthritis.

Another common group of symptoms of arthritis is carpal tunnel syndrome. This can be defined as a tingling feeling in the hands of the patient. It is basically a sensation similar to the feeling one gets when hit on the funny bone. People with arthritis are also at risk for Sjogren's syndrome, a disorder that can cause dryness in the patient's body. This dryness usually starts in the eyes but can be experienced in the nose, throat, and mouth too. Sometimes the patient's skin suffers from overall dryness. This dryness is often caused by the inflammation of glands, which stops them from releasing moisture as they would in their normal operation. Another characteristic symptom of arthritis is joint stiffness, especially in the mornings. This is a common problem that can cause pain after long periods of slowed activity, such as sleeping.

Arthritis is a rheumatic disease and therefore can cause symptoms that affect other organs of the body too. This will cause patients to experience different signs and symptoms, such as fever, gland swelling, weight loss, fatigue, malaise, and even symptoms stemming from abnormalities of organs such as the lungs, heart, and kidneys. The most common form of arthritis is osteoarthritis, but other major types include rheumatoid arthritis and gout.

The main symptoms of osteoarthritis are as follows:[31]

- Morning stiffness
- Joint pain after use
- Joint pain when the weather changes
- Joint swelling
- Inflexible joints

The symptoms of rheumatoid arthritis are listed below:

- Pain in the joints of the hands or feet
- Swelling of the joints of the hands or feet
- Pain in the body and joints after periods of rest
- Painful joints
- Swollen joints

PAIN

Introduction

Pain is fundamentally the arthritis patient's warning that something is wrong. The human body is a complex system of nerves that transmit signals to the brain. If there is an injury, the nerves in that area send a message to the brain, which interprets these signals as pain. Pain is often a signal to act. For instance, touching a hot stove generates pain. The brain then signals the hand to pull away. The pain from arthritis, however, is long-lasting and therefore quite different from conventional pain. While it still is a signal pointing to the fact that something is wrong, such pain is often not as easy to relieve.

As already mentioned, pain signals are transmitted through a complex system of the nerves to the brain. Sometimes, the arthritis patient's body reacts and stops the progression of these signals by creating chemicals called endorphins. Different factors cause the body to produce these chemicals.[32] An example includes the concepts of thoughts and emotions: if a mother and her sons are involved in a car accident, the mother will probably have a lot of pain, but as she is more worried about her children, her own pain messages may not reach her brain. Codeine is a pain-blocking medicine that produces a similar effect for arthritis patients.

A Deeper Look at Arthritis Pain

There are several different forms of arthritis, all of which are associated with extreme pain. Arthritis pain is special in that it is usually worst in the mornings (after the sufferer wakes up) and fades during the course of the day. This pain is also acute during periods of physical activity or exertion. In some cases pain might not be the main feature of the disease. This is especially true of elderly people, whose physical activity is usually less than that of younger people. This is also the case with children, whose natural response is to avoid using the pain-ridden joints.

Arthritis patients experience two types of pain:

- Acute pain is temporary and usually severe. The pain is felt in the joints themselves or in the areas surrounding the joints. The duration can be a few seconds or longer but diminishes as healing occurs. Examples of injuries that cause acute pain in general life include burns, cuts, and fractures.
- Chronic pain ranges from mild to severe. There is no agreed-on time range for the duration of chronic pain, which can last for days, months, years, or even a lifetime.

Chronic pain is most commonly associated with osteoarthritis and rheumatoid arthritis. The severity of the pain is dictated by a number of factors. The most important are the amount of damage occurring within the joint and the related swelling. Furthermore, activities affect pain differently, so some arthritis sufferers tell of pain in their joints after getting up in the morning, while others develop pain after overuse of the joint. Arthritis patients, however, typically have acute pain in the mornings when they get out of bed. The pain subsides gradually as the day progresses.

The most common form of arthritis, osteoarthritis, affects mainly the hands but also attacks any weight-bearing joints of the human body, causing pain. These joints include the hip and knee joints, among others. Osteoarthritis progresses when the cartilage degenerates with age. The pain associated with this type of arthritis is often persistent. Rheumatoid arthritis affects the hands, wrists, and knees in a chronic, long-term way. In some patients, other parts of the body, such as the lungs and blood vessels, may become inflamed over the years as well. Gout, the failure of the body to eliminate excess uric acid, affects the big toe, knee, and wrist joints over the long term.

Facing the Pain

Arthritis sufferers react differently to pain for several reasons. Physical factors include the sensitivity of the nervous system and the severity of the pain itself. Emotional and social factors include a patient's fears and anxieties about pain, previous experiences with pain, energy level, and attitude about the disease, as well as the way people around the patient react to pain. A clearer understanding of pain enables one to deal with it better. People with arthritis who understand their pain well are better able to deal with their condition. They can manage their pain with a lot more ease and, hence, face the disease more comfortably. There are several well-known methods of facing the pain of arthritis. The straightforward method involves the authorized use of prescription painkillers. This is not a preferred choice for most patients due to the side effects, which can cause other complications. Another method to deal with pain is meditation or otherwise engaging the mind in some interesting activity that can divert attention from the discomfort. Joining support groups can also help mentally by allowing the patient to share his or her feelings, and sometimes helplessness, with others in a similar position. A simple way of dealing with the pain is exercise, which is covered more extensively in chapter 19. Even though it might seem counterintuitive, regular light exercise helps the joints to relax in the long run. Unfortunately, the pain associated with arthritis can be lifelong and lead to mental health issues such as depression and stress. Physicians therefore recommend that patients manage their pain using the method they find most suitable.

SWELLING AND INFLAMMATION

Overview

The terms *swelling* and *inflammation* are used extensively in this chapter as they are key characteristics of arthritis. Nonetheless, swelling and inflammation are two different things from a clinical standpoint, though both are signs of arthritis. Doctors specifically look for them while examining a patient suspected of having a bone or joint disease. Sufferers of all joint disorders, including osteoarthritis, rheumatoid arthritis, and gout, exhibit similar symptoms or signs, such as acute pain in the joints, swelling around the joints, and inflammation of the suspected areas. [33]

Swelling at a Glance

Swelling is the enlargement of organs or other parts of the body, often resulting from fluid accumulation under the skin. Swelling is defined as a temporary enlargement or protuberance in the body caused by injury or disease and can also result from an underlying lump that causes blockage. This means that the fluid is unable to circulate well in the affected joint. There are many types of swelling from a medical viewpoint. The most common classification of swelling is according to the area of the body affected. Generalized swelling refers to swelling present throughout the body; swelling can also be localized to a specific part or organ. Generalized swelling, or massive edema, is very common. Slight edema is difficult to detect, whereas major edema is "straightforward" enough for patients and caregivers to work on. Congenital swellings are generally present from birth, but some may appear later in life. Traumatic swellings develop immediately after a trauma. Acute swellings are characterized by redness, local fever, pain, and impaired function of the affected organ.[34] Chronic swelling usually presents with inflammation but does not necessarily imply the existence of edema. Edema can be classified as pitting or nonpitting. When pressed, pitting edema leaves a mark in the skin that takes few seconds to disappear. In nonpitting edema, pressing on the affected area does leave an indentation. Both types are important and need to be fully understood so that doctors can deal with the swelling correctly.

A Look at Inflammation

Inflammation usually results from injury and illness. It produces redness and swelling either externally or internally. Inflammation results when tissue reacts to injury. This injury can be caused by the presence of pathogens. It is characterized by increased blood flow to the tissue, causing increased temperature, redness, swelling, and pain. The first reaction of the immune system to an infection or irritation is inflammation, and the presence of this inflammation is necessary for the healing of wounds.

Inflammation is acute or chronic in nature. Acute inflammation is the response of the body to invading (usually harmful) stimuli and results when plasma moves from blood to injured tissue. Prolonged inflammation, also called chronic inflammation, involves the movement of cells to the area of inflammation. Acute inflammation is usually short-term and appears a short time after the introduction of the injury-sustaining stimulus and vanishes after the stimulus in removed. A major danger of inflammation is that it results in pain, swelling, and redness in joints and other body parts. This can be a serious situation with permanent effects.

General Role of Swelling and Inflammation

Inflammation is the natural response of the human body when there is an injury to the tissue, whereas swelling is a cardinal sign of inflammation within the soft tissue, which causes the pain. The swelling associated with inflammation contributes in numerous ways to nerve compression and nerve entrapment. Inflammation plays a key role in a number of diseases, including arthritis, diabetes, and heart disease. The fact is that the inflammation associated with all these diseases is nearly the same. Doctors hope that developing a better understanding of this inflammation will help further treatments for the diseases in question.

Swelling and Inflammation in Arthritis

Arthritis entails inflammation of the joints. The common forms of arthritis known for high levels of inflammation are listed below:

- Gouty arthritis
- Psoriatic arthritis
- Rheumatoid arthritis
- Systemic lupus erythematosus

Arthritis is almost synonymous with swelling and inflammation of the affected joints. Any patient with arthritis experiences swelling and inflammation and needs knowledge about how to deal with them. There is no cure for arthritis, but promising treatments exist to relieve the pain associated with it. Inflammation is normally necessary for the body to heal, but during arthritis, the immune system attacks the body instead. The inflammation affects (1) the thin synovial membrane, (2) the tendon sheaths, and (3) the bursae. A closer look at the structure and makeup of a joint in the human body reveals that joints in the body are enclosed in a thin capsule. The *synovium* is the technical name for the lining of this capsule. This wall is very thin and consists of only a few cells. The onset of rheumatoid arthritis induces the production of TNF-M cytokines.[35] These chemicals produce the inflammation and also result in the thickening of the wall of the synovium. The joint swells, and damage to the cartilage occurs. If the reaction is especially acute and the cartilage gets very damaged, the bones will be more exposed to overuse.

The bones can very easily rub together and damage each other while the patient experiences excruciating pain along the way. The joints and inflamed tissues then become stiff, painful, and swollen. The most common form of arthritis is called osteoarthritis, in which inflammation plays a major role. During inflammation, increased blood flow and the release of chemicals result in the accumulation of white blood cells in the inflamed region. The inflammation within the joints can cause irritation, wear down the cartilage, and swell the lining of the joints. The following may confirm swelling and inflammation in arthritis:

- Results of X-rays and blood tests
- Location of painful joints
- Complete medical history and physical exam
- Presence of joint stiffness in the morning

Inflammation during arthritis can also affect internal organs when the sufferer has a major autoimmune disorder. There are a number of treatment options for inflammatory joint diseases, but it has to be kept in mind that there is never a total cure. Patients are usually administered medicines and therapies or undergo surgery. There are many drugs available on the market to manage pain and swelling in arthritis. These include anti-inflammatory pain relievers and other medications. Intermittent swelling in arthritis is common and most likely occurs as a result of active inflammatory synovitis, but in any healthy joint there is always a certain amount of fluid. When a joint is affected by arthritis (particularly inflammatory types) irregular amounts of fluid leading to swelling are noted.

Chapter Six

Diagnosing Arthritis

Medical diagnosis has two sides. The first is concerned with the doctor identifying the disorder. The second is evaluative in nature: the doctor tries to determine the severity of the disorder and devises a treatment plan. The diagnostic process usually involves medical tests and imaging. The process whereby the physician makes a diagnosis is highly cognitive. It is very much akin to putting a complicated puzzle together with the help of the results of clinical tests and professional experience. The first "diagnosis" is usually quite wide, but subsequent tests narrow things down.

EARLY DETECTION AND ACTION PLANS

Benefits of Early Detection

Both skills and technology are advancing while medical science is at a stage where initial presumptions can be made increasingly early in the disorder process. The field of arthrology as a whole is seeking to raise awareness and encourage early interventions among those affected by a disorder. The thinking behind early-detection techniques is that the earlier a disorder is diagnosed, the greater the chances of recovery. Managing a disorder, especially early in its course, may lower its impact on the patient's life. An early diagnosis depends on certain tests, and the types of tests required will depend entirely on the patient's age, health, gender, and risk factors. Risk factors might include family history, such as having a close relative with cancer, and lifestyle issues such as smoking. Cholesterol screening, for example, is recommended for people who have a family history of early coronary artery disease. There is a higher mathematical probability for success in the treatment of any disorder if it has been detected early.[1]

Early detection will also help the patient financially. This is because the cost of treatment can be considerably higher if a disorder is detected at an advanced stage. Early detection means shorter, targeted treatment with few side effects. Proactive screening programs are very useful in helping to identify problems early and prevent disorders. Although screening sounds very promising in helping to prevent some very common disorders, a good screening method has proved elusive for many important disorders. Cancer and tumors fall into this category. Doctors and clinicians are constantly on the lookout for better screening procedures for identifying disorders early because they understand the virtues of early detection not just for health but for the wallet as well.

Early Detection Is Key in Arthritis

Arthritis is a chronic disorder. There are millions of sufferers worldwide with no cure in sight. This means that arthritis patients are reliant on pain-relief methods to ease the disorder rather than a complete treatment. A particular form of the disorder, juvenile rheumatoid arthritis (JRA), is prevalent in children (see chapter 9). Children who develop JRA never outgrow it and must unfortunately learn to live with the resultant issues for life. Early detection of the disorder is key to preventing further damage to the body, which can include a breakdown of cartilage, chronic inflammation, and damage to surrounding muscles and tissues.

A University of Colorado professor[2] argues that drug-free pain remission is only possible if the disorder is treated in its early stages, possibly even before the onset of symptoms. This underscores the importance of early diagnosis in arthritis to leading a healthy life. Of note here is that the pain associated with arthritis is mostly experienced by older patients, but this is not a set rule. Young people often find that they experience excruciating pain too.

A lot of progress has been made in medical science in tackling both arthritis as a disorder and the associated pain. However, the majority of these treatments can only be effective if the disorder is diagnosed early. There are medications available that can slow or even stop the disorder from progressing completely, but these are only truly effective if patients start treatment early. The prerequisite for that is early detection. A number of surgical procedures in the early stages of osteoarthritis can be very beneficial to the recipient. In short, patients of arthritis and their caregivers need to be alert to the signs and symptoms and take immediate action after discovering any problems. If not handled at an early stage, the inflammation of joints will most likely damage the cartilage protecting the surface of the bones. Cartilage acts as a cushion between bones that does not allow them to rub together.[3] In the event of the cartilage being damaged, the bones will start rubbing against each other, causing the arthritis sufferer discomfort. The virtues of early detection in light of proper diagnosis of arthritis are therefore paramount. Early detection will stop further erosion and reduce the amount of pain suffered by the patient.

An example here posits the opposite situation: a female patient who discovers she has arthritis after the cartilage is nearly gone will experience pain in that particular joint for the rest of her life. Early detection is vital for arthritis patients since without it, they will probably have to bear pain for the long run. Pain medication could help in that scenario, but it has side effects.

What to Do if Arthritis Is Suspected

A patient will experience a number of signs and symptoms during the onset of arthritis, and if any of them is present, the patient should immediately seek help. One of the first symptoms of arthritis is not joint pain but fatigue. Patients, especially in very early stages of the disorder, often experience tiredness and fatigue even due to normal physical activity. This is especially true in the mornings when a person wakes up tired. In any form of arthritis, the patient is bound to experience joint pain. However, joint pain can stem from a number of reasons, including inadvertent injury. If the pain does not subside in few days' time, the patient must consult a doctor. If the pain is accompanied by swelling, redness, and inflammation, then there is a high probability that it is arthritis, and the patient should not delay seeing a physician or other health-care professional. It is also vital to present as much detail to the doctor as possible. For instance, the intensity of the pain can be a good indicator. Details such as the time of day when the pain is most acute and what makes the pain worse or better will help the doctor make the correct diagnosis quickly and effectively.

Feeling pain might warrant someone's suspecting he or she has arthritis. Pain in the joints can often be relieved with some moderate self-medication. One can use painkillers and think that he or she is getting better, whereas in actual fact the pain is only being suppressed temporarily. The underlying problem still exists and is probably getting worse. Self-medication should be kept to a minimum by anyone suspecting he or she has arthritis. The patient should quickly seek medical advice before it is too late. Furthermore, the first port of call can be the family doctor, who can do the initial screening and testing and might refer the patient to a rheumatologist if necessary. Rheumatologists are specialists in arthritis and can be trusted to have the latest knowledge and the skills required to deal with arthritis patients. Perhaps the most important thing to do if one suspects arthritis is to prepare mentally for a long ride.

CLINICAL HISTORY

A full clinical history is called an anamnesis in medical literature. Doctors use this process to gain useful information that will help in the diagnostic process. This information can be ascertained by asking direct questions of the patient and the people around him or her. The clinical history is a vital part of making a diagnosis and providing quality care. Symptoms are the sensations that the patient suffers and can describe to the doctor, whereas signs are observable instances of those symptoms. Both are part of the overall history-taking process.

Role of History Taking

A medical history is a comprehensive assessment of the factors affecting a patient's health status. This entails gaining useful information that will help form an accurate picture for the physician. The information can include cultural and family background or anything else the doctor feels will contribute positively to the diagnosis. The medical history is a crucial element in the entire medical process. It helps to determine the right prognosis and treatment plan for each individual. It can also act as a very useful teaching aid. The information obtained in this way, coupled with a medical examination, will assist in providing a reliable diagnosis.[4] Even if the initial formulation of the diagnosis is not complete, the entire history will be available for future reference. It can be used by another physician consulted by the patient or by the same doctor during a future visit of the patient. Medical history taking may be of an extremely comprehensive nature, usually associated with medical students learning the art, or it can entail iterative hypothesis testing, often associated with busy, practicing physicians.

Nowadays, one innovation in the medical profession is computerized history taking. In the years to come this could be crucial to time management for the doctors. Hospitals are already developing online tools and decision-support systems to aid professionals as much as possible.

Whatever the methodology or level of detail of history taking, some established norms are followed. While taking the general history of a patient, most health-care professionals will ask questions to ascertain the following:

- Identity and demographics
- Chief complaint
- History of the present illness
- Past medical history
- Review of organ systems
- Family disorder history
- Childhood disorders

- Social history
- Regular and acute medications
- Allergies
- Sexual, obstetric, and gynecological history

The medical history is an essential element of clinical record keeping. It is the foundation of an accurate diagnosis and fast patient recovery. There is no comprehensive and agreed-on standard for taking a medical history. It is therefore up to the medical practitioner to record the most comprehensive history possible to help others later. Some of the major reasons why clinical histories are extremely invaluable before and after diagnosis are as follows:

- They secure accurate information, which helps in providing specialized care to patients.
- They get information regarding the presence of specific medical conditions, such as a heart condition, diabetes, asthma, epilepsy, and allergies. Such information could be vital in a medical emergency.
- They prevent medical complications by ensuring that the correct medication is administered.
- They prevent lawsuits filed against arthritis caregivers who have maintained a thorough history.

DIAGNOSTIC TESTS AND SCREENING PROCEDURES

As the previous sections have made clear, it is vital to diagnose arthritis as early as possible. This helps in relieving the patient of the pain associated with the disorder. This section provides a thorough listing of the tests and other screening procedures involved in the proper diagnosis of arthritis.

Blood Tests Involved in Diagnosing Arthritis

When a patient presents symptoms and signs associated with joints such as joint pain, swelling, and inflammation, doctors usually suspect arthritis. Doctors who specialize in the diagnosis and treatment of arthritis and other rheumatic conditions are called rheumatologists. The first tools these doctors have at their disposal are blood tests to confirm the presence of the condition. There are six basic blood tests to confirm the presence of arthritis.

Rheumatoid Factor

Rheumatoid factor (RF) is defined as a binding antibody. These are different from normal antibodies in that they can bind themselves to the other antibodies.[5] Antibodies are normal proteins found in the blood that function within the immune system. However, RF is only found in about 1 percent of the population. The presence of RF is ascertained from a blood test usually used to diagnose rheumatoid arthritis. RF is present in approximately 80 percent of adults who suffer from arthritis. RF increases if the arthritis is prolonged in a patient. A presence of high levels of rheumatoid factor (in about the ninety-fifth percentile) strongly indicates the presence of rheumatoid arthritis. RF is nonetheless not exactly the best choice for detecting other major types of arthritis.[6]

Anti–Cyclic Citrullinated Peptide

The anti–cyclic citrullinated peptide (CCP) blood test, like the RF test, helps to confirm the presence of rheumatoid arthritis in a patient. The problem with the RF test is that a large number of patients who are positive for CCP do not actually have rheumatoid arthritis. Rheumatoid factor is less important from a diagnostic point of view than CCP. An abundance of the anti-CCP antibody in a patient's blood is a clear indicator of the presence of rheumatoid arthritis. Low levels of the antibody are usually ignored by doctors, but high levels, if present, can indicate a potential risk of joint damage.

Erythrocyte Sedimentation Rate

The erythrocyte sedimentation rate (ESR), or "sed rate" for short, is a test used to diagnose inflammation. It technically measures the speed at which blood cells fall in a tube. A high recorded value shows the presence of inflammation. A number of other factors can contribute to an elevated ESR, such as pregnancy, infection, or tumor. However, the most common reason for a high ESR is arthritis. The reason for this is simple: the ESR tests for inflammation, and if the patient is not suffering from any specific preexisting illness, then the high ESR shows the presence of arthritis. The test is usually the first one ordered by a doctor suspecting arthritis.

C-Reactive Protein

The C-reactive protein (CRP) test aims to numerically measure the concentration of a special type of protein in the blood. This protein is attributed to periods of inflammation or infection. It is quite similar to the ESR test in that it also confirms the presence of inflammation. Unfortunately, CRP is not specific enough in that it only points to the presence of acute inflammation, which could be the result of a number of disorders, including arthritis, cancer, heart attack, lupus, and tuberculosis. Therefore, the doctors usually use this test along with a number of other procedures to confirm the presence of arthritis in a patient.

Antinuclear Antibody

This is an important test in the diagnosis of arthritis. There is usually no antinuclear antibody (ANA) in the blood of a normal person, although exceptions exist. Low levels of ANA are present in an arthritis patient, whereas higher amounts of ANA are associated with other disorders.

Complete Blood Count

A complete blood count (CBC) measures the number of red blood cells, white blood cells, platelets, and other constituents in a blood sample. A low white blood cell, red blood cell, or platelet count indicates the presence of inflammation associated with arthritis.

Imaging Strategies Involved in Diagnosing Arthritis

Although blood tests are very effective in diagnosing arthritis, health-care professionals need to get a better idea of the damage to the patient's joints. Imaging techniques may give the doctor a clearer picture of what is happening to the joints. Three imaging techniques are often used.

X-ray

This imaging technique uses invisible electromagnetic radiation, or X-rays, to formulate an accurate picture of the internal structure of the body. X-rays are also called ionizing radiation.[7] They are most often used to picture bones and organs. An X-ray test is quite safe[8] as it uses a very small amount of radiation. The machine is extremely localized so that only the targeted area is affected. In evaluating arthritis, the doctor uses X-rays to rule out injuries and other joint disorders. These detailed pictures provide conclusive evidence to the physician of the presence of arthritis.

Computed Tomography Scan

This scanning procedure uses a mixture of X-rays and computing power. It takes cross-sectional pictures of the body that provide a very detailed look inside a patient. A computed tomography (CT) scan can capture images of the inside of the body very accurately. They are generally more detailed and better than general X-rays. They are very useful for providing a very clear picture of the bones and their shapes. The deterioration of the tissue is also very visible, which can clearly point to the presence of arthritis.

Magnetic Resonance Imaging

In diagnosing arthritis, a magnetic resonance imaging (MRI) scan can be helpful. While X-rays are used to observe dense tissue, MRIs are used mostly for observing soft tissue. The MRI scan provides very clear images of the body parts without using X-rays. MRI uses radio waves, a computer, and a large magnet to produce these images. This scan is used to detect the presence of a disorder but also has major significance in evaluating a patient's treatment. The scan is considered extremely safe by medical professionals, and a patient should have no qualms about having an MRI, especially provided its benefits related to arthritis.[9] (If a patient has any surgical clips, artificial joints, staples, or a cardiac valve replacement, having an MRI is not advisable.) The actual procedure takes only a few minutes and is quite simple. Edema of the bone marrow is another critical feature detected by MRI and associated with inflammatory joint disorder and could be a forerunner of erosion in the arthritis sufferer.

Other Screening Procedures in Diagnosing Arthritis

In addition to the aforementioned blood tests and imaging techniques, a few other specific procedures are involved in the diagnosis of arthritis.

Arthroscopy

This is a minimally invasive diagnostic procedure used for conditions of a joint. The procedure involves a small, lighted optic tube (arthroscope) that is advanced into a joint through a minuscule incision. Pictures of the joint's interior are shown on a screen. These are then employed to evaluate any degenerative and arthritic changes in the joint. Arthroscopy is effective in detecting bone disorders and tumors too. The doctors are better able to determine the cause of inflammation and bone pain using arthroscopy.

Ultrasound

This is a diagnostic procedure used occasionally to find inflammation before X-rays show damage. An ultrasound produces sound waves that are beamed directly at the human body. These beams strike the surface and are reflected back. The recording of this echo forms a detailed picture of material underneath the skin. This technology is especially good for looking at the interface between solid and fluid-filled spaces. This interface is the basis of arthritis. The erosion of cartilage between bones is the chief culprit and is accurately caught during ultrasound imaging.

Bone Densitometry

This is a very different sort of test in that it measures the density of the bone. Bone densitometry is also referred to as dual-energy X-ray absorptiometry (DEXA).[10] The technique is especially useful in diagnosing osteoarthritis.

Outside of arthritis, the most popular use of DEXA is in dealing with bone fractures.

PHYSICAL EXAMINATION FOR ARTHRITIS PATIENTS

To make a correct diagnosis of arthritis, the family physician or internist will also perform a thorough physical examination. The doctor will examine the patient's joints for redness, ease of movement, warmth, tenderness, and damage. Because some subtypes of arthritis, such as lupus, may harm internal organs, a complete physical examination that includes the nervous system, lungs, heart, abdomen, ears, mouth, eyes, and throat may be necessary. Laboratory tests may also be ordered to confirm the diagnosis. These can include tests of the blood, urine, and synovial fluid (lubricating fluid found in the joint). These tests are also useful later on for monitoring the disease and the effectiveness of treatments and medications. The doctor will look for visible signs of arthritis during a physical examination. The patient will be observed for signs and symptoms of arthritis, which include redness and warmth near the joint, bumps or nodules, tenderness, joint stiffness, fluid on the joint, the pattern of affected joints, and fever. As physical information is gathered, the doctor will then work on providing an accurate diagnosis based on the results, as well as the results of tests and X-rays performed. During the physical examination, the doctor may check the patient's range of motion to see how different it is from the typical range of motion for a certain joint. This is done to assess limitations caused by existing joint damage, joint swelling, muscle spasms, or pain.

It is necessary to disclose symptoms that have disappeared as well as symptoms that have increased in intensity. Symptoms that have gone away suggest that the treatment regimen is working; the opposite can be said of accrued symptoms. The keen observations of both the patient and doctor are relevant and form the basis for future decisions about treatment goals.

Chapter Seven

The Roles of Various Types of Physicians in Arthritis

The following sections will help arthritis patients become proactive and ask questions of their doctors to get the best treatment and diagnosis possible. Physicians will also ask detailed questions of patients concerning their symptoms and medical histories to correctly diagnosis their condition. Several tests and physical examinations also play a great role in the proper diagnosis and treatment of arthritis patients. The observations of the arthritis patient and the doctor are integral in determining the best options for the patient's treatment.

ROLE OF INTERNISTS AND FAMILY DOCTORS IN ARTHRITIS

Family practice physicians provide basic, primary care and see patients of all ages. They have broader experience in diagnosing and treating both children and adults. Family physicians spend their three-year training period studying the medical problems of children and adults, obstetrics, and surgery. They are qualified to treat everyone from babies to adults, but their training is not as extensive in one area as that of an internal medicine specialist. Special emphasis is placed on disease prevention and primary care for whole families, with consultations when appropriate.

Internal medicine doctors, or internists, spend three or more years learning about the medical problems of teens and adults. They are also educated in the basics of primary care internal medicine, which includes an understanding of wellness, mental health, substance abuse, disease prevention, and effective treatment of common maladies of the eyes, ears, skin, nervous system, and reproductive organs. They are able to address any problem, no matter how complex. Internists can also diagnose multiple medical problems that arise in one patient and are tied together. Most family doctors refer patients with puzzling medical issues to internists for diagnosis. Internists can also provide primary care as well as subspecialize in a variety of areas, including gastroenterology, rheumatology, and endocrinology. Internists do not typically see patients under the age of eighteen and usually have more hospital-based experience than family practice physicians.[1]

THE JOB

Typical Workday

Family practice physicians usually spend their days treating men, women, and children who either have a medical problem or are just generally concerned about their health. Their job is to treat illness as well as to answer health-related questions. A family practice physician guides patients on adapting healthy habits such as quitting smoking, reducing fatty-food intake, and even losing weight. They conduct physical examinations and can later refer patients to internists for peculiar medical conditions. Typically, family physicians see patients in a clinic up to five days per week. Some family practitioners take a day or two off from seeing patients at their clinic to check on patients living in nursing homes. In addition to their hospital and nursing home rounds and office hours, family physicians may also be on call at a hospital several nights a week and sometimes even over the weekend or during holidays. When on call, depending on the setup of the particular hospital, the physician can either admit patients over the phone or may have to be present at the hospital when paged.

Internists provide nonsurgical treatment of diseases. They perform physical examinations and gather information about a patient's medical history and current symptoms. Internists order tests and X-rays depending on the patient's medical problem and provide a diagnosis based on test results and physical examinations.[2]

Family Physicians, Internists, and Arthritis

Both family physicians and internal medicine specialists treat patients suffering from arthritis. As rheumatoid arthritis can often be initially mistaken for an injury, especially if it starts out in one joint, most sufferers will end up in a family physician's care. A family physician is qualified to treat arthritis patients unless the condition is extremely severe and requires a specialist or drastic surgical treatment. The family physician will take note of the patient's symptoms and medical history before ordering tests or X-rays to make a proper diagnosis. For moderate arthritis, family practice physicians might recommend medication and exercise or refer the patient to a physiotherapist. Many patients appreciate the support provided by family physicians for dealing with their arthritis.

If in acute pain or the usual treatment is unable to relieve their symptoms, patients might choose to see an internal medicine specialist. Internists will work to reevaluate the symptoms to find any other underlying problems or determine the severity of the condition. The optimal solution for providing the best medical care to an arthritis patient is for a team of physicians and internists to work together. However, if the symptoms are severe and the diagnosis points toward acute arthritic conditions, a rheumatologist might be recommended.

An orthopedist is an internist who specifically treats diseases of the joints, muscles, bones, and tendons. This specialist diagnoses and treats arthritis, back pain, and muscle strains along with common athletic injuries and "collagen" diseases. When surgery is being considered, internists and family physicians will recommend an orthopedist. Orthopedists are similar to family practice physicians and internists, except, if qualified surgeons, they perform major surgery on the joints. Orthopedists and physical medicine specialists often work closely to offer the best nonsurgical and, when necessary, surgical and postsurgical care to the patient.[3]

Prevalence and Statistics

According to the American Medical Association (AMA), as of 2010 there were slightly more than 246,000 primary care physicians in the United States.[4] This number, however, requires adjustment as it overestimates the number of practicing physicians. The AMA data in question include some retired physicians and others who have left the workforce. It also includes the substantial number of primary care–trained physicians who practice in non–primary care settings, such as emergency departments or hospitals. After the required adjustments, the correct number of practicing primary care physicians in the United States is estimated to be closer to 209,000. Of these, approximately eighty thousand are family practice physicians, and seventy-one thousand are internal medicine specialists.[5]

Patients Seen by Family Physicians

When people have a nonemergency health issue, they often see a family physician. Family physicians are trained to see a wide variety of patients, from those suffering from heart disease or diabetes to those with acute conditions such as infections and flu. Family physicians care for their patients in diverse environments, including their homes and areas not covered by other health-care providers. Most physicians still see their patients in a medical office, although they may also provide care in hospitals or other medical and rehabilitation facilities. Patients who start suffering from arthritis symptoms will usually end up at their family physician's clinic for diagnosis and treatment. In some cases, early arthritis may be mistaken for an injury, so family physicians focus on gathering information from their patient to make a precise diagnosis. Regardless of the original reason for the patient's visit, a family physician will ask many questions in order to assess the patient's overall health. This way, the family physician can come to a correct diagnosis even when the patient's symptoms are common or undefined. Arthritis patients are just one of the many patient types a family physician is capable of treating. Individuals who visit a family physician regularly for treatment are more likely to receive preventive services, better management of chronic illnesses, and decreased chance of premature death.[6]

Patients Seen by Internists

An internist who further specializes in rheumatic diseases is called a rheumatologist. These doctors are trained in the treatment and diagnosis of arthritis and other diseases of the bones, joints, and muscles. Also certified in internal medicine, a rheumatologist can provide consultations to a diverse group of patients who suffer from arthritis and other diseases related to the rheumatic system. This type of physician can treat arthritis, autoimmune diseases, osteoporosis, and pain disorders affecting the joints. There are more than one hundred different forms of these diseases, including rheumatoid arthritis, osteoarthritis, gout, lupus, back pain, and tendonitis.[7] Some of these are very serious diseases that can be difficult to diagnose and treat. Internists also see patients with soft tissue conditions related to the musculoskeletal system, and the specialty also interrelates with the rehabilitation of disabled patients, physical medicine, and physiotherapy. Patient-education programs and occupational therapy also fall under this specialty.[8]

QUESTIONS FOR THE FAMILY PHYSICIAN OR INTERNIST

Introductory Questions

While the doctor is usually the one who asks questions of patients to gain perspective on their symptoms, patients can respectfully and proactively take charge as well. The right questions asked by a patient can make the difference in how a disease is managed. Patients should feel free to ask questions about their diagnosis, medications, alternative or complementary therapies, and even their emotional and financial health. Engaging in a healthy dialogue with the doctor can educate patients about arthritis and the treatment options available. It will also give the doctor a better sense of how arthritis is affecting the patient's life. It is important that patients realize that their time with the doctor is limited and come to their appointments prepared.

Postdiagnosis Questions

Once the arthritis sufferer is diagnosed with arthritis, the doctor will provide information about the condition. Patients can ask their doctor about the following:

- What type of arthritis they have and whether it can affect other parts of the body besides the joints
- Which joints are affected and how severely
- What caused the arthritic condition and if it is hereditary
- What the best treatment options are for the kind of arthritis they have been diagnosed with
- What the risks of not treating their condition are
- How arthritis can affect them over the long term
- How quickly their condition will progress
- How much joint damage they already have
- Whether they currently need surgery or might in the future
- What to do if their symptoms worsen

Questions about Medications

The doctor might prescribe medication for managing arthritis pain and inflammation. It is important for patients to understand the medication and take it as directed. Arthritis patients can ask their doctors the following about their medication:

- Whether they need medication or could be treated effectively without it
- How often they will have to take the medication and for how long
- If there is any medication they can take on an as-needed basis, such as when they experience joint pain
- What type of drug is being prescribed and how it works
- Where they can get more information about the prescribed medication
- How the medication will make them feel
- How they can know if the medication is effective
- When they can expect improvements in their pain
- What the risks are of not taking the medication as directed or forgetting to take it
- Whether the medication has been tested on people with the form of arthritis they have been diagnosed with
- Whether the prescribed drug is habit-forming

- Whether the medication can be taken on an empty stomach
- Whether the medication can interact negatively with other medications they take
- Whether they should avoid certain foods, drinks, vitamins, herbal supplements, or over-the-counter drugs while taking the medication
- Whether they should avoid alcohol
- What "biologic" medications are, why they must be injected, and whether they would be helpful for the patients' arthritis

Questions about Therapy

Doctors often recommend physical therapy for the treatment of arthritis symptoms as it helps maintain or restore physical function. Other complementary and alternative therapies are also beneficial for arthritis patients. Patients can ask their doctors about the following regarding therapy:

- Whether they would benefit from physical therapy and could get a referral for a physical therapist
- Whether the patient should see other specialists, such as a rheumatologist, occupational therapist, orthopedic surgeon, or pain specialist
- Whether they should consider any complementary or alternative therapies
- Whether acupuncture can benefit their condition and help relieve joint pain or stiffness
- Whether hot and cold therapies, hydrotherapies, and mobilization and relaxation therapies work effectively
- Whether clinical trials or research support the alternative or complementary therapies
- Whether any herbs or supplements are recommended

Questions an Internist or Family Practice Doctor Might Ask

Correctly diagnosing rheumatic conditions can sometimes be difficult as some early signs and symptoms are common to many different diseases. The doctor will review the patient's medical history, conduct physical examinations, and obtain tests and X-rays to make a correct diagnosis and may even have to see the patient several times to make sure the diagnosis is accurate. The doctor will have to ask several detailed questions about the symptoms the patient is experiencing in order to make the right diagnosis. The past medical history and related information will give the doctor a clear idea about whether any other inherited conditions, and not necessarily a rheumatoid condition, might be causing the symptoms. It is vital for people suffering from joint pain to give the doctor an accurate, complete description of the symptoms they are experiencing as well as their family medical history. The doctor might then ask about the following to help in making a diagnosis:

- How long the patient has had the symptoms, if they have ever occurred before, and, if so, how they were treated
- How bad the symptoms are and if they come and go or are persistent
- If the symptoms affect the patient's feelings, home life, or work life, and, if so, to what extent
- Which part of the body experiences the pain and how it changes over time
- Whether the patient has any idea about what might be causing the symptoms and if any actions or movements make the pain better or worse
- Whether activity makes the pain more intense
- Whether the patient has had any illness or injury that may account for the pain
- Whether the patient has any other symptoms besides the joint pain
- Whether the patient is experiencing any other pain besides the joint pain
- Whether the patient experiences pain in more than one joint
- When the pain occurs and how long it lasts
- When the patient first noticed the pain and what he or she was doing when it occurred
- Whether the pain and other symptoms have been occurring for some time and why the patient finally came to see a doctor
- Whether the patient has a family history of arthritis or other rheumatic diseases
- Whether the patient is receiving medical care for any other medical problems
- Whether the patient has ever had surgery for another medical condition and if there were any complications
- Whether the patient takes any medications, supplements, or herbal remedies and, if so, how often
- Whether the patient has ever experienced an adverse reaction or allergy to any medication
- Whether the patient has had any recent infections
- Whether the patient smokes, consumes more than the average amount of alcohol, or takes any recreational drugs

As rheumatic conditions are very diverse and sometimes affect several different parts of the body, the doctor may ask many other questions about the patient's health covering various other topics. The doctor may also advise the patient to keep a journal to record the pain. While using medications and treatments, the patient should keep an account of how the affected joint looks and how its appearance changes over time. This will give the doctor insight into how the patient is responding to treatment. The patient should also record how the level of pain changes at different activity levels, how acute or minor the pain experienced is, what exactly he or she was doing when the pain started, and how long it lasts. Keeping a journal to record these occurrences will ensure that the patient has a complete record of his or her condition and level of pain and will remember details when questioned about them by a family physician or internist.

ROLE OF RHEUMATOLOGISTS IN ARTHRITIS

Rheumatologists are physician specialists who treat arthritis and autoimmune diseases. These include a medley of different musculoskeletal pain disorders and osteoporosis. The most prevalent among them are rheumatoid arthritis, osteoarthritis, lupus, and gout. These very serious diseases can last a lifetime as no known and reliable treatment exists for the majority of them.

BEGINNINGS

Educational Process of Becoming a Rheumatologist

Rheumatology is a specialist medical profession that focuses on the joints and tissue. After the completion of a medical degree and residency, aspiring rheumatologists must work in the public hospital system for some time, after which they can apply for further training and eventually get a fellowship. The foremost purpose of these fellowships is to prepare doctors for the specialties this discipline demands. This program usually takes around two to four years to complete. Pediatric rheumatologists require a further one to two years of fellowship after this. Every qualified rheumatologist usually seeks board certification in rheumatology and internal medicine from the American Board of Internal Medicine. These exams give the doctor an accreditation. As with other medical disciplines, rheumatologists really need to keep themselves up-to-date and should be aware of the latest developments in their field.

THE JOB

A More Detailed Description

A rheumatologist is a doctor who treats arthritis and other joint and muscle diseases. Rheumatology deals specifically with the study, diagnosis, and treatment of rheumatic and musculoskeletal conditions. Rheumatologists are specially trained medical doctors who deal with a variety of issues that involve joints, soft tissues, and connective tissues. They are therefore called specialists or specialist physicians.

A Typical Day for the Rheumatologist

Rheumatologists are chiefly responsible for the diagnosis and treatment of rheumatic conditions and arthritis. They review patient medical histories, perform diagnostic tests, and discuss treatment options with patients. They use many different tests, such as chemical pathology and X-rays. Rheumatologists treat patients with a variety of different conditions, such as arthritis, sports injuries, joint disorders, osteoporosis, and chronic fatigue syndrome.[9] They usually provide a range of different and specialist treatment options, such as medications and occupational and physical therapy. Many rheumatologists conduct research to gain a better understanding of the causes of conditions and to develop improved treatments.

Although rheumatologists perform a variety of duties and tasks in an average workday, their most important role is to diagnose and treat rheumatoid arthritis. They are also educators in the sense that they give patients a better understanding of the disease. Rheumatologists are active members of a patient's health care team. They receive referrals from other medical practitioners and can refer patients to other specialists. Many arthritis patients need physical therapy; some require psychological help to fight their disease. It is vital that the rheumatologist encourages patients by providing authentic evidence of how the disease can be overcome.

When Arthritis Sufferers Require the Services of a Rheumatologist

A patient finds himself sitting in a rheumatologist's clinic in one of two ways. Sometimes the patient's consulting doctor has referred him to the specialist fearing that the patient is suffering from a particular form of arthritis or joint disorder beyond the doctor's ability to treat. The doctor might have reached this decision merely by looking at the signs the patient is exhibiting or after reviewing test results. In either case, the rheumatologist is the specialist who can conduct further treatment. Sometimes, however, the patient feels the need to consult the rheumatologist directly. The main symptoms that should lead one to consult a rheumatologist include joint pain and swelling that has persisted for more than two weeks. These signs point directly to the presence of arthritis, and a rheumatologist should to be consulted as soon as possible. Another sign is tenderness that becomes worse with movement or activity. Joints that are red and warm indicate inflammation. A loss in range of motion could be another sign of the onset of arthritis. Other signs that should lead one to see a rheumatologist are unexplained fever, weight loss, extreme fatigue, or a general feeling of malaise. The presence of any of these conditions points to arthritis, and the patient is advised to consult a rheumatologist.

Figures

The number of rheumatologists has increased in recent years, but the retirement rate will surpass this growth. Researchers estimate that almost half of currently practicing rheumatologists will retire by 2020 and that by 2025 there could be a shortage of around twenty-six hundred rheumatologists in the United States.[10] The number of registered and practicing rheumatologists in the United States in 2005 was close to five thousand.[11] The breakdown by gender shows that the numbers are equal among male and female rheumatologists up to the age of forty-four, whereas above this threshold, there are more male practitioners. The number of rheumatologists joining the profession has grown by almost 40 percent—from 122 in 2000 to 168 in 2006.[12] However, the major issue with this healthy-sounding growth rate is that the retirement rate will outpace it heavily. Rheumatologists are already overloaded and struggling to make schedules work; the future is looking even bleaker. According to a 2005 investigation, of 400 available fellowships, only 366 were filled.[13] As the population ages, there is a high probability that more people will develop arthritis. This, coupled with a shortage of rheumatologists, means that the workload on these specialist doctors is likely to increase in the coming years.

Although rheumatologists' workload varies from region to region, the overall work requirements have increased steadily over the years due to a growing gap between supply and demand. More people are aging and developing arthritis, requiring more visits to the doctor. The average number of visits has also increased, and patients face a long wait both in the United States and the United Kingdom. The situation is becoming alarming as doctors have less incentive to become rheumatologists. This is because rheumatologists are among the least compensated of all medical practitioners. For the record, cardiac surgeons make the most money. Thus, the profession is not attracting a lot of young doctors, whereas the demand is growing daily, at least in the Western world. No dependable statistics exist on rheumatologists' workloads; however, the waiting times for arthritis patients, as well as the ratio of patients per rheumatologist, have increased steadily. Patients trying to make an appointment with a rheumatologist might have better luck getting in sooner if they are willing to take a less popular time slot, perhaps by taking time off work or reworking their schedule.

QUESTIONS TO ASK A RHEUMATOLOGIST ABOUT TREATMENT

The treatment of arthritis is not an exact science. No one set treatment plan can rid sufferers of this condition. The disease attacks the joints, and the patient suffers from pain, inflammation, and possible swelling. The strength of symptoms varies from patient to patient and also depends on the type of arthritis diagnosed. It is important for every patient to completely understand his treatment plan and options in order to gain the confidence to deal with the malady head on.

Pain relief medication is the answer in most cases. The rheumatologist often has to work with other doctors, such as the referring primary care physician and other doctors who have a history of treating a particular patient (the patient might feel more comfortable with his family doctor). In this capacity, the rheumatologist must advise other doctors constantly about the diagnosis and treatment options selected for the patient. The rheumatologist can also make further referrals that will help the patient. Therefore, it is vital to ask the right questions of the rheumatologist in order to get a complete picture of where the treatment is headed. Some of the most common questions [14] to ask the doctor are as follows:

- How long will the treatment last?
- What type of treatment will it be? Will it involve medication or regular hospital visits?
- Will the treatment entail any sort of chemotherapy or physiotherapy requiring consultation with another physician?
- Should any lifestyle changes be made in order to make the treatment as effective as possible?
- Will the medication or treatment have any side effects?
- Should particular patients not take the sort of medicines administered during the treatment of arthritis?
- How many people respond well to the medication and treatment?
- What can be done to make the treatment work better?
- If the primary treatment does not work, is a secondary option available?
- What kinds of tests are required, and will they be conducted regularly?
- How much will the treatment cost?
- What is the long-term effect of the treatment?
- Is weight loss needed?
- How often will the visits be?
- How can the tiredness associated with rheumatoid arthritis be cured?
- Is work or business permitted?
- Should certain foods or beverages be avoided as part of the treatment?
- Is exercise recommended or ill-advised?

• Where can more information about the disease and its treatment be found?

After a rheumatologist officially diagnoses a patient with arthritis, people react in a number of different ways. Some people take it on the chin and weigh up their options. Others suffer from feelings of helplessness and depression, which eventually worsens their condition. Pulling through a medical condition requires the minds of both the rheumatologist and the patient. Those who simply decide to give up become a burden on their families and the state. It is important that patients not lose motivation and stay focused on the light at the end of the tunnel. In order to do this, the patient must understand fully what is happening inside his or her own body so as to make lifestyle adaptations in a manner advisable for the affected joints. It is clearly important that patients have a good communicative relationship with their rheumatologist and that both parties trust each other.

More Questions

An arthritis patient should always ask the rheumatologist some additional questions:

• What is the diagnosis? Is it possible to explain it?
• What type of arthritis is present?
• How dangerous is it?
• Does a treatment exist?
• What is happening in the body as a result of arthritis?
• Can the body can take it and for how long?
• How long can a patient expect to experience symptoms?
• Will the disease ever get better?
• How many patients with similar symptoms has the doctor seen get better?
• Is the disease particular to some people, or is it universal in nature?
• Can normal life be resumed?
• Should counseling be sought?
• How can one feel positive about the situation?
• Are there are any support groups in the area?
• Do other people in the neighborhood suffer from the disease?
• Is the disease contagious in any way?

QUESTIONS FROM THE RHEUMATOLOGIST

It is common practice in arthritic science for rheumatologists to ask extensive questions of the patient in order to understand the symptoms better and place the signs in context. Every human being is different both psychologically and physically. Doctors need all the information they can get to make a correct diagnosis. This is only possible if patients are frank and open with the doctor and answer all questions to the best of their ability. The arthritis patient has to be precise, accurate, and succinct in explaining symptoms. Before making or while awaiting an appointment, it is a good idea to track signs and symptoms in a health log or journal. The arthritis sufferer should note the time of onset of symptoms, the level of pain and disability, and anything that triggers or alleviates symptoms. The more information offered, the better the doctor's ability to help. The patient should bring all written notes to the appointment and include a list of current medications, any allergies, and any other medical concerns that might be ancillary to the symptoms but could have some bearing on the treatment course decided on by patient and doctor.

Upon Initial Introduction

Some patients are initially uncomfortable talking to a rheumatologist they do not know, but the better patients understand arthritis, the better their chances of getting better. The most important thing in the initial consultation is for the doctor to understand the patient and context better.[15] The rheumatologist might ask questions such as the following:

- What is your profession?
- How would you rate your general health?
- How are you feeling today?
- What illnesses did you have as a child?
- Does your father or mother suffer from joint trouble?
- Have you suffered any broken bones?
- Have you ever experienced unexplained tiredness?
- How would you rate your body strength?
- Have you ever had a major disease?
- Do you regularly use any medicine?
- Have you got any allergies or other particular conditions?
- Have you ever had surgery?
- Do you know why you are here today?

Through the Course of Visitations

During follow-up visits after the initial diagnosis, the rheumatologist will likely have developed a personal rapport with the patient and will ask more incisive questions to determine the effect of the disease on the body and to ascertain whether the treatment is working. These questions are usually quite penetrative and aim to determine the effect of the disease on the patient's quality of life. This is important in order to prescribe the right dosage and decide whether to take an aggressive treatment approach. The rheumatologist will also ask questions relating to the sufferer's personal and family life in a bid to determine the severity of the disease. He or she might inquire about the patient's smoking and drinking patterns to determine the correct medication and judge if it will have the desired effect. [16]

Based on the level of comfort with the doctor that the patient has developed over time, questions during follow-up visits can include the following: [17]

- How bad is the pain, and where exactly does it hurt?
- At what time of day is the pain worst?
- How long do the bouts of pain last, and how is relief found?
- What exercises are currently in place?
- Is the current medication working?
- Is the sensation of pain dull or sharp?
- Is there ever any swelling of the joints?
- Is there any difficulty moving the joints?
- Are mornings very painful?
- Is any redness of the joints observed on a typical day?
- Is there any feeling of numbness?
- Is exhaustion frequent?
- Are the joints used more than average?
- Is the dosage appropriate for the severity of symptoms (based on what the patient thinks)?

ROLE OF ORTHOPEDIC SURGEONS IN ARTHRITIS

Orthopedics is a surgical field that specifically deals with ailments associated with the musculoskeletal system. As the name suggests, the musculoskeletal system integrates the two systems—namely, the muscular and the skeletal systems—that aid movement of the human body. While the underlying theory of orthopedic surgery may seem considerably simple, the process of becoming an orthopedic surgeon is highly complex.

THE JOB

The entire job of an orthopedic surgeon revolves around employing various tools in order to best treat the patient. The tools may be diverse in nature and may also consist of physical and medical means, in addition to the usual surgical apparatuses. The job incorporates examination, conservation, and restoration of function of a patient's limbs or vertebral column. Both the primary and secondary musculoskeletal problems experienced by an arthritis sufferer's central nervous system are dealt with, such as cancerous growths, wounds, degenerative disease, trauma, hereditary abnormalities, and contagions. An orthopedic surgeon reestablishes bodily operations through surgery, particularly targeting the ligaments, tendons, joints, bones, nerves, and muscles, and also uses objective, medicinal, and rehabilitative approaches whenever the need arises. Laser surgery is also performed to eliminate worn-out cartilage in the knees or other damaged regions. A surgeon normally performs shoulder arthroplasty for shoulder fractures resulting from rough sports or caused by osteoarthritis or rheumatoid arthritis.

Several work activities beyond treating patients are typical for every orthopedic surgeon. Orthopedic surgeons are responsible for accepting patient referrals from other doctors, carrying out physical examinations, and ordering processes such as MRIs, X-rays, and other tests. They are also required to see patients individually in order to continue with the all the complementary procedures, such as additional examinations or specified testing, in order to start treatment. All orthopedic surgeons must also notify support staff of surgery times. Moreover, the surgeons themselves are responsible for booking operating rooms in order to make sure that all support staff are notified and prepared for the surgery accordingly. Managing arthritis patients' charts and all required hospital records, as well as keeping records, is an orthopedic surgeon's responsibility. Once the procedure has been carried out, it is important for the surgeon to see the patient in order to monitor recovery and answer any questions that the patient may have. Specialized care, along with timely management of medical assistance, must be planned once the surgery is done. This means that the work of an orthopedic surgeon is not confined to the operating room. Other tasks must also be carried out to ensure proper treatment.

Orthopedic surgeons generally operate, but orthopedic practice is also largely about the nonoperative supervision of the musculoskeletal system. Aside from performing surgeries, an orthopedic surgeon also diagnoses a patient's disorder, taking into account clinical history and the results of the physical examination, X-rays, and other relevant tests. Based on the diagnosed condition, the orthopedic surgeon recommends an appropriate treatment, which may include specific medications, splints, exercises, injections, physical therapy, or surgery. An orthopedic surgeon also directs and monitors the patient's rehabilitation by initiating physiotherapy and exercise. Moreover, he or she provides information and gives advice for preventing deterioration in a patient's condition. Orthopedic surgeons have used technological advances—such as joint-replacement surgery, minimally invasive surgery, and keyhole, or arthroscopic, surgery, which allows surgeons to clearly view the inside of a joint—that have helped many patients over the years.[18]

ORTHOPEDIC SERVICES FOR ARTHRITIS

Arthritis patients will benefit a lot from seeking orthopedic services as early as possible. Medical experts can provide patients with professional aids and opinions through evaluations, consultations, and treatment programs.[19] It must be noted that early diagnosis and treatment of arthritis is highly important. Orthopedists can provide health rubrics to help arthritis patients live a better life. They can give patients information on their condition, physical training, and self-help instructions. They can also provide arthritis patients with referrals, nutritional guidance, and pain-management systems. They may also direct patients to educational events such as forums, lectures, and workshops where nutrition and appropriate therapies are discussed. When arthritis patients need surgery, orthopedists can also educate them beforehand about the procedure.[20]

The fast pace with which medical technology advances nowadays allows more complex operations to be performed on an outpatient basis, and patients already have the option of recuperating in their homes instead of the hospital.[21] Several orthopedic surgeries can now be offered in both inpatient and outpatient settings,[22] and medical pain-management teams come up with customized pain-control plans for each patient.[23]

Orthopedic Specialist's Arsenal

Arthritis can seriously impair mobility. Meticulous analyses of symptoms and a physical examination diagnose arthritis. X-rays show the severity of arthritis, while blood tests and other laboratory examinations aid in determining the type of arthritis.[24] From the diagnosis, an orthopedist comes up with a plan that will help the patient cope with the ailment. Over-the-counter drugs may be utilized in controlling pain and joint inflammation. Such anti-inflammatory medicines include aspirin, ibuprofen, and naproxen. Acetaminophen may also be used to alleviate pain. Orthopedists may also prescribe certain medicines after evaluating the patient's type of arthritis, its seriousness, and the patient's overall bodily health. Anti-inflammatory drugs may not be safe for patients suffering from ulcers, asthma, or kidney or liver disease, for instance. Cortisone injections into the joint may alleviate the pain and swelling for a time; however, injecting into the same joint repeatedly and frequently can damage it. Viscosupplementation (injection of hyaluronic acid preparations) may also be performed to help lubricate the joint. This operation is usually done on the knee.[25]

Addressing Mobility Issues

Orthopedists may also recommend exercises and physical therapy courses for arthritis patients. Canes, crutches, walkers, and splints may minimize the stress and strain on arthritic joints. Orthopedists may also educate arthritis patients about how to perform daily activities in a way that will lessen the stress on affected joints. Certain exercises and physical therapies may reduce stiffness and strengthen the weakened muscular tissues around the joint. In most cases, arthritis patients are still able to continue performing usual daily routines. Exercise schemes, anti-inflammatory medications, and weight-reduction programs for overweight patients are frequently employed to ease pain and stiffness and augment mobility. [26]

A Glance at Orthopedic Surgery

Generally, orthopedic surgery for arthritis only becomes necessary when nonsurgical treatment techniques fail to alleviate pain and other symptoms. The kind of operation performed depends on the type of arthritis the patient suffers from, its gravity, and the patient's overall health status. Surgical operations on arthritis vary and can include removal of diseased or damaged joint lining, realignment of joints, fusion of bones' ends in the joint to prevent joint motion to relieve joint pain, and replacement of the entire joint. Some varieties of arthritis, such as rheumatoid arthritis, are usually attended to not only by an orthopedic surgeon but by a team of health-care specialists that may comprise rheumatologists, physical and occupational therapists, social workers, and rehabilitation specialists. Orthopedic surgery often results in great pain reduction for people suffering from acute arthritis. It also results in relief and restoration of lost joint function. [27]

When orthopedic surgery is deemed necessary, orthopedic surgeons discuss the surgical options available with the patient. They point out the advantages and disadvantages of immediately undergoing or delaying surgery, assessing the patient's age, health, and level of activity. The orthopedic surgeon may also advise about appropriate alternative treatment options, explaining the benefits and risks of each and the possible results if the patient refuses to undergo treatment. Not all arthritis patients ought to have surgery, and it must be remembered that a referral to an orthopedic surgeon does not automatically mean that an arthritis patient will have orthopedic surgery. [28] If an orthopedist refers the arthritis patient for surgery before trying other methods to alleviate the pain, it might be worth getting a second opinion prior to opting for this route.

A statement published by the Healthcare Cost and Utilization Project (HCUP) of the US Agency for Healthcare Research and Quality shows that in 2005 more than 3 million musculoskeletal operations were performed, accounting for roughly 9 percent of the total hospitalizations in the United States.[29] The number of these operations increased by almost 25 percent from 1997 to 2005. Of all these orthopedic procedures, spinal fusions had the greatest increase at about 70 percent: 202,100 operations in 1997 to about 350,000 operations in 2005. During the same time span, increases were also seen in knee arthroplasties (approximately 70 percent) and hip replacements (more than 30 percent). Musculoskeletal operations were also done more on women and seniors. The evaluations were based on information from the 2004 HCUP and the 2005 Nationwide Inpatient Sample (NIS). The NIS also provided data from 1997 to 2005, with additional information obtained from the national census.[30]

Laminectomy

A laminectomy is performed by an orthopedic surgeon. It is an orthopedic spine surgery to take out the lamina, which is a part of the vertebral bone. Laminectomy has a number of variations and may range from minimal, requiring only a small skin incision to push muscles back instead of cutting into them, to more serious. The most conventional type of laminectomy takes out more than just the lamina; the posterior backbone and superimposing muscles and tendons may need to be removed entirely. This removal may also lead to the cutting of several back muscles attached to these structures. The recovery period may vary greatly depending upon the kind of laminectomy carried out. A minimal procedure may involve a recovery period of just a few days, whereas conventional open surgery may take several weeks or even months to heal completely. The success rate for laminectomy depends on several factors specific to the surgery, as well as the surgeon's technical expertise and selection of "proper" patients.

Laminectomy may be performed for several reasons. These include treating severe spinal stenosis by way of relieving pressure on the nerve roots or spinal cord, accessing a mass or tumor present in or around the spinal cord, or contouring the vertebral column in order to rectify a deformity, such as kyphosis, in the spine. A number of surgical tools may be needed to carry out the procedure. These include laser, surgical instruments, rongeurs, and drills. The most common reason for carrying out a laminectomy is to cure spinal stenosis.

FIGURES

The American Academy of Orthopedic Surgeons (AAOS) leads in providing musculoskeletal education to orthopedic and nonorthopedic surgeons alike internationally.[31] The AAOS conducts the biennial Orthopedic Surgeon Census, which aims at collecting relevant data pertaining to orthopedic practice and demographics. The AAOS employs the gathered facts and figures to come up with an accurate and updated report on orthopedic practice and subjects on practice management.[32]

The 2010 Orthopedic Surgeon Census shows that there are over twenty-five thousand orthopedic surgeons in the United States. Of this number, almost two thousand are candidate member practitioners (CMPs), 550 are CMPs who have applied for fellowship, about 2,000 are nonmember practitioners, approximately 17,800 are active fellows, and nearly 3,000 are emeriti.[33] Based on this same survey, the largest percentage of US orthopedic surgeons, approximately 40 percent of respondents, are in private practice in an orthopedic group setting, and 20 percent more work in a solo private practice setting. Moreover, 9 percent deliver services in a multispecialty group private practice, and another 9 percent are in academic practice and earn their salary from an academic institution. Eight percent work for a hospital or a medical center, 3 percent are in academic practice with their salary coming from private practice, 2 percent work for a pre-paid-plan health maintenance organization, 2 percent are in military practice, 1 percent work in public institutions (with salary coming from nonmilitary government entities), and an additional 1 percent serve as contracted employees. The last 2 percent of the respondents are classified as conducting "other" forms of orthopedic practice.[34]

Noteworthy Statistics

Approximately seven hundred physicians successfully accomplish orthopedic residency training annually in the United States. Around 10 percent of all current orthopedic surgery residents are women. An estimated 20 percent of these belong to minority groups. Approximately 20,400 orthopedic surgeons and residents are actively practicing in the United States as of today.[35] The 2011–2012 *Occupational Outlook Handbook* published by the US Department of Labor states that around 3 to 4 percent of all working medical doctors belong to the branch of orthopedic surgery.[36] A census carried out by the AAOS in 2008 estimated the number of orthopedic surgeons to be approximately 25,464. The majority worked in California (2,569), closely followed by Texas, Florida, and Illinois. Around 46 percent of orthopedists work as specialists, whereas 24 percent practice as general orthopedic surgeons; however, 30 percent refer to themselves as general orthopedic surgeons with a particular sphere of interest.[37]

Degree of Specialization

In terms of the degree of specialization among US orthopedic surgeons (based on a 2010 survey), a little over 45 percent are specialists, around 30 percent are general orthopedic surgeons with a specialty interest, and roughly 20 percent are generalists.[38] The same survey also asked the respondents to identify their primary or specialty area(s) of orthopedic surgery. The results[39] were as follows:

- 40 percent in arthroscopy
- 11 percent in foot and ankle
- 12 percent in adult spine
- 40 percent in adult knee
- Almost 40 percent in sports medicine
- Almost 18 percent in total joint
- 17 percent in hand
- Over 16 percent in shoulder and elbow
- 10 percent in trauma
- 1 percent in orthopedic oncology
- 5 percent in nonoperative practice
- 4 percent in pediatric orthopedics
- 3 percent in disability/legal-related orthopedics
- 30 percent in adult hip
- 3 percent in pediatric spine
- 1 percent in rehabilitation/prosthetics/orthotics

Of respondents, almost 7 percent said they had no specialty, and 2 percent identified themselves as having "other" specialties.

Orthopedic surgeons attend to many patients suffering from different types of musculoskeletal ailments, such as back pain, sports injuries, arthritic hips and knees, and stiff neck. These musculoskeletal problems have a great effect on Americans and the health-care system. Musculoskeletal problems account for more than 14 percent of the US annual health-care budget, with services including an approximate 135 million ambulatory health-care visits, more than 3 million hospitalizations, and nearly $245 billion in medical cost. Proper diagnosis and truly apposite solution programs for these conditions are provided by orthopedic surgeons, making consultation with one necessary.[40]

From the Eyes of the Orthopedic Surgeon

Orthopedic surgeons accept patients regardless of age: newborn babies, children, athletes, baby boomers, and the elderly. These patients may have problems ranging from bone and joint difficulties to damage to the muscles, ligaments, and tendons in any part of the body. Patients treated by orthopedic surgeons may suffer from any of the following problems, to name a few:[41]

- Back pain
- Sciatica
- Fractures and dislocations
- Growth abnormalities
- Pulled muscles
- Scoliosis
- Bowlegs
- Bunions
- Bone tumors
- Muscular dystrophy
- Finger and toe abnormalities
- Torn cartilage
- Cerebral palsy
- Clubfoot
- Unequal leg length
- Torn disks
- Torn ligaments
- Osteoporosis
- Sports injuries
- Rheumatoid arthritis
- Work-related injuries
- Tendon problems
- Osteoarthritis
- Bursitis
- Sprains and strains

Demographics of Procedures

The collective hospital costs for orthopedic operations in 2004 reached $31.5 billion, equivalent to more than 10 percent of the combined cost of hospital care in America. The three most common orthopedic operations were knee arthroplasty (the restoration or substitution of the knee), hip replacement, and spinal fusion (the joining of at least two vertebrae to rectify an unstable part of the spinal cord). These three operations also proved to be the costliest among musculoskeletal surgeries; the national bill for all three treatments amounts to more than $17.5 billion. In a span of nine years (1997 to 2005), musculoskeletal surgeries saw growth from 2.7 to 3.5 million. Spinal fusions led as the operation with the greatest increase in number from 202,100 in 1997 to 349,400 in 2005, roughly a 70 percent rise. Similarly, the number of knee arthroplasty operations and hip replacements also rose. Knee arthroplasty saw about a 70 percent increase from 328,800 operations in 1997 to 555,800 in 2005. Hip replacements rose by about 30 percent, from 290,700 operations in 1997 to 383,500 in 2005.[42]

Among the musculoskeletal operations done in 2004, more were per-formed on women than men, particularly knee arthroplasty and hip replace-ment. Knee arthroplasty was done 70 percent more often in females (roughly twenty surgeries for every ten thousand females) than in males (twelve sur-geries for every ten thousand males), while hip replacements were done 60 percent more on women (fifteen surgeries for every ten thousand females to almost ten surgeries for every ten thousand males). The gender difference among spinal fusion operations was not as great, although the number of operations on females was still a little larger than for males (10.9 surgeries for every ten thousand females against close to ten surgeries for every ten thousand males).[43]

Adult knee, at nearly 35 percent, is the most widely practiced orthopedic specialty, followed by arthroscopy, at 34 percent.[44] Sports medicine is at 33 percent, while total joint is at 28 percent, and both shoulder[45] and hip-re-placement surgery are at 25 percent. Surgeries related to ankle, foot, and spine are close to the end of the standing at 11 and 10 percent, respectively.[46]

These orthopedic procedures are more frequently done on older patients, usually in their late sixties, especially knee arthroplasties and hip replace-ments. Patients of spinal fusions, on the other hand, are generally younger, with their mean age tipping at fifty years. The number of knee-arthroplasty and hip-replacement operations is shown to surge with age, with respect to the following[47] :

- Knee arthroplasty operations are performed on the elderly at a much high-er rate, with eighty recorded operations for every ten thousand people age sixty-five or older compared to only twenty-five operations for every ten thousand people age forty-five to sixty-four.
- For hip replacements, approximately seventy operations are done for eve-ry ten thousand people age sixty-five and older compared to only about fourteen operations for every ten thousand people age forty-five to sixty-four.
- Spinal fusion operations, on the contrary, are performed more equally among different age groups, with considerable numbers done on people age eighteen to forty-four (roughly eight operations for every ten thou-sand). Twenty operations are done for every ten thousand people age forty-five to sixty-four, and eighteen operations are done for every ten thousand people age sixty-five and older.

Although there exists a global organization of orthopedic surgeons, the Inter-national Association of Orthopedic Surgeons,[48] there is no known worldwide demographic survey on orthopedics, although national data may be available for individual countries.

THE COMMUNICATIVE PROCESS

Before undergoing any surgical procedure, an arthritis patient needs to fully understand the consequences of the process, as well as its advantages and disadvantages. Therefore, it is necessary for a patient to ask his or her orthopedic specialist relevant questions regarding the procedure. These doctors are always willing to explain details and elucidate concepts that are still obscure to their patients.

Prior to Orthopedic Surgery

It is imperative that the patient understands the risks involved in an operation and its success rate. Significant topics a patient must bring up include the following:[49]

- Why the procedure is the recommended treatment
- Possible alternatives to the main recommendation
- Benefits of the operation regarding pain relief and mobility
- The duration of the benefits
- The specific name of the operation, both technically and popularly, and how it is performed
- Whether the operation will cure the ailment and whether further surgery(s) will be needed
- The frequency and total number of such procedures performed annually in the facility where the patient will have the same procedure
- The percentage of patients whose well-being improved after the operation
- The consequences of postponing the surgery
- Whom to consult if the patient wants a second opinion

The patient may also inquire about the following:

- Duration of the operation[50]
- Duration of the hospital stay following the surgery[51]
- What the discharge instructions to follow may be
- Duration of the recovery period
- Limitations while convalescing
- Whether assistance at home will be required after the operation and for how long
- Whether the patient will have any disability afterward and if physical therapy will be required.
- When the patient can return to work
- When he or she can drive a car again
- When he or she can engage in sexual activity[52]

- Whether there are writings or videos about the operation that the patient can review prior to the procedure
- Whether the doctor will confirm and mark the site of the surgery prior to the operation[53]

On Postoperative Activity

The patient will be under observation in the hospital for a specific period after the operation. The doctor or the nurse will review postoperative instructions with the patient, as well as special instructions about diet, rest, medication, follow-up consultations, and the use of any medical equipment such as a sling or crutches. During follow-up consultations, the doctor will provide additional postoperative instructions, and these may include discussions about rehabilitation, the removal of stitches, when the patient can drive or return to school or work, the use duration for the sling or crutches, and any pain medications, to name a few.[54]

During the course of the treatment, the orthopedic surgeon is likely to get a baseline assessment of the patient's strength and mobility before the operation. The assessment may include discussions about the patient and his or her problem, as well as family history, and tests to determine the patient's strength, motion range, and the stability of the injury. After the operation, the patient's physical therapy will most likely be divided into phases, the overall goal being for the patient to return to his or her activity level before the operation.[55]

Important Instructions

An individual may receive postoperative instructions, depending on the type of procedure performed. The primary factor common to almost all surgical procedures is the need for early mobilization as soon as the surgery is completed. The surgeon will most likely encourage some physical activity, as the muscles will be weak following illness and need to regain their strength. This is also important in order to metabolize residual traces of anesthetics and to fuel the healing process. The surgeon might also impart special instructions regarding pain control, exercise, wound care, and diet. While it is quite common for individuals who have just had an operation to feel a certain level of pain, it can be dealt with easily with the use of appropriate medicines. Just after surgery, the patient may need to receive pain-control medication through an intravenous tube so that the amount of medication taken can be regulated easily. Controlling pain may be quite a challenge for the surgeon as it is considerably harder to control pain than it is to prevent it. The pain medication prescribed is not addictive in the slightest, precluding worries about withdrawal symptoms. The surgeon may also prescribe blood-thinning medications and antibiotics in order to prevent blood clots from blocking the veins in the region that has been surgically treated. Nausea, loss of appetite, and constipation are common physical reactions to surgery. In order to aid the patient in excretion, urinary catheters may be fitted following the surgery. In addition, the surgeon may prescribe laxatives or stool softeners to assuage constipation. The surgeon may also instruct the patient to carry out several breathing exercises to dispel tautness in the chest and lungs.

The surgeon may also give instructions for proper care of the wound following an orthopedic surgery. The most common instruction is perhaps keeping the wound area free of moisture and as clean as possible. Medical staff at the hospital apply a dressing to the wound that will require changing as suggested by the surgeon. It is normally advised to refrain from bathing or showering until any staples or sutures have been completely removed. This is normally within ten days following the surgery. The surgeon may also recommend careful and regular monitoring of the body temperature to detect any abnormal changes. If suffering from inflammation in the leg after the surgery, the patient may be advised to elevate the leg slightly or to apply ice. Orthopedic surgeons are also likely to tell their patients to contact them if the wound starts to drain or turns crimson or if they experience symptoms such as shortness of breath, chest pain, or calf pain, three indications of a possible blood clot.

3

Many Faces of Arthritis

Chapter Eight

Rheumatoid Arthritis

Rheumatoid arthritis is a chronic inflammation of flexible joints that may affect tissues and organs. This disorder of the joints is one of the most common types of systemic inflammatory arthritis. To date, the root cause of rheumatoid arthritis is unknown, but the disorder is generally considered a systematic autoimmune disease that results when the immune system mistakenly attacks the host's own tissues and joints. Rheumatoid arthritis is named as such since it is one of the pathological conditions that characterize rheumatism, a general term used to refer to a wide range of conditions affecting the joints, tendons, bones, and nerves.

PREVALENCE AND STATISTICS

In the United States, nearly 24 percent of the adult population reports having doctor-diagnosed arthritis.[1] Between 2007 and 2009, 50 percent of people older than sixty-five had received an arthritis diagnosis. The case of juveniles is more staggering, with around 294,000 US children under the age of eighteen, or 1 in every 250, having some form of arthritis. The most common form of arthritis is osteoarthritis. However, other rheumatic conditions such as gout, fibromyalgia, and rheumatoid arthritis are quite common. In 2005, nearly 27 million adults had osteoarthritis. The figure for rheumatoid arthritis in 2007 among adults was around 1.7 million.[2]

There were approximately 3 million gout patients in 2005.[3] Doctor-diagnosed arthritis is more often reported by overweight subjects: wherein around 16 percent of nonoverweight adults report doctor-diagnosed arthritis,[4] roughly 30 percent of obese people report doctor-diagnosed arthritis. About 65 percent of adults diagnosed with arthritis are overweight or obese.[5] Thus, the likelihood of obese people developing arthritis is much higher for people who are not overweight.[6] The prevalence of rheumatioid arthritis in the Western world is between 0.3 and 1 percent, and a reasonable overall prevalence for definite rheumatoid arthritis is 0.8 percent in adults.[7]

SIGNS AND SYMPTOMS OF RHEUMATOID ARTHRITIS

Rheumatoid arthritis starts with the swelling of synovial cells. Synovia are relatively acellular areas with very vulnerable intimal lining that surround the joints. Other signs are accumulation of synovial fluid and development of lesions in the synovium, leading to damage to articular cartilage and fusion of joints. Rheumatoid arthritis affects the joints found between the fingers and the hands and between the toes and the feet. White blood cells such as CD4+ T cells, macrophages, and B cells sometimes form lymphoid aggregates with germinal centers.

Hyperplasia of the intimal lining ensues as macrophage-like and fibroblast-like synoviocytes grow. Serine proteases, metalloproteinases, aggrecanases, and other degradative enzymes weaken the extracellular matrix and soon damage the articular structures. As the disease progresses, it normally spreads to other joint areas, such as ankles, knees, hips, elbows, and shoulders. The symptoms are typically felt in the same joints on both the left and right sides of the body. Tissues of major organs such as the heart, lungs, and eyes may be affected. There is also a risk of nodular lesions, especially in subcutaneous tissues. The symptoms may fade then intensify from time to time, and flares may come and go with periods of relative remission when the inflammation and pain subside or disappear. In severe cases, rheumatoid arthritis can lead to deformed and dislocated joints.

RISK FACTORS

Gender, genes, age, and smoking are known to be risk factors for rheumatoid arthritis. Some experts think that genes could play an indirect role in triggering this autoimmune disorder since they can make living organisms more susceptible to environmental health risks that may cause rheumatoid arthritis. Women and older people are generally more susceptible to rheumatoid arthritis.

Gender and Age

Women are more prone to rheumatoid arthritis than are men, and people from age forty to sixty have a higher risk of developing the disease.[8] Women are also at greater risk of suffering fracture than men when age is taken into account. The risk of bone fracture does not surface in male rheumatoid arthritis patients until they get old, whereas their female counterparts are at higher risk, even those under the age of fifty.[9]

Genes

Family history is deemed a possible risk factor for rheumatoid arthritis based on the theory that predisposition to the disease is genetic. However, no conclusive studies identify specific genes associated with the disease, although convincing pieces of evidence warrant further research. In 1987, Peter Gregersen and colleagues found a string of five amino acids that seem to be unique to rheumatoid arthritis patients. The team proposed that this string within the major histocompatibility complex (MHC) may be playing a big role in developing susceptibility to the disease. The team called this string the "shared epitope."[10]

Gregersen, now director of the Feinstein Institute's Robert S. Boas Center for Genomics and Human Genetics, and other members of the North American Rheumatoid Arthritis Consortium (NARAC) are responsible for building a massive genetic database containing profiles of more than one thousand people with rheumatoid arthritis as well as their family members. Gregersen's team also accessed the Epidemiological Investigation of Rheumatoid Arthritis (EIRA) database. The two databases gave researchers more than three thousand genetic specimens for their studies. In 2007, Gregersen's team announced the discovery of variants of STAT4 and TRAF1-C5 genes, which seem to be contributing to higher risk of rheumatoid arthritis.[11] Prior to this, Gregersen had found strong evidence that the PTPN2 gene is associated with a twofold risk of developing rheumatoid arthritis and other autoimmune disorders. This was followed by the discovery of PADI4, which is believed to be a major risk factor among the Asian population, although less so among people of European descent. People with two copies of STAT4 are twice as likely to develop lupus and have a 60 percent increased risk of incurring rheumatoid arthritis as compared with people who do not have a copy of the genetic variant. TRAF1-C5 consists of two genes found lying close to each other on chromosome nine. It is still unknown which of these genes is a risk factor. Research findings suggest that having this variant at chromosome nine results in a 35 percent increased risk of getting rheumatoid arthritis.

Gregersen's 1987 discovery got a major boost in 2011 with the release of collaborative research studies from other research partners. The research validated and advanced Gregersen's 1987 study. The collaborating teams used a fine-mapping strategy to examine genetic samples derived from twenty thousand people. Genetic variants in the MHC of people with rheumatoid arthritis were compared with versions of genes found in patients who do not have this disease. The study identified positions in two amino acids from the shared epitope and discovered two more amino acids that may be risk factors as well. These amino acids are found in key immune system proteins called human leukocyte antigens, or HLAs, specifically at the base of the peptide-binding groove, which have the ability to detect and bind to foreign bodies. [12] The findings are expected to pave the way for the discovery of rheumatoid arthritis's autoantigen, or the material that causes the immune system to attack the tissues and joints.

Smoking

Smoking is also associated with increased risk of developing rheumatoid arthritis. One-third of cases involving the common forms of this joint disorder can be attributed to smoking. The risk is estimated to be 50 percent higher among smokers who have genetic predisposition for disease. [13]

The correlation between smoking and higher risk of rheumatoid arthritis is not as pronounced as the effect of smoking on lung cancer susceptibility. Rather, the risk of rheumatoid arthritis due to smoking increases in a way similar to that of heart disease caused by smoking. Rheumatoid arthritis is more likely to develop in people who smoke longer and more frequently. It has been proposed that smoking causes proteins to change and triggers an immune system attack on healthy tissues and joints. The pace of development and reaction may differ depending on genetic factors. A study [14] showed that smoking can also affect the efficacy of rheumatoid arthritis treatments. Smokers with rheumatoid arthritis are less likely to respond to methotrexate (MTX) and tumor necrosis factor (TNF) inhibitors as compared with patients who are nonsmokers. The ten-year study proved that those who have never smoked in the past have good response rates to these medications. The researchers examined the records of approximately fourteen hundred individuals participating in the EIRA in 1996 and 2006. The age of the patients ranged from eighteen to seventy. They entered the population-controlled study ten months after the onset of symptoms. The results showed that after three months of MTX treatment, current smokers showed less improvement compared with those who had never smoked. The smoking group had a 27 percent response rate, while the nonsmoking group had a 36 percent rate. In the TNF inhibitor study, 29 percent of smokers had a good response rate, compared with 43 percent among nonsmokers. Past smoking history showed no correlation to MTX or TNF inhibitor response rate. Around 14 percent of smokers responded well to medications after three months, compared with 34 percent of patients who had never smoked. The researchers underscored the need for further studies to determine if smoking cessation prior to initiating treatment would improve the response rate.

DISTINGUISHING CHARACTERISTICS OF RHEUMATOID ARTHRITIS

Hands and Fingers

The joints connecting the fingers to the hands and the toes to the feet are usually affected first. Several types of deformities are associated with rheumatoid arthritis, such as Z-thumb (a deformed metacarpophalangeal joint marked by a squared appearance), swan neck deformity (the joint nearest to the fingertip turns toward the palm), ulnar deviation, and boutonniere deformity. These conditions are not specific to the rheumatoid type of arthritis. They may also manifest in cases of osteoarthritis. Rheumatoid arthritis can still be distinguished from noninflammatory joint disorders such as osteoarthritis in which signs of swelling and morning stiffness are less remarkable and stiffness only lasts for an hour. At the onset of rheumatoid arthritis, pain may be asymmetrical, but the condition usually turns symmetrical soon. The rheumatoid nodule, also known as the cutaneous nodule, is the most common defining characteristic of rheumatoid arthritis. Pathologists call this inflammatory reaction "necrotizing granuloma." Rheumatologists do not yet know how the pathological process starts, but it may be basically the same as that of synovitis since both have similar structural symptoms. Various forms of vasculitis can be experienced by people with rheumatoid arthritis. Benign microinfarcts may develop around the nail folds. In severe cases, patients may experience livedo reticularis, a purplish discoloration of the skin due to damaged capillaries.

Rarities

The following rare skin symptoms are associated with rheumatoid arthritis:

- Palmar erythema, a reddening of the palm as a result of pathological and physiological factors
- Atrophy of digital (finger) skin, a condition characterized by thinning of digital skin
- Erythema nodosum, an inflammatory disease characterized by red bumps under the skin
- Sweet's syndrome, an acute case of neutrophilic dermatosis marked by erythematous plaques, lesions, fever, and sometimes blisters with an annular or arciform pattern
- Pyoderma gangrenosum, a type of noninfectious dermatosis causing tissues to become necrotic, leading to deep ulcers
- Lobular panniculitis, an inflammation of subcutaneous adipose tissue characterized by tender skin nodules

TECHNIQUES AND RESEARCH

Rheumatoid arthritis is detected mainly based on physical symptoms, radiographic indication of joint damage, and patient history. Rheumatoid arthritis is difficult to detect at an early stage, and most treatments available today offer only temporary relief. Some conditions that mimic the early signs of rheumatoid arthritis include crystal-induced arthritis, osteoarthritis, systemic lupus erythematosus, psoriatic arthritis, Lyme disease, reactive arthritis, ankylosing spondylitis, and hepatitis C. Laboratory tests and radiographic imaging are normally used to distinguish rheumatoid arthritis from such conditions. Initial diagnosis can be quite challenging, and it may take nine months from the onset period for the disease to be effectively diagnosed. The discovery of an effective cure for rheumatoid arthritis depends on clear understanding of the root causes of the disease. Research studies aimed at understanding the pathology of the disease have made significant progress over the past decades, thanks to advances in biotechnology and genetic engineering.

Physical Diagnosis

Due to the difficulty of diagnosing rheumatoid arthritis in its early stages, the American College of Rheumatology and the European League against Rheumatism collaborated to revise the recommended screening protocol for classifying rheumatoid arthritis. Modern drugs for managing rheumatoid arthritis, such as the disease-modifying antirheumatic drug (DMARD) methotrexate and recent biologic agents, have greatly improved patients' quality of life. This is partly due to early administration of therapeutic intervention, which not only improves response rate but also mitigates joint damage and disability. The collaborative initiative aims to allow drug researchers to enroll patients during the early stage of the disease by setting a standardized and more comprehensive assessment procedure for detecting early rheumatoid arthritis. Rheumatoid arthritis cannot be diagnosed with a single test. Several physical symptoms and laboratory results have to be taken into consideration. The 2010 classification system assigns the following scores when weighing the signs of rheumatoid arthritis for clinical trial purposes. This screening procedure is aimed at patients with at least one swollen joint and synovitis that cannot be better explained by another disease:

- One point when two to ten large joints are involved
- Two points when one to three small joints are involved, regardless of the presence of a large swollen joint
- Three points when four to ten small joints are involved, regardless of the presence of a large swollen joint
- Four points when more than ten joints are affected

- Two points for the presence of low-positive rheumatoid factor (RF) or low-positive anticitrullinated protein antibody (ACPA)[15]
- Three points for elevated, high-positive RF or high-positive ACPA
- One point for high erythrocyte sedimentation rate (ESR) or C-reactive protein (CRP) value
- One point for cases lasting for six weeks or longer.

The new diagnostic criteria agree with the latest understanding of the disease and treatment techniques. Unlike the 1987 criteria, the 2010 system does not emphasize the destruction of joints since this is what early detection is meant to prevent. In medical practice, however, the 1987 criteria are still widely applied and require the presence of at least four of the specified conditions in a certain period.

Laboratory Tests

To confirm that certain physical symptoms indicate rheumatoid arthritis, laboratory tests may be required. RF is a highly recognized indicator of rheumatoid arthritis. This can be measured via latex fixation/immunoturbidimetry, which determines the levels of different immunoglobulin isotopes: IgM RF, IgA RF, and IgG RF. The normal RF sensitivity for rheumatoid arthritis ranges from 60 to 90 percent. As the disease progresses, seropositivity likewise increases. Specificity is relatively low (between 70 and 80 percent), and those who suffer from other forms of rheumatism have high RF levels. Clinical findings show that the elevation of either IgG RF or IgA RF, or both, in people who also have IgM RF and joint disease is a significant indicator of rheumatoid arthritis. These combinations are rare in other cases of rheumatic disease in which there is a presence of IgM RF. IgA RF and IgG RF are, however, not highly sensitive, and their use in diagnosing rheumatoid arthritis is quite limited. Anti-CCP sensitivity is more specific than RF when diagnosing rheumatoid arthritis. As compared with RF marker, anti-CCP is considered equally sensitive and more specific. Combining the two markers provides greater sensitivity than either marker alone. Based on a study involving more than 550 patients with suspected rheumatoid arthritis, anti-CCP was present in thirty of eighty-seven subjects who had no elevated level of three RF isotypes (IgM, IgA, and IgG by enzyme-linked immunosorbent assays).[16]

Prognosis

It is possible for RF and anti-CCP to be detected years prior to the manifestation of symptoms. A study involving blood donors estimated the sensitivity of anti-CCP levels in the prognosis of rheumatoid arthritis to be between 29 and 37 percent, with a specificity of about 98 percent.[17] With the passage of time, the level of sensitivity increases. Anti-CCP testing may also be useful in the future diagnosis of rheumatoid arthritis in patients suffering from undifferentiated arthritis. Rheumatoid arthritis may progress or remain stable. Some patients eventually suffer from progressive joint damage; others have a self-limiting condition. Predicting the course of progression would be a big help in the proper prescription of DMARDs and prevention of misdiagnosis. An elevated RF level suggests higher risk for progressive joint damage. Very high titers can indicate severe joint conditions. Rheumatoid nodules, Felty's syndrome, peripheral neuropathy, vasculitis, skin ulcers, and IgA and IgG RF positivity in the early stage of rheumatoid arthritis may be signs of a more severe disease and higher risk of radiographic progression. Anti-CCP testing can predict the course of progression for a ten-year period following the onset of the disease. Research findings show that baseline anti-CCP (67 percent) and RF (69 percent) had similar sensitivity for prediction of radiographic advancement at five years, but anti-CCP markers had significantly higher specificity, at 56 percent compared with 24 percent for RF.[18]

Patients positive for anti-CCP but negative for RF may still be susceptible to rheumatoid arthritis, although the risk is lower in patients with positive RF and negative anti-CCP test results. People who have negative results on both markers have minimal risk of developing rheumatoid arthritis, but negative test results on both assays do not rule out existing rheumatoid arthritis. People with elevated RF and chronic hepatitis C virus or other polyarticular arthritis-induced infections are likely to be diagnosed with rheumatoid arthritis if the anti-CCP test result is positive. Abnormal ESR and CRP levels may indicate progression of rheumatoid arthritis, although these conditions can also be caused by other diseases. The level of disease activity is relatively low when ESR and CRP are at normal levels. When CRP and ESR findings are discordant, CRP seems to be a more reliable indicator of disease activity. One study showed that a high CRP level may be a predictor of long-term progression of rheumatoid arthritis.[19]

Gut Microbe as a Prognostic Marker

The Mayo Illinois Alliance for Technology-Based Healthcare reported that gut bacteria could play a role in rheumatioid arthritis when they exceed the normal count. Mayo conducted a study involving genetically engineered mice with a predisposition for rheumatoid arthritis. The findings showed that the immune response of mice to gut bacteria seemed to mimic the gender risk trends found in humans as female mice were prone to develop rheumatoid arthritis. Through genomic sequencing technologies, the alliance rendered solid evidence regarding the potential role of gut microbe as a prognostic biomarker for rheumatoid arthritis.[20] The research is the first to offer strong evidence that bacterial infection may have a role in the development of rheumatoid arthritis.

MODERN RESEARCH FINDINGS

Genetic engineering has played a key role in recent discoveries of possible ways to cure rheumatoid arthritis. Biologics have become the preferred treatment for rheumatoid arthritis, but several of these medications lose effectiveness over time and are more expensive than standard medications such as DMARDs. Introduced in the 1990s, biologic treatments mimic the natural antibodies to control inflammation. These medications are usually prescribed when cheaper drugs do not work or as a substitute for drugs with side effects. Response rates also vary from patient to patient.

PS-372424

Recent work on possible rheumatoid arthritis treatments focuses on controlling inflammation at the immune system level. A study on the PS-372424 compound demonstrated potential capacity to prevent white blood cells from finding their way to the joints. By preventing these cells from reaching the joints, bone damage can be prevented or mitigated. The study involved mice that were genetically engineered to possess a human-like immune system. The compound was able to prevent activated T cells from damaging the joints. Only the T cells implicated in the disease were affected. The compound binds to receptor CXCR3, which only the activated T cells possess, and thus causes no harm to other white blood cells. The mechanism has the advantage of being more specific and perhaps safer since it does not compromise the entire immune system. The compound opens the possibility of completely preventing the onset of inflammation that leads to rheumatoid arthritis.[21]

MMP-9

An enzyme called MMP-9 that belongs to a class of proteins has also been the subject of a study with the aim of developing treatment for autoimmune diseases. The enzyme performs critical roles, such as facilitating wound repair, but it triggers autoimmune problems when synthesized excessively. The research team used a vaccine to induce the immune system of mice to synthesize antibodies that can target the enzyme. The technique works in the same way as injecting a vaccine containing dead virus to trick the immune system into killing live virus. In this experiment, the mice received an artificial metal zinc-histidine complex. Blood samples derived from the laboratory mice had antibodies with structural and functional similarities to matrix metalloprotease (MMP) inhibitors. Dubbed "metallobodies," these antibodies can bind tightly to MMP-2 and MMP-9 in both mice and humans. The novel technique has the potential to treat autoimmune diseases such as rheumatoid arthritis and regional enteritis, or Crohn's disease. [22]

Anti-Interleukin-6 Receptor Antibody

Another study showed that anti-interleukin-6 (IL-6) receptor antibody can remarkably slow down the progression of joint damage even if the rheumatoid arthritis has been active. [23] After a year of treatment, rheumatoid arthritis patients taking methotrexate and placebo got an average score of around 21.7 on the clinical disease activity index, whereas patients who took tocilizumab (Actemra) in addition to methotrexate got a mean score of 20.2. The remarkable difference between the two was evident in the progress of the disease as shown in radiographic findings, with a mean change of 1.2 points for the first group and 0.4 points among tocilizumab patients. Recent data revealed that tumor necrosis factor inhibitors can slow down or prevent radiographic progression even in people who have been symptomatic or those who chronically develop a high level of acute phase reactants. To determine if the same is true with IL-6 inhibition, the researchers drew data from a randomized trial involving 531 patients divided into two groups: those who received methotrexate plus placebo and those who received methotrexate and tocilizumab. Those who were randomized to get placebo demonstrated significant association between worsening of radiographic scores and disease activity indices at the first year, whereas those receiving tocilizumab showed low correlation between X-ray progression and any disease variables, including swollen joint counts, CRP levels, and the simplified disease activity index. Erosion scores differed significantly between the two groups throughout the duration of the study, with the placebo group reporting a change of 0.65 points while the second group had 0.25 points. Corresponding changes in the narrowing of joint space were 0.53 and 0.14 points, respectively. The data indicates that tocilizumab interferes with the progression of radiographic progression of rheumatoid arthritis irrespective of disease activity. [24]

Anti–Tumor Necrosis Factor Agents

Clinical tests confirm the efficacy of anti-TNF agents in terms of slowing the progress of rheumatoid arthritis. The biologic agent is assumed to work by suppressing osteoclasts in joint lesions. More cytokines regulating matrix degradation may be involved as suggested by the results of several animal studies. Recently, experts discovered osteoclast-mediated bone resorption that is controlled by the receptor activator of nuclear factor kB ligand (RANKL), which is found in a wide range of cell types, such as T cells and synoviocytes, that play a role in the development of rheumatoid arthritis. Findings suggest that these cells have a role in osteoclast maturation and activation in the presence of cytokines such as TNF-α and M-CSF. Those with rheumatoid arthritis have a high level of soluble decoy receptors to RANKL, but their number normalizes following intake of TNF inhibitors.[25]

Side Effects

When the prescribed dosage is followed, anti-TNF drugs do not expose patients to higher risk of infection, according to a study published in the *Annals of the Rheumatic Diseases*.[26] When doses exceed the recommended level however, anti-TNF agents double the risk of developing infections. These findings were drawn from the analysis of data from eighteen trials involving eighty-eight hundred patients with rheumatoid arthritis, with an average follow-up period of about one year. Those who were treated with anti-TNF agents with the right dosage did not experience higher risk of death and other severe adverse conditions such as infections, nonmelanoma skin cancers, lymphoma, or noncutaneous cancers. Those who took two to three times more than the recommended dose were more likely to get serious infection, although their risk level fell as the trial progressed.

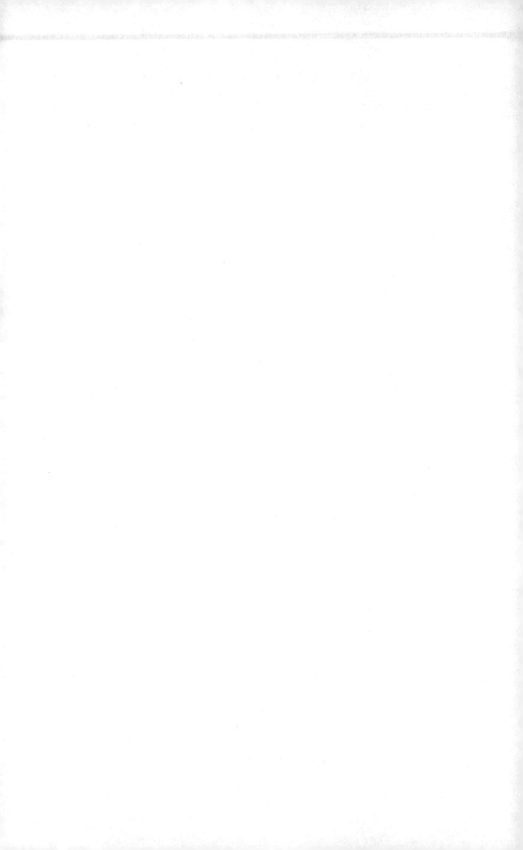

Chapter Nine

Juvenile Rheumatoid Arthritis

In order to fully grasp the meaning of the term *juvenile rheumatoid arthritis* (JRA), one needs to look at its component words. *Juvenile* refers to the state of being young, childish, or infantile. *Rheumatism* describes any painful condition related to the motor system of the body. This pertains to joints, muscles, and soft and connective tissues. As discussed previously, the prefix *rheuma* originates from the Greek word *rheuma*,[1] which pertains to the flowing of a river or stream. *Arthritis*, on the other hand, is a term concerned just with joint disorders. The term again originates from the Greeks: *arthron* means "joint," and *itis* means "inflammation." A joint is where bones meet, such as the shoulder, hip, and knee joints and the minor joints of the hands and feet. Joining the words to form the phrase "juvenile rheumatoid arthritis," one can conclude that it is a joint disorder found in youth. Indeed, arthritis is not a disorder exclusive to the elderly population.

INTRODUCTION TO JUVENILE RHEUMATOID ARTHRITIS

Children age sixteen and younger who experience joint disorders suffer from juvenile rheumatoid arthritis. Children can complain about aches in their joints, which can have multiple causes. However, if the pain persists for six weeks or more,[2] or there is swelling on or around the joints, the child might be suffering from JRA. Arthritis is a chronic condition and lasts a long time. It causes inflammation of one or more joints, sometimes retarding bone development and growth. Two important questions arise from the discussion so far: (1) Why categorize juvenile arthritis as a disease separate from that experienced by adults? and (2) Why can the two not be considered the same and treated as such when a joint disorder is the core problem? To answer these questions, the following section explains some major differences between adult and juvenile rheumatoid arthritis.[3]

Quick Facts and Statistics

The majority of patients suffering from JRA outgrow the disease, a finding that is very rare in the adult forms of arthritis. Rheumatoid arthritis in adults is a single disease with different manifestations, while JRA has distinct subtypes and is much rarer than arthritis in adults. JRA patients, more often than not, have negative rheumatoid factor (RF) in their blood, while 70 to 80 percent of adults with rheumatoid arthritis have positive RF in circulation. JRA interferes with proper growth of the bones, while that is not the case for adults, whose bones are already fully grown and developed. Due to these and other age-related factors, juvenile arthritis is termed a separate disease and dealt with accordingly.

There are three major subtypes of JRA, which can be determined by following the pattern of the disease in its first six months, considering how many joints are involved, and testing for certain types of antibodies present in the blood. These include the following:[4]

- Oligoarticular JRA: In this kind of JRA, only a few joints are affected. It usually affects large joints such as knees, shoulders, and elbows. *Oligo* means "few." When only one joint is affected, it is called monoarticular arthritis. This type is not very severe.
- Polyarticular JRA: This form of JRA affects five or more joints, usually in the hands and feet. A typical symptom is the swelling of fingers and toes. This type of JRA is often symmetrical, meaning that if a joint is affected on one side of the body, the same joint is affected on the other side as well.
- Systemic JRA: This type of JRA causes swelling, pain, and limited motion in one or more joints. It also causes inflammation of internal organs such as the heart, spleen, and liver. Typically it causes fever and a pink rash. Fever comes at the same time every day. It is sometimes referred to as Still's disease.

Oligoarticular and polyarticular JRA are more common in girls than boys. However, systemic JRA affects both sexes equally. Approximately 50 percent of children suffering from JRA have the oligoarticular type, 30 percent have the polyarticular type, and 20 percent suffer from the systemic type. Some important statistics (from the same source) about the prevalence of JRA are listed below. These statistics give insight into the magnitude of the problem and the number of people suffering from it.[5]

- One out of every one thousand children is affected by JRA worldwide.

- Young girls are more susceptible than boys to the disease.
- The disease is most common among Caucasians.
- JRA is one of the most common childhood diseases in the United States.
- Approximately 294,000 children are affected by JRA in the United States.
- Ambulatory care visits for JRA and other pediatric arthritis conditions number, on average, 827,000 annually.

A new term for JRA has recently gained popularity: *juvenile idiopathic arthritis* (JIA). *Idiopathic* is a medical adjective used to indicate that a condition arises spontaneously or without known cause. Since there are not many known causes of juvenile arthritis, the term JIA came into existence. Research suggests that JIA patients have a condition called autoimmune process.[6] This is when the immune system of the body becomes overactive and inappropriately starts attacking joint tissues as if they were harmful foreign bodies. There is speculation that autoimmune processes have a variety of triggers. At the top of the list are certain bacteria and viruses. Contrary to popular belief, there is scant evidence of children with food and other allergies developing arthritis. However, some research suggests the roots of the disease are genetic. If one family member has been diagnosed with an autoimmune disease, it is very likely that others, especially siblings, will have it too. Diagnosing JIA is not an easy task. Most doctors use a combination of blood tests, X-rays (to rule out fractures or cancer), and physical examination. Physical examination of the child is considered the most important of the three. This is discussed in detail later in the chapter.

DISTINCTION

Since more than a hundred different forms of arthritis are known and being treated, it is important to know what major factors distinguish one type from the others and how they affect the patient so that the problem is diagnosed properly and treated accordingly. Symptoms and features[7] typically related to JRA include the following: Persistent joint pain, inflammation, and swelling can occur. Joint inflammation over a long period causes permanent and irreversible damage to cartilage and bone. Morning stiffness of joints or stiffness after a nap has been observed, but the morning stiffness gradually improves after the patient wakes up. A child with JRA might exhibit irritability and refusal to walk or even use a specific joint. The patient might also suffer from recurrent fever with temperatures exceeding one hundred degrees. Fever usually occurs at the same time daily. A pale red or pink rash in the form of spots is typical in systemic JRA and usually appears on the chest and thighs and sometimes on other parts of the body. The rash usually accompanies fever spikes.

Bone Characteristics

Joints affected by JRA are mostly the knee and the joints in the feet and hands. Anemia, a red blood cell deficiency, is a common feature of polyarticular JRA. Remissions and flare-ups are a common feature of JRA. Periods when no symptoms appear (remissions) may be followed by periods when the severity of the symptoms peaks (flare-ups). Bone growth can be adversely affected. Growth can proceed either too quickly or too slowly, causing one limb to become longer than the other; joints may grow unevenly, advancing out to one side. Overall bone development and growth might be slowed to a considerable extent.

Soft Tissues

Muscles and other soft tissues around the affected joints may weaken. Weight loss and loss of appetite in children suffering from JRA are very common. Irritation and disease of the eye, which is composed of soft tissue, is a typical feature of JRA. Symptoms include blurred vision or even complete loss of vision in extreme cases, as well as excessive tearing, sensitivity to light, and redness in the eyes. Uveitis is the term for inflammation of the uvea of the eye. Another serious form of eye inflammation caused by JRA is iridocyclitis, a form of anterior uveitis. This is a serious problem and can lead to scarring of the eye and vision loss. Initially, there may be no noticeable symptoms of an eye problem. Resultant sleep disturbances are frequent among JRA patients. Children often face difficulty falling asleep and awaken several times during the night. Daytime sleepiness, mood swings, and fatigue are also common. A child suffering from JRA should have regular eye exams to detect any early changes in order to prevent damage.

Solid Outgrowths

In some subtypes of JRA, nodules develop on some parts of the body such as the elbows. Nodules are small bumps that receive a lot of pressure and become extremely uncomfortable or painful for the patient. Swollen lymph nodes are also an outcome of JRA, especially in the neck, under the jaw, or in the groin. Patients may feel heat or a burning sensation in the joints as a result.

SIGNIFICANCE OF KNOWING THE DISTINGUISHING
FEATURES

Symptomology

The characteristic symptoms and features explained above are only possible outcomes of JRA and represent a major part of why it is important to know the distinguishing features of the disease. Not all sufferers experience all symptoms, and not all experience the same intensity. Symptoms differ from child to child and from subtype to subtype. Some patients may have longer remissions and fewer and shorter flare-ups, while others may have the opposite. Patients and caregivers must also realize that persistent joint inflammation, pain, and stiffness are common to all types of JRA; they are mostly present in all patients and are typical signs of arthritis among children below the age of sixteen. Sensitivity to any changes in a child's gait, mood, and sleeping habits can be very beneficial to timely diagnosis and treatment. Contrary to what one might expect, children may not complain about the pain; they may learn to live with it rapidly.

The Overlooked Burden

JRA may affect the physical presentation of the young patient and can impact his or her emotional and social presentation. This is another reason why it is important to understand the distinguishing features of the JRA sufferer. Slower or faster bone growth can cause a limp or cause one arm or leg to become longer than the other, and uneven joint growth creates a different joint shape, especially in the elbows and knees. If joints of the hands and feet are affected, fingers and toes can become malformed, and hands and feet can swell. Some medicines used in the treatment of JRA can cause weight gain due to water retention and make the face rounder. These changes in physical appearance, along with the child's inability to participate in some physical activities, can create an emotional burden for him or her and cause extreme depression and stress. Others find it difficult to accept sufferers' different physical appearance and, more often than not, stare at them, making them feel uncomfortable. Children with JRA feel left out and alienated. This stress is thought to further increase inflammation and joint pain. Proper emotional support from family and at school and an understanding of the child's feelings and limitations can help the JRA patient cope better with the disease.

It has been observed that very young children with rheumatoid arthritis find it relatively easier to adjust than those in their teens. The teenage years can be a challenging enough experience without having to cope with a chronic, crippling, and life-altering disease. School life is affected, as is the social environment. JRA can turn children into loners with few friends, and like adults with arthritis they can suffer from depression and insomnia. Adults, however, are better able to express and share their feelings with their doctors. Children tend to internalize their feelings of despair, which makes the situation worse. Teenagers are known to be worse at handling their emotions as they are frequently depressed and disturbed. Parents must make sure that they join a local support group, have understanding teachers at school, and can continue some form of physical activity during remissions. Different studies suggest that overly authoritarian parents of teenage JRA patients can worsen the situation. Having enough autonomy in tasks such as socializing and physical activity can improve quality of life for these children, which is another reason why knowing the distinguishing features of JRA is important.

TECHNIQUES

Medical History

A detailed medical history and physical examination[8] can help immensely in the detection of JRA. A doctor can ask several questions of the child or the parents that will help diagnose the problem. These questions may include the following:

- When exactly did the symptoms first begin to appear?
- Which joints are affected?
- Do the joints feel stiffer in the morning?
- Is the child limping?
- Has there been weight loss?
- Has there been a loss of appetite?
- Can the child bear weight on the affected joints?
- Is there a family history of arthritis?

Answers to the above inquiries will provide the doctor with very useful information and make diagnosing JRA much easier.

Physical Examination

The components of the physical examination for JRA include the following:

- Careful inspection of the affected joints
- Evaluation of body temperature to record fever
- Examination of the skin to look for rashes
- Observation of the lymph nodes to look for any swellings

During such an examination the doctor notes the kind of joint inflammation, other signs such as fever or rash, and the number and location of affected joints. This information is deterministic in the diagnosis of JRA.

At the Lab

Some laboratory screening tests[9] for JRA are listed below.

Antinuclear Antibody Test

This test looks for certain antibodies present in the blood of a child suspected of having JRA. The presence of such antibodies increases the likelihood that the young patient will develop iritis, an eye inflammation thought to cause permanent damage to the eye. Some children with JRA have an increased risk of developing iritis. By helping to determine the likelihood of iritis, this test tells doctors if they must regularly check the eyes of JRA sufferers who are more susceptible to iritis in order to prevent permanent damage.

Rheumatoid Factor

Another blood test is done to see if rheumatoid factor is present in the blood of the child. RF is an antibody that determines whether the child is likely to carry the disease into adulthood or not. This antibody attacks healthy body tissues and causes damage. Presence of RF in a child is a surefire indication of JRA.

Other Tests

The erythrocyte sedimentation rate (ESR) test assesses the degree of inflammation and assists in determining the subtype of JRA present. The term *complement* refers to a group of proteins in the blood. A complement test is done to measure the level of complement in blood. Low levels of complement are associated with immune system disorders such as JRA. Sometimes urine analysis can indicate kidney disorders that are again associated with immune system issues. White blood cell count is another screening technique for JRA. An increased number of these specialized cells indicates possible infection, while a decreased amount suggests possible rheumatoid disease in the child. In arthrocentesis, fluid is extracted from around the affected joint via syringe and analyzed for diagnosis. A hematocrit measures the level of red blood cells in the blood. Decreased levels of red blood cells, known as anemia, are associated with rheumatoid diseases in children.

Treatment as a Technique

Once JRA has been detected, treatment is immediately started. The treatment approach is twofold: (1) to reduce pain and enable the child to lead as normal a life as possible, and (2) to prevent any permanent and irreversible damage. Treatment for JRA includes physical therapy and medication. Physical therapy is used to keep the joints flexible, which makes them less stiff and painful. Swimming, certain forms of aerobics, stretching exercises, and other physical activities that a therapist suggests can be a major help in the fight against JRA. Doctors and therapists may also suggest splints and other devices to ensure proper bone growth, a major concern in juvenile rheumatoid arthritis. Shoe lifts or inserts may be advised for children with unequal leg lengths. Increased intake of vitamin D and calcium is also advised. Massages, hot baths, and acupuncture are thought to temporarily relieve the pain and provide some comfort to the youngsters. Medication is prescribed according to the intensity of the disease and the subtype.

RESEARCH

JRA research focuses on the causes, prevention, and treatment of the disease. While research so far has not been able to specify particular causes of JRA, advances show that both genetic and environmental factors, such as viruses and bacteria, are responsible for causing the disease. Recent research suggests that JRA is associated with a virus called human intracisternal A-type particle (HIAP).[10] Antibodies against this virus have been found in a high percentage of JRA patients. HIAP technology is now being used to develop diagnostic tests and treatments for the disease. In terms of possible genetic causes, the human leukocyte antigen (HLA) haplotype gene is thought to determine the subtype of JRA in the patient. The National Institute of Arthritis and Musculoskeletal and Skin Diseases (NIAMS) set up a research registry for families in which two or more siblings have JRA.[11] The purpose of this registry is to study sibling pairs and focus on the genes that seem susceptible to the disease. The aim is to eventually use gene therapy and other gene treatment to treat such disorders.

The Current Situation

For quite some time, JRA has been considered an autoimmune disease, which basically means that the youngster's immune system starts manufacturing antibodies that attack healthy tissues of the body, resulting in inflammation and tissue damage. Recent research, however, has shown that not all cases of JRA are autoimmune related; some are caused by autoinflammatory disorders. Such disorders do not involve antibodies; rather, white blood cells, which attack harmful substances in the body, malfunction and cause inflammation for unknown reasons. Autoinflammatory disorders cause fever and rash. Areas of current research for JRA include the following: [12]

- Long-term effects of the drug methotrexate and corticosteroids
- Causes of sleep problems among JRA sufferers
- Causes and treatment of potential anemia in JRA patients
- Effectiveness of calcium supplementation in increasing bone density of the patients
- Long-term impacts of recurrent pain in children
- How exactly interleukin, a chemical involved in inflammation, influences the growth of new blood vessels in the joint tissues and causes them to overgrow
- Comparison of the effects of using (1) intravenous methylprednisolone, a corticosteroid medicine, and intravenous cyclophosphamide, which suppresses the immune system, and (2) intravenous methylprednisolone alone.

There is still no known way to prevent JRA. Scientists and doctors are always searching for more effective treatments with fewer side effects. In addition to research, clinical trials and controlled-environment case studies can help us understand many new aspects of the disease and its treatment. Anyone suffering from JRA can voluntarily participate in such clinical trials and case studies.

Chapter Ten

Osteoarthritis

The prefix *osteo*[1] derives from the Greek word for "bone." The term *arthritis*, however, concerns joint disorders. A joint is where bones meet, such as the shoulder, knee, and hip joints and the minor joints of the feet and hands.

OVERVIEW

In osteoarthritis, cartilage, the thin, smooth tissue providing a cushion between two bones that allows ease of movement, begins to break down. This causes the bones to react in those areas, and the ends of the bones begin to thicken and grow into external bone growths called osteophytes, or bone spurs. These outgrowths hinder normal joint movement. Bits of bones or cartilage move loosely in the joint space, and the joint may lose hyaluronic acid, which affects the joint's shock-absorbing capabilities. Cartilage is 60 to 80 percent water; osteoarthritis causes the cartilage to lose its fluid content, and this is when the damage begins. The synovial membrane, the thin inner lining of the joints, gets irritated and produces excessive amounts of synovial fluid, which in turn causes visible swelling around the joints.[2] Cysts begin to develop just below the damaged cartilage. Inflammatory proteins called cytokines may be released, causing pain, swelling, and damage. When the cushioning factor of the cartilage is completely lost, bones start to rub painfully against each other; sometimes a grinding sound can also be heard. Unfortunately, once damaged, cartilage cannot be repaired or regenerated. Osteoarthritis usually affects joints in the hands, neck, and spine or larger weight-bearing joints, such as the hips and knees.

There are two types of osteoarthritis: primary and secondary. Cartilage damage is the core issue behind both, and the symptoms and treatment are

153

also the same. Both types differ in terms of the causes behind the cartilage damage.[3]

QUICK FACTS AND STATISTICS

In recent years the incidence and reporting of osteoarthritis have increased many fold. Some interesting facts and statistics about osteoarthritis include the following:

- Before age forty-five to fifty, men and women are equally likely to develop osteoarthritis. After this age bracket, more women than men develop osteoarthritis, with 18 percent women and 9 percent men above the age of sixty-five affected by osteoarthritis worldwide.[4]
- Nearly 30 million adults in the United States have osteoarthritis, with more female than male sufferers.[5]
- It is estimated that by 2020, 20 percent of Americans (around 70 million people) will have reached the age of sixty-five and be at a risk for osteoarthritis.[6]
- Farming for ten years increases the risk of osteoarthritis by 9.3 times.[7]
- Caucasians have a higher risk of developing osteoarthritis than Asians.[8]
- African American women are twice as likely as Caucasian women to develop osteoarthritis of the knees. The reason for this difference is unknown, but recent studies support this fact.[9]

DISTINCTION

The signs and symptoms of osteoarthritis contribute to the detection and, ultimately, the appropriate treatment of the disease. Symptoms vary from patient to patient. Some may have severe pain with no X-ray evidence of joint damage, while others may feel very little or no pain, no matter how visible joint damage is in X-ray imagery. The symptoms get worse gradually and if the joint is overused.

Distinguishing Characteristics of Osteoarthritis

Some of the typical symptoms present in osteoarthritis patients are described herewith. Joint pain is felt when the affected joint is moved and worsens with higher levels of activity. Therefore, it is worst in the evening. Pain is usually relieved with sufficient rest but is originally brought about by a change in the weather. It also worsens when the patient is in a cold environment. Pain may worsen with stressful life events such as the loss of a loved one. Back and neck pain and stiffness can occur. The stiffness is felt in the affected joint after a nap or long period of inactivity, which might include sitting in one place for more than two hours. This is called the gelling phenomenon. The stiffness usually disappears within half an hour with slight movements that warm up the joint. Furthermore, movement becomes limited and inflexible. The osteoarthritis sufferer is unable to move the joint fully in all directions. A grinding is heard and felt when the affected joint is moved as the bones rub against each other due to lack of cartilage cushion. This sensation is usually felt while the patient is bending, kneeling, or climbing stairs (in case of hip or knee osteoarthritis). Bony outgrowths or spurs may form around the affected joints and seem to protrude from the joint area, giving the appearance of swelling. Joints feel tender when even mild pressure is applied. The following sections discuss the joints commonly affected by osteoarthritis.

Knees

Osteoarthritis most commonly affects the knees. People with excess upper-body weight, repeated injuries, or knee surgery tend to develop the condition. The knee area becomes curved outward, causing bowleggedness. People with knee osteoarthritis may start limping. The knee joint becomes unstable, increasing the risk of falling, especially among elderly people.

Hips

Hips are a common site for osteoarthritis. Obesity and inactive lifestyle are major causes of osteoarthritis of the hips. Pain due to hip osteoarthritis spreads to the groin, buttocks, and inner thighs. The ability to rotate, flex, or extend the hip may be completely lost. Activities that involve bending, such as putting on shoes and dressing, can become arduous.

Thumbs and Fingers

Osteoarthritis may develop at three locations in the hands: (1) the base of the thumb where the thumb and the wrist come together, (2) at the end joint closest to the finger, and (3) at the middle joint of the finger. Bone enlargements caused by the bony spurs of the degenerated joint may develop around the small joints at the ends of the fingers. They are called Heberden's nodes,[10] for a renowned British doctor. Another type of bone enlargement occurs at the middle joint of the fingers and is called a Bouchard's node, for a prestigious French doctor. Heberden's and Bouchard's nodes may or may not be painful, but both limit finger movement and are typical physical features of osteoarthritis. They are also thought to be genetic. Many females in one family may have these nodes at once.

Base of the Big Toe

Osteoarthritis at the base of the big toe can cause significant pain and often disability. Pain can radiate to the outside of the foot, the ankle, and possibly the knee. Motion is limited, and walking is also adversely affected. This can be caused by a combination of biomechanics and trauma.

Cervical Spine

Osteoarthritis of the cervical spine causes pain in the neck and back. Spurs can irritate the spinal nerves, causing severe pain and numbness throughout the spine. In severe cases, it can affect bladder and bowel movements.

SYMPTOMOLOGY

Osteoarthritis is not an inflammatory type of arthritis, which means that it is not characterized by joint inflammation such as that observed in rheumatoid arthritis, in which inflammation is the first and foremost indicator of the disease. A patient suffering from osteoarthritis experiences only a mild form of inflammation later in the course of the disease, and that too is impermanent. Rheumatoid arthritis, on the other hand, produces significant and visible joint inflammation. The joint becomes swollen and red, a clear indication of underlying inflammation and usually the first important sign of the disease.

Stiffness

Morning stiffness of the affected joints is experienced in both osteoarthritis and rheumatoid arthritis. In osteoarthritis, this stiffness goes away in half an hour or less with slight warm-up movements of the joints and a warm bath. [11] In rheumatoid arthritis, the stiffness can persist for up to several hours. Joint stiffness in rheumatoid arthritis is also much more pronounced and significant than in osteoarthritis.

Areas of Impact

Osteoarthritis is a localized disease, unlike rheumatoid arthritis, which is a systemic ailment. Osteoarthritis is caused by the loss of cartilage in the joint and manifests only in the affected joints; system-wide symptoms are absent. Rheumatoid arthritis, on the other hand, is an autoimmune disease and has body-wide symptoms, including fever, skin rash, and fatigue. It can also affect internal organs and several joints concurrently. Rheumatoid arthritis affects joints on both sides of the body symmetrically, but this is not necessarily the case in osteoarthritis. Osteoarthritis usually affects larger load-bearing joints. Rheumatoid arthritis is more common in the smaller joints of the hands and the feet.

Pain and Disease Progression

Pain is common in both rheumatoid arthritis and osteoarthritis, but it is more crippling in the former. Pain in osteoarthritis is caused by excessive use of the joint and improves with rest. Pain is at its worst in the mornings after waking for rheumatoid arthritis patients, while it is worst in the evening for osteoarthritis patients. Rheumatoid arthritis spreads rapidly throughout the body with visible symptoms that can worsen immediately after the first symptoms appear, but osteoarthritis progresses slowly over a long period with age and causes permanent changes to the bone structures around the affected joints.

TECHNIQUES

Detection Process

Osteoarthritis cases are on the rise. More and more people around the globe are coping with this problem, but proper detection can help reduce the number of osteoarthritis cases. Many screening techniques are used to diagnose the disease. The right diagnosis of osteoarthritis at the right time can prevent complications. No single test can confirm osteoarthritis. Usually, doctors use a combination of tests in screening for and diagnosing the condition. An osteoarthritis patient must visit a physician on first noticing symptoms such as pain in the joints, stiffness, loss of flexibility, spurs, or a grinding sensation between bones.

The following sections discuss how screening is conducted.[12]

Medical History

First, the doctor takes the patient's medical history. He or she will ask questions related to injuries, surgeries, and past medical conditions. These questions may be asked verbally, or the patient may be given an extensive questionnaire to fill out. The doctor will typically ask the following questions:

- What is your age and gender?
- Which joints hurt and for how long have they been hurting?
- Do the joints get stiff in the morning and how long do they remain stiff?
- Does osteoarthritis run in the family?
- Does the pain become worse after activity and improve after rest?

Physical Techniques

The following procedures help the doctor determine the patient's chances of getting osteoarthritis.

Physical Examination

The physical examination may include the following:

* Pressing the joint to check for pain
* Moving the joint in all directions to check its flexibility
* Listening for crackling or grinding sounds when the joint moves
* Looking for swelling around the joints

X-ray

X-rays of the joints can show clear signs of cartilage damage or reduction, which can indicate osteoarthritis. A decrease in joint space may suggest cartilage reduction. There may be an abnormal increase in bone density and bony spurs, cysts, or visible erosion, indicating osteoarthritis. However, it must be remembered that the absence of these conditions in an X-ray does not rule out osteoarthritis; nor does their presence alone confirm it.

MRI

If an X-ray report suggests osteoarthritis, an MRI scan is done to take a closer look at the details of the joints as well as the nature of the damage.

Blood Tests

Blood tests are done to rule out rheumatoid arthritis and other diseases with similar symptoms. Rheumatoid arthritis is confirmed by the presence of rheumatoid factor in the blood. Also, an increased level of uric acid in the blood might distinguish osteoarthritis from gout.

Body Mass Index

The doctor determines the patient's body mass index to see if excess body weight is exerting pressure on the affected joints. Overweight people experiencing joint pain are quite likely to have osteoarthritis.

Joint Fluid Analysis

The doctor usually extracts fluid from the affected joint and analyzes it to rule out other causes of pain and swelling. The presence of cartilage cells in the fluid indicates osteoarthritis.

Techniques for Doctor Visits

While visiting a doctor for screening, the osteoarthritis patient should remember the following important points. Patients must bring any previous X-ray reports, recent blood test reports, and medical records related to prior injuries or surgeries. This will save the time and cost of conducting new tests and help the doctor reach a diagnosis more quickly. The patient should also try to recall all previous joint-related mishaps in his or her lifetime. Usually, patients only remember the most recent injury, but the actual underlying cause may date further back. Considerable evidence supports the notion that a timely diagnosis can save the osteoarthritis patient a lot of pain and prevent possible disability.

Misdiagnosis of Osteoarthritis

Sometimes osteoarthritis is not accurately detected. There are several reasons for diagnostic pitfalls. [13]

Misinterpretation of the Patient's Pain

The pain may be due not to osteoarthritis but to some other form of arthritis or an injury. Sometimes pain is really due to osteoarthritis but is wrongly perceived as stemming from an injury or other form of arthritis. The pain may originate from one joint and be referred to another joint; for example, osteoarthritis of the hip may be causing pain in the knee. Careful localization and characterization of the pain through medical history and physical examination is necessary for an accurate diagnosis.

Misinterpretation of the Deformity

Deformity in osteoarthritis is caused by degeneration of the joint cartilage. However, such deformities can be caused by other diseases that cause similar symptoms, such as swelling, limited mobility, and crystallization, or "gelling," of joint fluid. This can be a major cause of misdiagnosis.

Misinterpreting X-rays

Sometimes the early stages of osteoarthritis are visually absent in an X-ray printout. Other times, decreased joint space stems not from loss of cartilage but some other disease. These confusions can lead to a misdiagnosis.

More on Misdiagnosis

Once the diagnosis is done, medications and other treatments are started. Doctors may suggest some form of exercise to keep the muscles from wasting. These include swimming, stretching, and yoga. Showers in the morning help reduce morning stiffness. Keeping the joints warm can also help reduce pain. Maintaining a normal body weight is also helpful in controlling the symptoms of osteoarthritis.

Treatment as a Technique

Osteoarthritis is chronic, that is, indicative of a lifelong disease. The disease itself is incurable, but treatments are available to improve its symptoms. Bone structure will remain the same once initially changed due to the disease. Doctors can prescribe medicines and therapies that can reduce pain significantly. Although surgery can bring some improvement, basic structure, once altered, is difficult to restore to its original form. That, however, does not mean that the patient has to live with the pain. Symptoms can be treated, and disability can be minimized. Since osteoarthritis is bound to develop to an extent with age, not much can be done to prevent or cure it completely. For the most part, osteoarthritis is a mild disease with a limited number of observable symptoms affecting only a single joint.

For some patients, the condition can become severe and result in the loss of mobility and disability. Surgery may be the only treatment. Surgery replaces the diseased joint with an artificial one and restores normal mobility and use of the joint for the osteoarthritis patient. In the elderly, many joints are usually affected. Elderly patients stop using affected joints due to extreme pain, which leads to muscle wasting and becomes a major cause of balance loss and falls. Due to the loss of hand or arm movement, assistance may be required several times during the day. Simple household chores, such as handling utensils, may become arduous. When the hip joint is affected, there might be difficulty in bathing, dressing, and undressing. This can cause stress and depression when patients feel they have to rely on others for even the smallest tasks. Proper counseling and support can prevent these feelings, which can further aggravate the problem.

RESEARCH

Experts continue to seek the exact causes of osteoarthritis and to understand the factors that increase risk for developing the condition in younger people. They are also striving to find new and better treatments for the symptoms to provide sufferers with as much relief as possible. Research suggests that 800 mg per day of chondroitin sulfate (derived from fish or other animals) can significantly reduce pain and improve movement in osteoarthritis of the hand.[14] Chondroitin helps the cartilage retain its moisture. Usually osteoarthritis is diagnosed after an X-ray is done, which happens only after the patient notices and complains about persistent joint pain. By then, most of the joint damage is done, and treatment focuses on reducing pain. In order to make a difference, intervention through medication needs to take place at an early stage. For this purpose, an early diagnosis is essential. Researchers have found a way to detect osteoarthritis at an early stage. A special MRI is used to determine the concentration of molecules known as glycosaminogly-cans (GAGs) in the joint cartilage.[15] It is known that the concentration of GAGs diminishes in osteoarthritis. Therefore, a dip in the concentration of GAGs suggests upcoming osteoarthritis. The loss of GAGs is potentially reversible in the very early stages. For now, scientists know that MRI for GAGs can be helpful for patients who suffer from arthritis in one joint and are at high risk of developing osteoarthritis in other joints. The technique is gradually becoming popular.

Chapter Eleven

Psoriatic Arthritis

Psoriatic arthritis is an inflammatory type of arthritis caused by a chronic skin disease called psoriasis.[1] Psoriasis causes patches of red, irritated skin on which flaking silver or white scales develop. To define psoriatic arthritis, one must understand that the word *psora* means "itch" in Greek; therefore, *psoriasis* means "itchy." As discussed throughout this volume, the term *arthritis* concerns joint disorders, wherein the prefix *arthron* means "joint" and the suffix *itis* means "inflammation" in Greek. Thus, the term *psoriatic arthritis* refers to joint inflammation caused by the itchy skin disease called psoriasis. Psoriatic arthritis is also called arthritis psoriatica, psoriatic arthropathy, or arthropathic psoriasis. Patients with the condition are first diagnosed with psoriasis, then with psoriatic arthritis, usually within a span of ten years. The severer the skin symptoms, the greater the chance of developing psoriatic arthritis. In some rare cases, patients develop arthritic symptoms before the skin condition, and in other extremely rare cases, only arthritic conditions develop with very little or no skin disease.

INTRODUCTION

Connections

The relationship between psoriasis and psoriatic arthritis is still not understood completely. Not everyone with psoriasis will develop arthritis, but people with psoriatic arthritis will have psoriasis too. Psoriasis and psoriatic arthritis are autoimmune diseases,[2] which means that the body's immune system starts attacking healthy cells and tissues as if they were harmful foreign bodies. In psoriasis, the body's immune system sends out signals telling the skin cells to grow rapidly, resulting in thick red patches that ultimately shed flakes. This immune response is thought to extend to the joints and lead to inflammation and swelling. The cause is still a mystery. Synovium lines the joints and produces synovial fluid, which lubricates the joint and helps in its movements. In an autoimmune disease, the white cells attack synovium and result in its malfunctioning. This causes synovium to produce thick, sticky synovial fluid, causing swelling and inflammation. This ultimately damages the joint cartilage, narrowing the space between bones.

Psoriatic arthritis can cause permanent joint damage and disability if not properly managed and treated in a timely manner. Psoriasis and psoriatic arthritis are thought to be caused in some cases by a certain genetic makeup. Those with the genetic marker HLA-B27 are at greater risk for developing both psoriasis and psoriatic arthritis. Other possible causes are deep cuts and traumatic sunburns. It is believed that physical trauma can erroneously provoke the body's immune system. Other environmental factors such as bacterial or viral infections can also initiate a faulty immune response in people with an inherited tendency toward psoriasis. Emotional stress can worsen psoriasis and increase the risk of psoriatic arthritis. Alcohol use and smoking have also been found to trigger psoriasis. Hormonal changes may aggravate the condition, increasing the chance of developing psoriatic arthritis. Allergic reactions to medications can stimulate inherent psoriasis, and disorders such as autoimmune deficiency syndrome (AIDS) can reduce the effectiveness of the immune system.

Types of Psoriatic Arthritis

Psoriatic arthritis is classified into five different types:[3]

- Symmetric psoriatic arthritis: This is the most common type of psoriatic arthritis. It affects the same joints on both sides of the body symmetrically, much like rheumatoid arthritis, although it is milder. It can sometimes be disabling and affects more women than men. It is usually accompanied by severe psoriasis.
- Asymmetric psoriatic arthritis: This type of arthritis can affect any joint anywhere in the body but is more common in fingers and toes. It can result in irregular shaping of the entire digit due to inflammation (dactylitis). This type can affect one or more joints per hand or foot, and the number of affected joints on the left versus right hand or foot is often unequal. Asymmetric psoriatic arthritis is the mildest form of psoriatic arthritis.
- Psoriatic spondylitis: This type of arthritis affects the spinal joints, causing morning stiffness of the back and neck. One or both sacroiliac joints (joints linking the spine and pelvis at the lower back) can be affected. Psoriatic spondylitis may also attack connective tissues such as ligaments.

It can cause immense pain and difficulty walking and can eventually disable the patient.

- Distal interphalangeal predominant: The distal joints of the fingers and toes (closer to the nails than the wrists or ankles) are affected in this type of psoriatic arthritis, which can sometimes be confused with osteoarthritis. However, nail changes in psoriatic arthritis, such as discoloration, detachment, and white patches, can distinguish the two. It is very rare and usually affects men only.

- Arthritis mutilans: This is the most severe and destructive form of psoriatic arthritis and can cause disability. Fortunately, it is very rare. It attacks and can completely destroy the minor joints of the feet and hands. It sometimes shortens the affected fingers and toes. This condition is also known as opera glass hand.

Some interesting facts about psoriatic arthritis that highlight the significance and widespread prevalence of the disease are listed below:

- Approximately 7.5 million Americans, or roughly 2 percent of the total US population, have psoriasis.[4]
- Of patients with psoriasis, 10 to 30 percent develop psoriatic arthritis.[5]
- Approximately 1 million people in the United States have psoriatic arthritis.[6]
- Around 40 percent of psoriatic arthritis patients have a family history of either psoriasis or psoriatic arthritis, or both.[7]
- Almost 90 percent of people who experience psoriatic arthritis notice nail involvement first.[8]
- Caucasians are more prone to developing psoriatic arthritis than African Americans.[9]

DISTINCTION

Physical Signs and Symptoms

It is important to know the typical symptoms of a disease. These help in both diagnosis and treatment. As stated earlier, most (not all) psoriatic arthritis patients have psoriasis. Psoriasis causes red patches of skin covered with silvery white flakes and dry, cracked skin that may bleed.[10] Patches can range from small spots to areas with major scaling. When the symptoms of psoriasis become aggravated and include joint inflammation, the condition is called psoriatic arthritis. Symptoms may range from mild to severe and differ from patient to patient. Patients may experience periods of remission, when the symptoms completely go away or improve considerably, followed by periods of extreme flare-up, when the symptoms are at their worst. This can sometimes make diagnosis difficult. Usually, the symptoms worsen as the disease progresses. Typical signs and symptoms of psoriatic arthritis include the following: [11]

- Inflammation leading to painful, swollen, hot, and red joints.
- Sausage-like appearance of swollen fingers and toes.
- Nail changes, including discoloration and development of yellow spots and tiny depressions, or pits. Nails may loosen and digress from the nail bed or develop fungus. This is one of the first noticed symptoms of psoriatic arthritis.
- Inflammation of muscles, tendons, and the area around the cartilage, usually occurring on the heels or the soles of the feet. Psoriatic arthritis can cause difficulty in walking and climbing stairs. When inflammation occurs in the muscles of the chest wall, it can cause immense chest pain and shortness of breath.
- Joint stiffness at its worst in the mornings or after long periods of sitting. Stiffness improves with movement.
- Pain in the affected joints. The intensity of pain varies among patients and sometimes from day to day.
- Acne.
- Inflammation of the front of the eyes, also called conjunctivitis. Inflammation around the pupil can also take place. Known as iritis, this is a painful condition that gets worse with bright light and can lead to permanent blindness.
- Stiffness and pain in the back and neck.
- Inflammation around the heart leading to shortness of breath and even heart failure in severe cases.
- Skin lesions anywhere on the body. Common spots for such lesions are inside the belly button, between the buttocks, and behind the ears. Patches of red, irritated, and itchy skin develop. They are covered with white or silvery scales that keep shedding.

TECHNIQUES

Overview

Successful treatment can only begin after a disease has been correctly diagnosed. A large number of people throughout the world are coping with psoriatic arthritis. It is a long-lasting disease with no cure. Treatments are aimed at reducing the symptoms of the disease once it has been diagnosed. Symptoms include both the skin issues and the joint problems. Both can be sources of extreme discomfort and pain for the patient. In order to diagnose psoriatic arthritis, doctors use a number of screening techniques as no single test can confirm the condition. Diagnosing psoriatic arthritis can be a tricky business because the symptoms come and go and are common to other diseases. Diagnosis is usually based on elimination method.

Screening Techniques

An important aim of screening is to distinguish between the more than one hundred different types of arthritis. Symptoms sometimes overlap; for instance, joint pain and inflammation are common features of most types of arthritis. Therefore, only careful screening can diagnose the disease correctly. Then further action, such as administering medication and physical therapy, is possible. Immediately on noticing symptoms of psoriasis, a person must visit a doctor.

The following sections discuss screening and testing for psoriatic arthritis. [12]

Medical History

First, the doctor takes a medical history, either by asking questions directly or having patients fill out a detailed questionnaire. Typically, the questions asked include the following:

- When were the symptoms first noticed?
- Has any member of the family had similar symptoms?
- Does any immediate family member (father, mother, sibling, or child) have psoriasis?
- In which joint(s) is the pain felt?
- Are the joints stiff in the morning?

Knowing the patient's medical history can help the doctor reach an accurate diagnosis in a short time. Evidence suggests that an early diagnosis and appropriate treatment thereafter can prevent potential disability. Therefore, a patient must fully cooperate with the doctor and relate his or her medical history correctly and with as much detail as possible.

Physical Examination

A physical examination done by the doctor is crucial to psoriatic arthritis diagnosis. In the majority of cases, symptoms of psoriasis, when coupled with arthritis symptoms and related complaints by the patient, can confirm psoriatic arthritis. The physician looks for red patches of inflamed skin with a scaly surface. If they are not visible on the exposed portion of the skin, the physician may look for them in hidden places, such as the scalp, umbilicus, genitalia, and perianal areas, where psoriasis can go unnoticed. If psoriasis is found on the skin of the patient, the fingers and nails are examined next. Psoriatic arthritis usually affects the nails of the patients at an early stage of the disease. The physician may also examine the joints to look for any tenderness, swelling, stiffness, and inflammation.

X-ray

X-rays of the affected joints reveal the extent of joint damage. They sometimes help distinguish between different types of arthritis. Psoriatic arthritis has an erosive effect on the bones, giving rise to a classic "pencil-in-cup" deformity: Changes in the joint space and signs of deformity may not be visible on an X-ray in the early stages of psoriatic arthritis.

Blood Tests

Blood tests are mostly done to rule out other conditions. A test for rheumatoid factor (RF) is done to differentiate between rheumatoid and psoriatic types of arthritis, as RF is present in the former and absent in the later. If RF is found in the blood, psoriatic arthritis is ruled out, and further testing is done to confirm rheumatoid arthritis. An erythrocyte sedimentation rate test is used to determine the degree of inflammation. Blood tests may also reveal the presence of the genetic marker HLA-B27 in almost 50 percent of the people with psoriatic arthritis. This almost always confirms psoriatic arthritis.

Fluid Extraction

A small amount of fluid is extracted from the affected joint and analyzed to help distinguish between gout and psoriatic arthritis. If the patient has gout, there will be a high amount of uric acid in the extracted fluid.

Bone-Density Scans

Bone density scans are done to check for bone loss, a characteristic of psoriatic arthritis.

APPROACHES VERSUS MISDIAGNOSES

Direct Treatment

Topical corticosteroids are the most common medication used to treat psoriasis found in a psoriatic arthritis sufferer. These medications suppress the immune system, which slows down skin cell turnover. This results in reduced inflammation and itching. Vitamin D analogues are also used to slow skin cell production. Salicylic acid is used to reduce scaling. Disease-modifying antirheumatic drugs (DMARDs) are also used to treat psoriasis, as they block or suppress some activities in the immune system, curbing abnormal outgrowths in the skin. These include methotrexate, sulfasalazine, cyclosporine, and leflunomide. Physical therapy and simple exercises are advised to relieve the pain. Warm showers in the morning can ease stiffness. Most importantly, psychological treatment must accompany treatment of the physical symptoms because stress is known to exacerbate both the skin and the joint disease.

Misdiagnosis of Psoriatic Arthritis

Sometimes patients with psoriatic arthritis are misdiagnosed due to a misinterpretation of the symptoms. Psoriatic arthritis can be confused with either rheumatoid arthritis due to its inflammatory nature or with gout due to the similar physical appearance of the joints. Psoriatic arthritis is less frequently misdiagnosed as osteoarthritis. A misdiagnosis or late diagnosis can hinder successful treatment and increase the risk of disability many fold. In order to help the physician reach the correct diagnosis, the patient must also prepare for the screening day. He or she should know the diseases that run in the family and bring old medical records and any recent X-ray or blood test reports. This will inevitably save time. Once a patient has been diagnosed with psoriatic arthritis, treatment is begun to ease the psoriatic and arthritic symptoms related to both the joints and the skin.

RESEARCH

Researchers are focusing on finding causes as well as treatments for psoriasis and psoriatic arthritis. In recent years, more attention has been given to research on psoriasis than ever before. Obesity[13] has recently been added to the list of the risk factors for psoriatic arthritis. A study suggests that people with psoriasis who are obese in their early adulthood are at greater risk for developing psoriatic arthritis. The study found that body mass index at age eighteen could actually predict psoriatic arthritis among psoriasis patients. While researching the causes of psoriasis, researchers found that one specific gene variation,[14] the HLA-CW0602 antigen found on chromosome six, is a major genetic cause of psoriasis. Many DNA sites other than chromosome six are being observed scientifically to discover the determinants of psoriasis. Much progress has been made in order to discover different treatments for psoriasis.

The immune system sometimes increases the production of a skin protein called tripartite motif-containing protein 32 (trim32).[15] This skin protein consequently produces a substance referred to as CCL20,[16] which triggers the production of psoriasis-inducing immune cells in the skin. This discovery will help develop better treatments that focus on skin cells rather than suppressing the immune system as a whole. Researchers are also busy studying the relationship between psoriasis and psoriatic arthritis as well as between psoriasis and other dangerous conditions, such as heart disease, diabetes, and hypertension. A network of laboratories and clinics is conducting these comparative studies. Recently, a subset of immune cells called gamma-delta-T cells[17] has been found to trigger the thickening and scaling of skin in psoriasis. This can be a step toward finding safer medicines for treating psoriasis.

Chapter Twelve

Septic Arthritis and Reactive Arthritis

Septic (infectious) arthritis and reactive arthritis are two arthritic disorders that result from an infection. Though related in their etiology and their characteristic of causing arthritic joints, the way the infection triggers each condition differs. The main difference between the two conditions may be further clarified with an examination of the terminology used for each.

ORIGIN OF TERMINOLOGY

The term *septic* derives from *sepsis*, which pertains to systemic compromise due to the spread of infection;[1] thus, the term *septic arthritis* is at times used interchangeably with *infectious arthritis*. Reactive arthritis was previously known as Reiter's syndrome, named for the late German physician Hans Conrad Julius Reiter, who was instrumental in the identification and description of the condition.[2] The term *Reiter's syndrome* has lost popularity due to exposure of Reiter's Nazi Party affiliation and his prosecution at Nuremberg as a war criminal for alleged participation in the forced human experimentations at the Buchenwald concentration camp. A group of doctors campaigned for the renaming of Reiter's syndrome as reactive arthritis back in 1977.[3] The condition may also be known as arthritis urethritica, polyarteritis enterica, or venereal arthritis. The term *arthritis urethritica* reflects its tendency to occur after a genitourinary infection; the term polyarteritis enterica stems from its tendency to affect multiple joints and to occur after a gastrointestinal infection; the term venereal arthritis was coined due to its tendency to occur after a known venereal infection. The main difference between reactive and septic arthritis is that septic arthritis is caused by an infection of the joint. Reactive arthritis is instead an autoimmune response in reaction to an infection in another part of the body. Each disorder is discussed in further depth in this chapter.

OVERVIEWS, MICROBIOLOGY, AND PREVALENCE

Septic Arthritis

Septic arthritis is an infection resulting in an arthritis characterized by purulent invasion and intense pain at the infected joint.[4] This condition may also be known as suppurative arthritis, due to its characteristic of producing purulent substances, or pus, as well as bacterial arthritis, even though the condition may at times be of fungal or viral origin instead of the more common bacterial origin. The causative infectious agent in septic arthritis can spread to the joint from other previously infected areas of the body. The infection may affect only a single joint without affecting other parts of the body, but it may still spread to other body parts. Septic arthritis commonly affects the knee or wrist and may also affect other joints, such as the ankle, hip, elbow, and shoulder. The infection infiltrates and damages the joint, causing severe pain, suppuration, heat, and swelling. This severe form of arthritis also develops along with sudden onset of fever, chills, and joint pain.[5] If the sufferer of some forms of septic arthritis does not seek rapid medical attention for diagnosis and treatment, the joint may incur irreversible and permanent damage in a period of days. Therefore, the situation should be regarded as a medical emergency.

Gonococcal arthritis is the most prevalent form of septic arthritis in the United States.[6] This class of septic arthritis is less prevalent in other areas of the world, such as Western Europe, where it is presently uncommon. The causative organism behind this form of the condition is the Gram-negative diplococcus bacterium Neisseria gonorrhoeae, which is most likely spread to the joint systemically due to disseminated gonococcal infection. This specific condition can manifest either as arthritis-dermatitis syndrome, which is a bacteremic infection accounting for 60 percent of gonococcal arthritis cases, or as an arthritic infection localized in a single joint, which accounts for the remaining 40 percent of cases.[7]

Reactive Arthritis

Reactive arthritis is an autoimmune condition caused by the body's immune response to an infection. The causative infection is not located in the affected joint itself (cross-reactivity).[8] The triggering infection is usually or often already in remission by the time the patient presents with arthritic symptoms, making it difficult to ascertain the initial cause. Cultures taken from the synovial fluid of the joints affected by reactive arthritis will characteristically yield negative results, indicating the cause is not a direct infection of the joint but instead may be due to overstimulation of the autoimmune response or to the depositing of bacterial antigens in the joints in an unknown manner. Though the mechanism of reaction from the infection is still unknown, it is said that reactive arthritis often manifests within one to three weeks after a known infection.

Microbiology of Arthritis

The etiology of septic arthritis is commonly bacterial in nature; mycobacterial, viral, and fungal arthritis occur in rare cases.[9] The pathogen responsible for septic arthritis must reach the synovial membrane of the joint. The microorganisms are usually carried to the joint by the bloodstream from an infectious source such as an infected wound or abscess located elsewhere in the body; they can also be introduced by skin lesions or trauma penetrating into the joint, or they can extend from an infection in adjacent body tissue, such as infected soft tissue or bones suffering from an osteomyelitic condition. As bacteria are the most common cause of septic arthritis, various strains may be the culprit behind the condition. *Staphylococcus aureus* is the common causative pathogen in adults, while *Streptococcus* is the second-most likely causative pathogen in this group.[10] *Neisseria* gonorrhoeae is the most prevalent causative microorganism in young adults, although it is now thought to be rare in Western Europe.[11] Moreover, Haemophilus influenzae, once the most prevalent causative pathogen in children, is now declining in areas where *Haemophilus* vaccinations have been introduced.[12] *Escherichia coli* (*E. coli*) is the most likely causative microorganism among the elderly, the seriously ill, and users of intravenous drugs. *Salmonella*, *Brucella*, and tuberculosis are the causative pathogens behind septic spinal arthritis.[13] Pseudomonas aeruginosa, the bacterium responsible for endocarditis, has also been identified as a causative pathogen for septic arthritis in children who have suffered a wound penetrating directly into the joints.[14]

Reactive arthritis may also be caused by bacterial infection. It is triggered by a recent prior infection; the most common culprit in the United States is the genital infection *Chlamydia trachomatis*. The bacterium known as *Ureaplasma urealytium*, a pathogen of the urinary tract, is also known to trigger the condition. The condition may also be triggered by bouts of gastrointestinal infection or food poisoning from *Salmonella, Shigella, Yersinia,* and *Campylobacter*, which are all enteric bacteria genera.[15] The infection is not located in the ailing joint and may no longer present elsewhere on the body by the time the reactive arthritis develops. Other microorganisms may still be behind a case of reactive arthritis, but evidence indicating that they are the actual cause is still circumstantial.[16]

Prevalence of Septic Arthritis and Reactive Arthritis

Young children, older adults, and individuals with artificial joints are at greater risk than the general population for developing septic arthritis. Those with artificial joints may be infected with different organisms in comparison with the general population and may present with slightly different symptoms.[17] In general, if an individual affected by septic arthritis seeks medical attention and treatment within a week after symptoms first appear, a full recovery is likely. On the other hand, individuals aged twenty to forty years, and men more so than women, are more likely to be affected by reactive arthritis. Caucasians are more likely to be affected than individuals of African American descent due to the frequent occurrence of the HLA-B27 gene within the white population.[18] Patients infected with the human immunodeficiency virus (HIV) also have an increased risk of developing this condition.[19] Arthritis makes it extremely difficult for affected individuals to remain physically active, and they become bound to their homes. These individuals are at increased risk for obesity, depression, and heart disease due to inactivity and anxiety from worsening disability.

IMMUNE SYSTEM'S ROLE IN ARTHRITIS

Septic arthritis and reactive arthritis are both conditions that involve an immune system response. However, septic arthritis is the result of the body's normal immune response to an actual infection present in the ailing joint. Reactive arthritis, on the other hand, is the result of the immune system's abnormal response to what it believes is an infection present in the joint but which is actually an infection in a part of the body outside the joint; this mistaken response, which may be due to misinterpretation or oversensitivity, is considered abnormal, and therefore reactive arthritis is classified as an autoimmune disease. An overview of the human body's immune system can better explain the mechanisms behind these two conditions.

Overview of the Human Immune System

The human immune system is an intricate defense system designed specifically to defend against the many different types of pathogens. A pathogen is any organism, usually living, that can cause disease. Pathogens include bacteria, which are single-celled organisms capable of living outside the body; protozoa, which are single-celled organisms that live in and are spread through water; pathogenic proteins, which are multicelled organisms that can only reproduce inside another, more complex living organism; fungi, which are plantlike multicelled organisms that take nutrition from other living organisms such as plants and animals; viruses, which are multicelled organisms that invade and reproduce inside another microbial organism; and parasites, which are full, complex organisms that feed off the nutrients of another complex organism and tend to live in the intestinal tract or bloodstream of the host. In theory any these organisms can cause septic or reactive arthritis, but parasites are very unlikely to cause these conditions, and bacteria are the most prevalent culprits. In the event that a pathogen passes through the body's outer physical barriers, such as mucus and the skin, and penetrates the internal structures of the human body, the immune system kicks in. [20]

What Goes Wrong with the Immune Response

Septic arthritis is really the result of damage caused by the invading organisms and the normal immune response of the body to the infection in that specific joint or set of joints. In septic arthritis, the macrophages ingest a pathogen that has infected a joint. They then degrade the pathogen into antigens and relay them to the helper T cells in the lymph nodes. The T cells then create antibodies specific to the antigens. The inflammatory response also releases histamine, which increases the blood flow to the affected joint to cause swelling, redness, and pain, which in turn causes stiffness and difficulty moving the joint, leading to arthritic symptoms. Meanwhile, the invading organisms cause damage to the joints. Such damage incurred by the joints may be irreparable if medical attention is not sought immediately. Suppuration, which is the result of the white blood cells' fight against the invading microorganisms, may also contribute to the arthritic condition. The fever response, which triggers the release of pyrogen, may also contribute to the degeneration of the joint. Although the exact etiology of the condition is still uncertain, reactive arthritis, unlike septic arthritis, is caused by a faulty immune system response. The condition occurs in the absence and aftermath of an actual infection located in a part of the body outside the affected joints.

Two theories of the mechanism behind reactive arthritis exist for the purpose of explanation. The first theory speculates that antigens are deposited in the affected joint; the second theory speculates that the immune system has become faulty in detecting the actual presence or absence of pathogens and creates an exaggerated immune response in the joints even though there is no infection or the infection is located elsewhere in the body. According to both theories, the immune system believes there is a current infection in the joint and releases histamine and pyrogen to produce inflammation and fever. The inflammation causes joint stiffness, pain, and immobility—all arthritic symptoms. The absence of an actual pathogen may mean that the inflammation and fever will last for an uncertain period, but it also means there will be little to no damage to the affected joint.

DISTINGUISHING CHARACTERISTICS

The main characteristic differentiating septic and reactive arthritis from other types is that the former mainly results from infection. This means that they will most likely present with fever. The main difference between reactive and septic arthritis is that, in the latter, infection of the joint itself is the cause of the suppuration leading to the arthritis. Reactive arthritis is not caused by an infection of the joint itself; rather, the inflammation is caused by an autoimmune response due to an infection located in another part of the body; this is known as cross-reactivity.[21] Septic arthritis will most likely affect an individual joint (monoarthritic) if only one joint is infected. Due to the possible systemic nature of reactive arthritis, it will most likely affect several joints (polyarthritis). Septic arthritis will also most likely yield positive culture results and present with suppuration, unlike reactive arthritis, which may not yield the same results due to the absence of an infection at the actual site of arthritic symptoms.

TECHNIQUES AND RESEARCH

Diagnostic Techniques

The diagnosis of both septic and reactive arthritis is made through a clinical examination conducted by a duly licensed and qualified health professional, who may require other examinations such as blood tests and radiology to create a differential diagnosis. However, radiographs (X-ray) and sonographs (ultrasound) are mostly used only to assess and monitor the severity and progression of the condition. Magnetic resonance imaging is also an effective diagnostic tool. The history of the current disorder may guide diagnosis, with the following significant markers:

- Speed and time of onset
- Pattern and symmetry of joint involvement
- Aggravating versus relieving factors
- Quality and severity of pain

Rheumatoid arthritis is generally worse in pain and stiffness during mornings; by comparison, osteoarthritis is usually aggravated after strenuous activity, such as exercise. There is no diagnostic test to rule out septic arthritis completely; however, it should be considered whenever a patient presents with rapid onset of joint pain. Usually it only affects one joint (monoarthritis), but a few joints can be affected simultaneously in cases involving *Staphylococcus* or *Gonococcus* infections. The affected joints may present with pain, swelling, redness, and warmth, often affecting joints in the limbs instead of deep joints such as the hips and shoulders. A fever of above 38.5 degrees Celsius and history of septic arthritis may also be indicative of the ailment.

The Gram stain can indicate, but cannot rule out, septic arthritis.[22] Gram stain and culture of fluid from the joint and blood test serums can also indicate a positive diagnosis when yielding elevated neutrophils, erythrocyte sedimentation rate (ESR), C-reactive protein (CRP), and white blood cell count. Being a sort of systemic autoimmune disorder, reactive arthritis can be expected to cause polyarthritis, which is a multiple-joint arthritic condition. The affected joints may also present with pain, swelling, redness, and warmth. Swab samples taken from the urethra, cervix, urine, or throat can be cultured in an attempt to identify the causative organisms. Blood tests and synovial fluid cultures may also be done to reveal elevated ESR and CRP to support the diagnosis. A blood screening may be done to identify the presence of the gene HLA-B27, which is present in an estimated 80 percent of all patients suffering from reactive arthritis.[23]

Treatment Techniques

The main goal of treatment for both septic and reactive arthritis is to identify and eradicate the causative pathogen with the appropriate antibiotics. In the meantime, the treatment is symptomatic. Medications such as antibiotics, nonsteroidal anti-inflammatory drugs, steroids, and analgesics can help decrease inflammation in the joint, resulting in decreased pain and joint damage.[24] Reactive arthritis may require immunosuppressants in addition to the above medications to reduce oversensitivity of the immune system. Extreme pain, redness, and swelling may require drainage by needle puncture to alleviate these signs of inflammation. Surgical replacement of the joints may also be needed in eroding types of arthritis such as certain strains of septic arthritis. Surgical debridement, or arthrotomy, is usually indicated for infections involving prosthetic joints. Individuals for whom surgery is contraindicated will have to undergo long-term trial antibiotic therapy.[25]

Chapter Thirteen

Enteropathic Arthritis

Great-intestinal (enteric) health is essential to a productive and successful life. Hence, arthritis sufferers must take proper care of their bodies from a digestive standpoint. As the years pass, working professionals employed in offices are becoming less concerned about their digestive health due to a lack of time. In performing their everyday activities and meeting other commitments, some forget about maintaining good health, especially getting regular exercise or at the very least eating a balanced diet on a proper schedule. As a result, one reads about people dying of several illnesses of the digestive system. If their death histories are traced, we find that most did not bother to consult a doctor due to their busy schedules.

OVERVIEW

Enteropathic arthritis sufferers must bear in mind that a simple failure to take proper care of their health will result in several diseases that have been causing death around the world. General arthritis comes in different types, and enteropathic arthritis is one of them. Enteropathic arthritis is characterized by an inflammatory condition affecting the spine and other joints.[1] This type of arthritis is common among people suffering from ulcerative colitis and Crohn's disease. The term *enteropathic arthritis* is new to medicine, and the reader should be familiar with it. Hence, the upcoming sections provide an idea of what enteropathic arthritis is, its nature and symptoms, possible tests required, and other information. This chapter also aims to increase public awareness of this kind of arthritis in an effort to decrease its prevalence.

Origin of Terminology

A thorough understanding of the topic requires basic understanding of the term *enteropathic* and, more particularly, its origin. *Enteropathic* comes from the Greek words *enteron* meaning "intestine," and *pathos*, meaning "suffering." Thus, enteropathic arthritis is a form of arthritis related to the intestines.

Digestive System's Role in Arthritis

Most people know that their bodies are composed of several systems that work hand in hand. If one of these systems fails, the body will not operate normally, and this will result in problems, including diseases. The digestive system is one of the systems responsible for maintaining the body. This system also plays an important role in avoiding arthritis. Knowledge of how one's digestive system works is necessary to fully understand the digestive system's relation to arthritis.

Arthritis patients need enzymes in order for food to be properly processed into nutrients for absorption during digestion. If the human body fails to produce enough enzymes, this will result in poor digestion. Improperly digested food will lead to the development of endotoxins. Endotoxins are chemicals toxic to the human system that are generated by an improper pH and inadequate numbers of digestive enzymes and microorganisms. Their presence destroys the lining of the digestive tract, causing several abnormalities in the body, including arthritis. Thus, the level of risk for arthritis depends on the functioning of the digestive system. It is thus necessary to maintain proper good health in order to avoid arthritis. Eating healthy food can be one way of doing this.

DISTINGUISHING CHARACTERISTICS OF ENTEROPATHIC ARTHRITIS

Preliminary Differences

Arthritis is considered a complex disease. General arthritis comes in different forms and types, and each more or less shares common features, making it difficult to ascertain which particular type has afflicted a patient. Despite the common features among different types of arthritis, it is important to consider the differences between enteropathic arthritis and the other forms of arthritis to have a better understanding of both.

One major difference lies in the symptoms. Enteropathic arthritis is somewhat related to the intestines; hence, gastrointestinal symptoms usually occur. Once a person is suffering from this kind of arthritis, he or she will experience stomach pain, diarrhea, constipation, and vomiting. This makes enteropathic arthritis different from other types of arthritis.[2] Research shows that joint manifestations occur in conjunction with gastrointestinal disease in enteropathic arthritis.[3]

Another difference is that both the bowel disease and the arthritis have to be treated in this type of arthritis. If one can only treat the bowel disease, this type of arthritis cannot be medicated wholly. If only the arthritis is treated, the bowel disease will trigger recurrences of arthritis. Nonsteroidal anti-inflammatory drugs, often used to treat arthritis, cannot be used since they worsen bowel diseases. That said, treating both the bowel disease and the arthritis is highly recommended because addressing the joint problems alone can trigger the bowel disease and will not lead to a complete cure. Various medical experts suggest that this type of arthritis can be cured using anti–tumor necrosis factor drugs such as Humira, Remicade, and Cimzia.[4]

Individuals suffering from Crohn's disease or ulcerative colitis are likely to have this kind of arthritis. These two diseases are autoinflammatory conditions in the bowel that can be toxic.[5] Studies reveal that enteropathic arthritis is more prevalent among individuals with Crohn's disease. Currently, there is no known cure for enteropathic arthritis.[6] In the United States, this is now the priority among medical experts and other medical professionals who are looking for an effective drug to cure this type of arthritis. Medications and therapies are available to manage the symptoms of both the arthritic and bowel components of the disease, which can alleviate the sufferings of those afflicted with it.

Duration of the Disease

Enteropathic arthritis has also no estimated duration. According to medical experts, treatment of this type of arthritis depends on prompt medication. Healthy lifestyle is also important and includes eating a considerable amount of fruits and vegetables. Drinking enough water can also aid in curing the disease since proper water intake can encourage proper digestion. On the contrary, if improper medication is administered, the illness might become serious, meaning that it will take longer for the disease to be fully treated.

In terms of infections, there is no substantial difference between enteropathic arthritis and the other types. Infections depend on how disciplined a person is in taking prescribed medications. Laxity in following the doctor's advice will prolong recovery time.

TECHNIQUES AND RESEARCH

Introduction to Screenings

Medical experts around the world have seen the complex intricacies involved in diagnosing enteropathic arthritis. As a matter of fact, this type is crucial in the sense that both the bowel diseases and the arthritis have to be treated, or the sufferer's problems will surely worsen. Yet doctors might have a difficult time identifying enteropathic arthritis considering the aforementioned complexities. Toward this end, several diagnoses are required in order for an expert to conclude that a sufferer is really suffering from this disease. Doctors usually employ a number of screening techniques in determining whether a particular sufferer has enteropathic arthritis so that medication can be prescribed immediately. Before proceeding to the various tests, doctors usually conduct a short interview with the sufferer regarding the different signs and symptoms experienced prior to the consultation. This step is necessary in order for the doctor to have an initial idea of what is really happening to the sufferer.

Screening for Anemia

The first screening technique that doctors employ usually involves investigation for signs of anemia, or a below-normal level of hemoglobin.[7] Hemoglobin is the protein found in red blood cells, which are responsible for carrying oxygen to all parts of the body. Anemia is common among people diagnosed with enteropathic arthritis. To further determine if a sufferer is anemic, doctors study the blood counts and any remarkable changes in hemoglobin. In this process, the sufferer's cooperation is required so that the best remedy can be applied immediately.

Blood Tests

Doctors also conduct blood tests to check the enteropathic arthritis patient's iron levels. The term *blood test* refers to a process of examining the blood of a particular person with the purpose of determining whether it contains impurities. Blood tests are essential in assessing the physiological and biochemical conditions of the human body. In relation to enteropathic arthritis, blood tests are conducted to further assess the condition of the sufferer—that is, whether he or she has an iron deficiency, which is somehow related to anemia. A person with low iron is more likely to be anemic.

Erythrocyte Sedimentation Rate Test

Erythrocyte sedimentation rate (ESR) is a blood test that has been used for many years in detecting conditions associated with acute and chronic inflammation. This procedure is considered easy and inexpensive. ESR is generally used, however, in conjunction with other tests because its results are nonspecific, meaning that doctors cannot pinpoint the exact location of the inflammation based merely on this test. Still, this test is essential in diagnosing enteropathic arthritis because its result can be used to support the doctor's diagnosis.

C-Reactive Protein Test

C-reactive protein (CRP) is also a nonspecific test. Medical professionals use it to spot inflammation, especially if there is notable suspicion of tissue injury or infection with enteropathic arthritis. Again, this test cannot pinpoint the exact location of the inflammation or determine its possible causes. CRP, however, is not an effective diagnostic procedure to determine the complete health of a person. Nevertheless, its results, together with signs and symptoms and other tests, can be used in determining whether an individual has an inflammatory disorder that might be acute or chronic. [8]

Although the CRP test is considered nonspecific, it is essential in determining whether an individual has a severe bacterial infection as determined by the signs and symptoms discussed by the doctor and patient at an earlier stage. The CRP test is also essential during the treatment phase for enteropathic arthritis because, by conducting a series of these tests, the doctor can conclude whether the applied treatment is effective. The degree of effectiveness depends on the level of CRP: a lower CRP level indicates that the medication is working because CRP levels drop as inflammation subsides.

Examination of Spinal and Sacroiliac Joints

The sacroiliac joint is found between the ilium and the sacrum of the pelvis. In humans, the sacrum supports the spine and is in turn supported by an ilium on each of its sides. The joint is a synovial joint that provides an interlocking effect of the two bones. [9] The human system comprises two sacroiliac joints, one on the left and the other on the right. These joints, which vary from one person to another, often match each other. [10]

To further determine the enteropathic arthritis patient's condition, the doctor usually examines the spinal and sacroiliac joints. The relevance of examining them is important, considering that arthritis is by nature a joint abnormality. On discovering indicators of abnormalities, the doctor will recommend tests to further diagnosis.

Colonoscopy

A colonoscopy provides an interior look at the colon and rectum of the enteropathic arthritis sufferer. The doctor uses a flexible tube called a colonoscope that has the ability to snip off polyps.[11] As the name suggests, the colon is the main focus in this kind of screening technique. During a colonoscopy, patients are usually given a light sedative and pain medication to help them stay relaxed. The amount of sedative and pain medication depends on the particular situation and needs of the patient. This screening test is necessary to diagnose enteropathic arthritis because it focuses on the colon, which is usually where gastrointestinal problems occur.

Synovial Fluid Aspiration

Synovial fluid is a clear fluid secreted by membranes in joint cavities, tendon sheaths, and bursae. This fluid is essential because it functions as a lubricant in the human joints. Once a joint disorder occurs, synovial fluid is removed and examined as it may contain indicators of disease, such as white blood cells or crystals. Synovial fluid analysis is essential in diagnosing enteropathic arthritis. Procedurally, a sterile needle is inserted through the skin into the joint space. After extracting the synovial fluid, the doctor will examine it using recommended medical procedures and techniques in order to further assess the enteropathic arthritis patient's condition. Whether the individual suffers from this form of arthritis depends on the color of the synovial fluid.

ADVANCES IN ENTEROPATHIC ARTHRITIS RESEARCH

Medical research is so vast that medical experts always keep an eye on new discoveries in arthritis. These are important developments in the medical field. Yet findings are always changing, and the results of one study might be overturned by another in a matter of days. This reality does not hinder medical experts in searching for the best breakthroughs in the field of medicine and, more specifically, related to enteropathic arthritis. The Arthritis Foundation released a noteworthy report,[12] and based on its assessment, the current severity and risk of arthritis and the future of biologic medications in treating major forms of arthritis stand among the top ten significant arthritis advances of 2008. This alone indicates that advocates in the medical and scientific field have become alarmed by the rising number of arthritis sufferers. Enteropathic arthritis, being new, is also one of the Arthritis Foundation's concerns. Toward a similar end, an article maintains that spondyloarthropathies and enteropathic arthritis share distinct clinical and radiographic features, as well as a common genetic predisposition.[13] This is important to further devise a better alternative in curing enteropathic arthritis in the years to come.

In October 2010, updates on the genetics of spondyloarthritis, ankylosing spondylitis, and psoriatic arthritis were also published.[14] Updates include a description of spondyloarthritis as a group of inflammatory rheumatic diseases that share common genetic characteristics. The article also states that the genes of a particular patient suffering from ankylosing spondylitis are being identified, and these are being compared with recent candidate genes from others identified as suffering from enteropathic arthritis. Experts support the idea that individuals having either axial or peripheral arthritis will most likely experience enteropathic arthritis.[15] Enteropathic arthritis occurs before or after the onset of intestinal symptoms. Peripheral arthritis is also considered episodic and asymmetric and most frequently affects the knee and ankle. These are some of the advances in the field of enteropathic research that experts have released. At present, there are still no advances focused on an absolute cure for enteropathic arthritis. Nevertheless, the advances mentioned may be useful in coming up with a mechanism that can totally cure enteropathic arthritis in the coming years.

Chapter Fourteen

Related Manifestations

Arthritis is connected to many clinical syndromes, of which this chapter explores three. A *syndrome* is an association of several clinical and recognizable features that are either signs or symptoms. Medical signs are features observable by someone other than the arthritis sufferer, whereas symptoms are features reported by the patient.

DISEASES AND SYNDROMES

The Difference

The main difference between a disease and a syndrome is basically the symptoms that each produces. A disease may be referred to as a medical condition with clear and defined signs and symptoms, while a syndrome has a number of symptoms with no known cause and, in most cases, suggests the possibility of an underlying disease or developing disease. A disease has three basic factors: (1) a defined number (group) of symptoms, (2) a known biological cause, and (3) a consistent change in anatomy. Whereas the mechanisms behind the occurrence of syndromes are a mystery, the causes of diseases are easily identifiable. The general treatment of syndromes is symptomatic, whereas with a disease, the underlying causes (which are known) are treated. At times a syndrome may indicate the presence of several diseases, or several different diseases could cause the same syndrome. These terms are used somewhat loosely. For example, even though AIDS has a known cause, the human immunodeficiency virus (HIV), it can be called a syndrome. Others would say that HIV is a disease since it causes a set of symptoms and because one can have an HIV infection without having AIDS. The terms *disease* and *syndrome* therefore overlap substantially, and their meaning often depends on context.

SJOGREN'S SYNDROME

Also known as Mikulicz disease or Sicca syndrome,[1] this is a disorder in which the immune cells attack and destroy glands that otherwise produce tears and saliva, causing dryness in the mouth, nose, throat, skin, and eye. An autoimmune disorder, Sjogren's syndrome affects the immune system, and instead of the system fighting off foreign substances, it attacks the body's own parts.[2] The syndrome may also affect the lungs, kidneys, blood vessels, digestive organs, and nerves.[3] Primary Sjogren's syndrome occurs without the presence of any other autoimmune disease, while secondary Sjogren's occurs with rheumatic diseases such as arthritis, lupus, and some forms of scleroderma.

Prevalence

There are various statistics as to the prevalence of this disease (syndrome). According to the National Institutes of Health (NIH), about 1 to 4 million people live with Sjogren's in the United States.[4] Of these cases, 90 percent occur in women. The disorder is listed as rare by the NIH's Office of Rare Diseases. According to research done in Japan, Sjogren's syndrome is less common in men than in women.[5] This research investigated the salivary gland manifestations in men with Sjogren's syndrome and compared the results with those for females. Though the syndrome can be contracted at any age, symptoms are more prevalent after the age of forty-five.[6]

Arthritis and Sjogren's Syndrome

While joint degeneration is a major symptom of Sjogren's, the syndrome's relationship to arthritis is still not clear. Patients who have no other rheumatologic diagnosis but do have symptoms of Sjogren's have primary Sjogren's syndrome. A large number of Sjogren's patients have also been found to have rheumatoid arthritis, which is considered a major risk factor for Sjogren's. Since there is no known cure for Sjogren's, the symptoms can only be managed. Some of the drugs prescribed for rheumatoid arthritis have shown great results in the treatment of Sjogren's syndrome.

Symptoms of Sjogren's Syndrome

Symptoms include the following:

- Dry eyes
- Sore tongue
- Difficulty chewing, swallowing, and even talking
- Dry and burning throat
- Tooth decay
- Oral yeast infection

Diagnosis of Sjogren's Syndrome

A full doctor's examination is necessary to confirm the diagnosis, but the following tests will still be used:

- Special ophthalmologic or dental tests
- Tests for elevated immunoglobulins and high levels of other blood proteins
- Rheumatoid factor
- Sjogren's syndrome A (SSA) anti-Ro and Sjogren's syndrome B (SSB) anti-La (antibodies found in Sjogren's patients, though not all Sjogren's patients test positive for them)
- Antinuclear antibody test

A minor salivary gland biopsy for diagnostic purposes may be carried out, which might include parotid gland biopsy if malignancy is suspected and biopsy of an enlarged lymph node to rule out pseudolymphoma or lymphoma.

Treatment of Sjogren's Syndrome

The treatments for Sjogren's vary from patient to patient, depending on the part of the body affected. The doctor will help patients relieve symptoms, especially dryness. If one has excessive dryness—such as overall dehydration and dryness of the skin—inflammation can take place throughout the body. This may also include nerve, skin, lung, and kidney problems, as well as disorders of the connective tissue and the digestive system. A person with extraglandular problems may be prescribed medications, which may include nonsteroidal anti-inflammatory drugs (NSAIDs) for joint or muscle pains, saliva- and mucus-stimulating drugs for nose and throat dryness, and corticosteroids or disease-modifying antirheumatic drugs (a type of immunosuppressant) for lung, blood vessel, kidney, or nervous system problems.

If hoarseness develops due to throat inflammation as a result of dryness or coughing, one ought to avoid further strain on the vocal cords. Sjogren's patients should not clear their throats before speaking but instead sip water, chew gum, or suck on candy. They may also be asked to laugh or hum to gently pull the vocal cords together. For vaginal dryness with painful intercourse, vaginal moisturizers help restore moisture. Some forms of water-soluble lubricants can make intercourse more comfortable. Depending on the patient's symptoms, the doctor may also suggest medications to increase the production of saliva for dry mouth. These drugs include pilocarpine (also called salagen and used for glaucoma) and cevimeline (Evoxac), which helps in saliva and tear production. These drugs do have side effects, however, including, among others, sweating, abdominal pain, flushing, and increased urination. Specific complications are also addressed since mostly symptoms are treated. Patients who develop arthritis symptoms are given NSAIDs or other arthritis medications. Those with yeast infections of the mouth are treated with antifungal medications. Other treatments include the use of immunosuppressant drugs that treat malaria, such as methotrexate and cyclosporine.

FELTY'S SYNDROME

Felty's syndrome was first described in 1924 by Dr. Augustus Felty. The symptoms of this potentially serious condition are similar to those of rheumatoid arthritis. Felty's syndrome is described by the presence of certain conditions, including an enlarged spleen (splenomegaly), rheumatoid arthritis, and a low white blood cell count. Associated symptoms are pain, swelling, and stiffness of the joints, most commonly in the joints of the hands, feet, and arms. Felty's syndrome is sometimes characterized by the triad of (1) rheumatoid arthritis, (2) splenomegaly, and (3) granulocytopenia, when the number of granular white blood cells is decreased. Although many patients with Felty's syndrome are asymptomatic, some develop serious and life-threatening infections secondary to granulocytopenia.

The causes of Felty's syndrome are still unknown. Some patients with rheumatoid arthritis are found to develop the syndrome, but most do not. Since the white blood cells are fashioned within the bone marrow, patients with Felty's have been found to have active bone marrow function and to be producing white blood cells despite the low level of circulating white blood cells. Therefore, white blood cells are getting stored disproportionately in the spleen of Felty's patients. People suffering from Felty's syndrome often report symptoms of mild inflammatory joint disease caused by synovitis. Usually, the patient's history reveals a long preceding period of active and aggressive joint disease, which can be confirmed by physical examination and plain radiography. Some patients present with so-called burned-out (quiescent) joint disease. A lack of active joint disease should not dissuade clinicians from considering a Felty's diagnosis. Other patients with Felty's syndrome commonly present with bacterial infections of the skin and respiratory tract. An aggressive level of immunosuppression directed at the underlying rheumatoid arthritis may contribute to susceptibility to infection.

Felty's Syndrome and Arthritis

Felty's syndrome is regarded as a rare complication of rheumatoid arthritis since it is characterized by neutropenia (low neutrophil amounts) and splenomegaly. Despite its rarity, it is a serious disease in its own right and a model for investigating the genetic determinants of rheumatoid arthritis susceptibility. As it is a polygenic disease, the development of rheumatoid arthritis hinges on various environmental factors.

Symptoms of Felty's Syndrome

The following symptoms are common to Felty's syndrome:

- Eye problems, including dryness and irritation due to concurrent Sjogren's syndrome and red, painful eyes due to episcleritis (inflammation or irritation of the eye sclera)
- Infections due to neutropenia (lung and skin infections are most common)
- Weight loss
- Fatigue
- Anorexia
- Left-upper-quadrant pain

Symptoms related to rheumatoid arthritis, including joint swelling, pain, stiffness, and deformity, are also common in Felty's syndrome.

Diagnosis of Felty's Syndrome

Clinical diagnosis is based on the features of unexplained neutropenia and splenomegaly in a patient with rheumatoid arthritis. Relevant investigations carried out to establish the syndrome include the following:

- Radiography (ultrasound or CT scan to check splenomegaly)
- Bone marrow biopsy (sometimes required to differentiate Felty's syndrome from other diseases, such as granular lymphoma or low-grade non-Hodgkin's lymphoma)
- Full blood count (for neutropenia)
- Test for autoantibodies
- Anti–cyclic citrullinated peptide antibody test
- Test for inflammatory markers (ESR and CRP)
- Liver function test (to check for raised liver enzyme levels in case of liver involvement)

Some patients with Felty's syndrome have more infections, such as pneumonia and numerous skin infections, than the average sufferer. Increased susceptibility to these infections is owing to the low white blood cell counts typical of Felty's syndrome. This syndrome can be further complicated by the emergence of ulcers in the skin of the legs. Finally, 95 percent of patients with Felty's syndrome are found to be positive for rheumatoid factor.[7]

Treatment of Felty's Syndrome

Treatment is not always necessary beyond managing the underlying rheumatoid arthritis to a certain level. Patients with severe infectious diseases may benefit from injections of stimulating factor that boost the white blood cell count. The best-known treatment for Felty's syndrome is simply to control the underlying rheumatoid arthritis. Immunosuppressive therapy for rheumatoid arthritis improves granulocytopenia and splenomegaly. This verifies that Felty's syndrome is an immune-mediated disease.[8] Most of the traditional medications used in the treatment of rheumatoid arthritis have been employed in addressing Felty's. Treatment for patients with Felty's often includes physical therapy, occupational therapy, a good exercise plan, weight loss, joint rest, medication to control inflammation, and removal of the spleen. Other treatments may include aurothioglucose and immunosuppressive agents such as methotrexate (Rheumatrex) and cyclophosphamide (Cytoxan), as well as colony-stimulating factors for anemia and low white blood cell counts that include filgrastim (Neupogen) and sargramostim (Leukine).

If an urgent correction for neutropenia is unnecessary, most practicing rheumatologists use the above drugs first when treating Felty's. They are usually combined with folic acid to minimize adverse effects. The potential for leukopenia limits the use of cyclophosphamide, although it may have a role in some cases. Physicians have more experience using cyclophosphamide for rheumatoid vasculitis and other serious rheumatoid arthritis extra-articular manifestations than for Felty's. For this reason, it is not an initial choice of therapy. Due to its adverse effects, penicillamine is being used less frequently for rheumatoid arthritis and has never been a first-choice therapy for patients.[9]

Initial treatment and management of patients with Felty's syndrome and life-threatening infections should always include administration of a growth factor. Long-term use of G-CSF appears to be well tolerated, although hypersensitivity vasculitis and flare-ups of the underlying rheumatoid arthritis in these patients have been reported. At high doses, corticosteroids can increase the granulocyte count, partly through demargination. This effect does not persist when tapering the patient to a typical low dose (less than 10 mg) used for rheumatoid arthritis articular disease. Empiric administration of high-doses of intravenous methylprednisolone is often prescribed, but the effectiveness wanes over time. Long-term usage of high-dose corticosteroids could further increase the risk of infection. Corticosteroids should probably be viewed as a second-line treatment modality but never the first.

BEHCET'S SYNDROME

Behcet's syndrome is also referred to as Behcet's disease, Behçet syndrome, morbus Behçet, and Silk Road disease. A rare immune-mediated condition, Behcet's syndrome is often characterized by a triple-symptom complex of recurrent lyaphthous ulcers, genital ulcers, and uveitis. It is a multisystem disorder of unknown etiology probably first described by Hippocrates around 400 BC.[10] It is named after Turkish dermatologist Hulusi Behçet, who in 1937 described a syndrome of recurrent aphthous ulcers, genital ulcerations, and uveitis leading to blindness. The etiology of Behcet's syndrome has yet to be found. The syndrome is more profound in individuals of Mediterranean and Asian descent than those of European origin. Both the environmental and inherited (genetic) factors, such as microbial contaminations, are thought to be the major players leading to the development of Behcet's syndrome. Behcet's syndrome is noncontagious and mainly affects people in their twenties and thirties. Diagnosing this illness can take a long time because the symptoms come and go, and in most cases it takes months or even years to acquire all the symptoms. Behcet's is not associated with cancer, and links to tissue types are not certain. It does not follow the usual pattern of other autoimmune diseases, but one study has revealed a possible connection to food allergies, particularly to dairy products. In America, an estimated fifteen to twenty thousand people[11] have been diagnosed with the disease, and in the United Kingdom, there is one case estimated for every one hundred thousand people.[12] Men are more frequently affected than women globally, but in the United States, females are more affected than males.[13]

Relationship between Behcet's and Arthritis

Arthritis is one signs of Behcet's disease, and the two combined are know as Adamantiades-Behçet's disease or Adamantiades syndrome.[14] It occurs in more than half of all patients known to have Behcet's and causes swelling, pain, and stiffness in the joints, particularly in the ankles, knees, elbows, and wrists. This kind of arthritis, resulting from Behcet's syndrome, usually lasts for a few weeks and does not cause any permanent damage to the joints.

Symptoms of Behcet's Syndrome

Behcet's syndrome involves inflammation of the blood vessels. The disorder can cause a wide range of symptoms, but rarely does someone with the disorder experience them all. The most common symptoms include the following:

- Mouth sores: These affect almost all patients with this disease. They are identical to canker sores and are the very first signs that an individual notices, though they may occur long before any other sign manifests. At times they may be painful, preventing the patient from eating. They last for between ten and fourteen days.
- Genital sores: These affect more than half of Behcet's patients. They commonly occur on a man's scrotum and a woman's vulva. The sores are very similar to mouth sores and are very painful. After a few outbreaks, they may result in scarring. [15]
- Skin sores: These are the most recognizable manifestations of Behcet's disease. The sores look similar to red or pus-filled bumps or bruises. They are raised and typically appear on the legs and upper torso.
- Uveitis: This involves inflammation of the back or middle part of the eye, which includes the iris. It is found in many people with Behcet's.

Serious complications can include blood clots, meningitis, inflammation of the digestive system and blood vessels, and blindness. Treatment focuses on the treatment of symptoms, reducing pain, and preventing serious problems.

Diagnosing Behcet's Syndrome

The diagnosis of this disease is currently a difficult affair as no specific tests can confirm its presence. The physician will perform an examination to rule out other conditions with similar symptoms. The full diagnosis may take a long time since all the symptoms may not surface for months or even years. The final diagnosis is based on discovery of recurrent oral ulcerations in conjunction with any two of the following: skin abnormalities, eye inflammation, and genitalia ulcerations. A detailed skin test known as a pathergy test can also indicate the existence of the syndrome. This evaluation involves pricking the skin of the forearm with a sterile needle. The test is deemed positive for Behcet's syndrome when the puncture produces a red nodule greater than two millimeters in diameter after twenty-four to forty-eight hours. Even after establishing all these determinants, the physician must rule out other conditions with comparable symptoms, such as reactive arthritis and Crohn's disease. The Behcet's patient may be advised to visit an eye specialist to identify possible complications related to eye inflammation. The patient should also visit a dermatologist who may biopsy the genital, oral, or skin lesions to help set the Behcet's apart from other disorders.

Treatment of Behcet's Syndrome

The treatment of Behcet's syndrome depends on the harshness of the symptoms and the part of the body affected in an individual patient. For mouth and genital ulcers, steroid (cortisone) gels and creams such as Kenolog in Orabase can be helpful. Oral and genital ulcers healed and were reported as less frequent in nine of twelve patients treated with Trental (pentoxifylline).[16] Joint inflammation can require nonsteroidal anti-inflammatory drugs or oral steroids. Colchicine and oral injectable cortisone are exploited for inflammation involving the skin, eyes, joints, and brain. However, bowel disease is addressed with oral steroids and sulfasalazine. Persevering treatment of eye inflammation is important. Behcet's sufferers with eye symptoms or a history of eye inflammation should visit an ophthalmologist routinely since partial blindness may occur if the condition goes neglected for too long.

Research[17] has also confirmed that official management of resistant eye inflammation with new biologic drugs hinders tumor necrosis factor (TNF), a protein with a major role in starting inflammation. These TNF-blocking drugs, including etanercept and infliximab, can also be useful for major oral ulcerations. Noteworthy problems of the eyes, arteries, and brain can be difficult to approach and require powerful prescriptions that suppress the immune system, known as immunosuppressive agents. Recent studies[18] suggest that administering thalidomide benefits certain patients with Behcet's syndrome by preventing and treating ulcerations of the mouth and genitals. Some observed side effects of thalidomide include (1) nerve injury (neuropathy), (2) irregular fetal development, and (3) hypersedation.

4

Resolutions

Chapter Fifteen

Initial Approaches to Rheumatic and Joint Problems

Problems of the joints of the human body are considered chronic, meaning that they have a long duration and are incurable. There are more than one hundred different types of joint problem, some of which cause swelling and pain in the joints, while others may affect multiple organs. The causes of joint problems vary from old age to general wear and tear, autoimmune disorders, infection by viruses and parasites, and genetic and environmental factors. The exact causes of many forms of joint problems are not yet fully understood by the medical community, which makes it difficult to find a cure.

DIFFICULTY IN INITIALLY APPROACHING JOINT PROBLEMS

Complexity

The complexity of joint problems increases due to the fact that they come in so many different forms, each with different symptoms and affecting a different part of the body. Studies indicate that race, gender, age, and genetic factors also play a part in making some groups more prone to some forms of joint problems, while some types seem to run in families. Joint diseases are therefore extremely complex, and so far only a few are curable, though in most cases proper medication and therapy can keep the disease under control.

Research and Clinical Trials

Scientists all over the world are investigating many new treatment methods for joint problems, including new drugs that can provide relief for the painful symptoms and prevent worsening of the matter at hand. Genetic research and engineering may also bring about new methods of diagnosis and perhaps a full treatment and cure. At this time, a variety of medications such as pain-killing, anti-inflammatory, and antirheumatic drugs are used to relieve symptoms and slow the progression of the disease. Apart from medication, some new forms of therapy, such as biological treatments, work by stopping chemicals in the blood from triggering joint problems. Most medications, however, involve some side effects and should be used only after proper consultation with a doctor. In advanced cases, the patient may also need surgery to reduce pain and correct damage to the joints. Surgical procedures may include replacement of the damaged joint, removing the inflamed lining of the joint cavity, removing bone to relieve pain, releasing trapped nerves, fusing a joint, or repairing damaged tendons. While none of these methods can fully cure or halt the disease, they can send it into remission.

AVOIDANCE AND SELF-CARE AS INITIAL APPROACHES

Prevention Means Avoidance

The best way of dealing with joint problems is to avoid, at least partially, any modifiable risk factors related to joint problems, coupled with timely diagnosis and treatment. Modifiable risk factors are those that can be prevented or changed. One of the most common modifiable risk factors for joint problems as reported is obesity.[1] Obesity leads to increased pressure on the joints and hence may contribute to the onset of joint problems. Controlling body weight through healthy eating and regular exercise can act as a preventive measure against the disease. Another common risk factor is joint injury. Care should be taken to avoid joint injuries, and any injury that occurs should be provided timely treatment.

Risk factors include frequent and repetitive joint movement, such as kneeling or stooping, which also put extra pressure on the joints and may contribute to the occurrence of the disease. Infections, which can lead to joint problems, should also be brought to the attention of a health-care professional immediately. Another important modifiable risk factor is smoking. Smoking increases the probability of developing joint problems as well as their severity. According to a study conducted by Swedish researchers[2] between 1993 and 2006, nonsmokers are 50 percent more likely to respond well to treatment than smokers.

Appropriate management of joint problems through medical treatment and a proper health-care regimen can help the patient lead a relatively painless and healthy life. It is very important for the patient to understand the disease, participate in the treatment, and handle the emotional side of joint problems positively. Joint problems may have a negative emotional impact on the patient, who may feel angry or frustrated due to the change in lifestyle that the disease brings in its wake. Studies[3] indicate that patients suffering from depression are more likely to experience joint pain flare-ups. A positive outlook, open communication, support from family and friends, involvement in social activities, and even joining support groups can help the patient come to terms with the condition and continue to lead a healthy and active life.

Self-care

Self-care[4] is critical in that today's fast-paced lifestyle leaves people rushed and tired, with little or no time to exercise or maintain healthy eating habits. Increased consumption of fast foods, addiction to smoking and alcohol, sedentary lifestyles, mental and physical exhaustion, and inadequate sleep and rest all contribute to a decline in our health and well-being. Joint problems are only one outcome of such a lifestyle. While some of these factors may be unavoidable in today's world, it is important to be aware of their negative effects and to make the required lifestyle changes. It is essential to incorporate healthy habits into day-to-day living in order to maintain a healthy body and mind. In case of joint problems, a light exercise regimen, eating the right foods, and regular rest and sleep can significantly reduce pain and other symptoms and prevent progression of the disease.

Following some simple self-care rules can also go a long way in controlling joint problems. For instance, people who work in an office environment that involves long periods at a desk should avoid sitting in one position for too long. Bending and flexing the legs, moving the neck from side to side, rotating the wrists, and taking brief breaks to get up and stretch the body are simple measures that can prevent the occurrence of joint problems and help keep the disease under control. Patients with any joint problem, be it arthritis or some other issue, should also focus on leading as normal a life as possible. This means taking part in social activities, meeting with friends, joining support groups if required, finding a suitable hobby, and even practicing meditation. Such activities keep patients from focusing excessively on their pain and other negative aspects of a life with joint problems and thereby help them develop a positive outlook. An optimistic attitude, acceptance of the situation, and a positive spirit are as important as any medication in the treatment of joint problems.

One must keep in mind that while not all joint problems are fatal, they are serious and debilitating issues that can strike people of all ages, races, and genders. Although long-term ailments with mostly no cure, they can be controlled through timely diagnosis and treatment. It is therefore important that any symptoms of joint problems, such as pain or inflammation, be brought to the notice of a health-care professional as soon as possible. Joint problems can have a serious emotional impact on the arthritis patient, who may feel angry and upset because of acute pain, loss of mobility, and the resulting impact on lifestyle. It is therefore important that the patient understand the topic, be involved in the treatment, and follow a proper self-care regimen. Family, friends, and other support groups can significantly contribute to the patient's overall health and mental well-being. With proper care and medication, sufferers of joint problems can continue to lead healthy, independent, and active lives.

WHAT TO DO IN CASE OF AN EMERGENCY

Arthritis problems are usually chronic though not life threatening. In the absence of timely treatment, however, a problem with a joint can become an extremely painful condition and have a very negative effect on overall health, well-being, and lifestyle. If left untreated, some joint problems may impair movement to the point of causing disability and also affect vital organs, thereby creating life-threatening situations. Recent studies also suggest that people with problems in their joints are more prone to heart disease and stroke. According to research conducted by scientists at Copenhagen University,[5] arthritis patients have a 40 percent higher risk of developing heart conditions. Therefore, rather than accepting joint problems such as arthritis as an inevitable part of ageing, individuals should be vigilant and take note of any symptoms that may indicate a potentially critical situation.

Examples

Some more serious manifestations of joint problems,[6] that might require hospitalization, are as follows:

- Septic joint problems such as septic arthritis are considered a medical emergency when they cause excruciating pain because of potential serious damage to bone and cartilage. Septic joint problems can cause septic shock, which can be fatal. The infection can get out of control during an emergency if not addressed promptly.
- A severe gout attack can be excruciatingly painful, and the patient should be given immediate medical attention.
- Atlantoaxial subluxation with spinal cord damage, such as that seen in rheumatoid arthritis, is a problem in which the vertebrae of the cervical spine are misaligned. There is potential for nerve damage, paralysis, and even death.
- Renal crisis, such as that seen in scleroderma, means that the kidney has been affected. This may cause a decline in kidney function and in some cases even heart failure.

- Digital ulcers and gangrene sometimes occur with scleroderma. Digital ulcers are sores that appear on fingers and toes and in other joint areas. They are painful and susceptible to infection.
- Amaurosis fugax is a sudden, painless, temporary loss of vision.
- Pulmonary-renal syndrome involves bleeding in the lungs and kidney damage. It also involves vasculitis.

It is essential to monitor the condition of the patient carefully and be on the lookout for emergencies or warning signs that may indicate complications arising out of joint problems or the side effects of medication. Some specific symptoms that warrant immediate medical intervention, even initially, are listed below.[7]

- Lack of improvement: If there is no significant improvement of joint symptoms with treatment, changes in medication may be required; in extreme cases, surgery may be needed. A lack of improvement may indicate that the treatment or medication is not working or that there are additional complications.
- Fever: While mild fevers can easily be dismissed when it comes to arthritis pain, it should be kept in mind that individuals with joint problems are susceptible to infections. It is therefore advisable to consult a doctor in case of fever (a natural reaction to infection) to ensure that the situation does not deteriorate any further and complications are avoided.
- Numbness or tingling: Sometimes swelling of the joints may press upon the nearby nerves, causing numbness or a tingling sensation. Called nerve entrapment, this problem should be treated as early as possible. These symptoms may indicate a very dangerous condition known as vasculitis, which is basically inflammation of the blood vessels.
- Eye redness or rashes: Also a symptom of vasculitis, this condition should be brought to the doctor's attention as soon as possible.
- Vision loss and problems with red and green color distinction: In rare cases, some drugs used to address joint-related emergencies can cause injury to the retina, imparing the patient's ability to distinguish between red and green. In such cases, the medication should be stopped immediately.
- Nausea and vomiting: Some types of medications used in joint-related emergencies also cause nausea and vomiting. As this can lead to dehydration, the doctor should be consulted on the apprearance of these symptoms. The medication may need to be reduced or stopped.
- Dizziness or light-headedness: This may be a serious side effect of prescribed drugs. If any such symptom is noticed, a doctor should be notified immediately.

ACTION PLANS

In the context of initial approaches to joint problems, the patient should immediately consult a health-care professional and share the details of symptoms, even if they do not seem related to joint problems. If the conditions are severe, it is advisable to go to the nearest emergency room or contact emergency help centers (for instance, by dialing 911). The doctor will then evaluate all the symptoms and may advise further tests, including MRI, CT scan, X-ray, blood tests, and antibody tests, to determine the appropriate course of treatment. If required, other specialists, such as a rheumatologist, orthopedic surgeon, chiropractor, or physical and occupational therapist, may also need to be consulted.

Things to Avoid

In case of any emergency, it is important for the patient to avoid ignoring critical, painful symptoms. Doing so will only aggravate the condition and may cause joint damage and disability. While it is alright to indulge in some mild exercise, strenuous, high-impact exercises, such as jogging and weight lifting, should be avoided since they put extra pressure on the joints. At the same time, the patient should avoid a sedentary lifestyle and continue to do some light exercises to keep his or her body weight under control. Staying in one position for too long or moving in ways that place extra stress on the sore joints must also be avoided.

IMPORTANCE OF SEEING A DOCTOR REGULARLY

What Warrants a Visit

Aches and pains are the joints' way of signaling that something is wrong, and it is unwise not to heed them.

Pain as a Warning Signal

Pain is usually only a symptom of an underlying medical condition, and it is not only advisable but essential to consult a doctor to diagnose and treat the problem. Pain from joint problems can occur for several reasons,[8] the simplest being a recent injury. In the absence of injury, joint pain can be a symptom of a variety of diseases. While joint problems are among the most common causes, joint pain can also be caused by other serious medical issues, such as diabetes, bone cancer, and tumors projecting into the joints. Some common causes of joint problems include the following:

• Injuries such as joint overuse, dislocation, or torn ligaments

- Infectious diseases such as dengue fever, hepatitis, Lyme disease, measles, and mumps, as well as joint septis and osteomyelitis (bone infection)
- Diabetes
- Sickle cell anaemia, a serious blood disorder
- Typhus, a disease cause by a bacterial infection
- Synovial sarcoma, a tumor near a joint

Clearly, joint pain can stem from a variety of serious diseases, many of which may be life threatening. Ignoring the pain will not make the underlying cause go away and will only increase the severity of the condition, making it more difficult to treat. In extreme cases, a delayed diagnosis may mean that it is too late to treat the disease, resulting in a potentially fatal condition. A person experiencing joint problems must therefore always consult a doctor if any unexplained pain persists for more than a week, especially if accompanied by fever, weight loss, or other unexplained symptoms. It is necessary to identify the underlying cause of the pain and to obtain proper treatment and medication at the initial stages.

Benefits of Check-ups

In case of joint problems, a regular check-up routine has many benefits. First of all, initial check-ups ensure that the entire problem is monitored and appropriate measures are taken to arrest it. Periodic check-ups enable the doctor to spot any signs of aggravation of the condition. They also allow the doctor to verify whether the prescribed medication is having the desired effect or any change or alternate method of treatment (such as surgery) is required. In addition, many joint medications have severe side effects. Regular consultation ensures that any such side effects are detected and the medication is stopped or altered. Regular check-ups also enable the doctor to ascertain if any new symptoms have developed that may indicate a new complication. Thus, the doctor and patient can together work out an effective management program that can help the patient deal with the long-term consequences of living with joint problems such as arthritis.

Relief of Pain

Whether joint pain results from sudden injury, gradual joint problems, or more serious conditions, such as those listed above, periodic check-ups are advised to ensure that the ailment is fully cured or kept under control. Periodic consultations give the doctor an opportunity to monitor the current status of the pain and prescribe the required treatment. They also help give the patient an understanding of both the condition and measures to keep it at bay. Further, some medications prescribed for joint pain may have serious side effects, which again necessitates regular communication with the doctor so that any drugs causing adverse side effects can be discontinued and alternative treatment given. Timely check-ups are also essential to identify symptoms that may be warning signs of a more serious condition. These warning signs may indicate deterioration of the patient's condition or a new illness or complication. Only a qualified health-care professional can study these symptoms and take appropriate action to prevent a serious outcome in the future.

Dangers of Initial Neglect

It is important to remember that arthritis progresses over time, which is a key reason not to neglect it. The patient should understand that treatment for joint problems such as arthritis is long-term and may last for the rest of the patient's lifetime. It is therefore essential to have regular consultations with the doctor to assess the state of the disease at any given time and to get the appropriate care. Not following a regular check-up routine can cause the disease to progress. Severe or advanced joint problems cause joint crepitance (squeaking and crackling noises when the joint is moved), inability to lift objects, and failure to bend or straighten a joint. Over a period, joint problems may cause physical deformation and eventually lead to permanent joint damage and disability.

Depending on the severity of the disease, check-ups can be done as often as every two to three months or every six to twelve months. During the check-up, the doctor will assess the current condition of the patient based on the severity of pain, the duration of pain or stiffness, the number of inflamed or painful joints, how well the patient is functioning at the given time, and any other symptoms related or unrelated to joint problems that may have developed since the previous check-up. The doctor will also examine whether there are any side effects of prescribed medication and may recommend further tests if required. Based on the results of the above, the doctor will then suggest a course of treatment, which may include medication (chapter 16), physiotherapy, or surgery (chapter 17).

Chapter Sixteen

Pharmacological Treatments for Arthritis

Pharmacology concerns the science of treatment using drugs. In the case of arthritis, a variety of prescription and nonprescription medications aim at relieving symptoms and arresting the progression of the disease. The commonly prescribed medications for arthritis can be broadly classified as analgesics (painkillers), disease-modifying antirheumatic drugs (DMARDs), biologics, corticosteroids, and nonsteroidal anti-inflammatory drugs (NSAIDs).[1]

Biological Treatments for Arthritis

Biologics comprise a relatively new form of therapy that involves the use of biological response modifiers (BRMs), substances produced naturally in the body in small amounts. They fight infection and disease. Using modern scientific techniques, it is now possible to artificially produce large quantities of BRMs, which can be used for treatment of arthritis. Biological drugs act as suppressors of cytokines, or substances that trigger the immune system and increase inflammation in the arthritis-affected joints. As with other forms of treatment, biologics also cause some side effects, such as fever, nausea, and skin reactions; in rare cases they may reactivate prior ailments, such as tuberculosis and hepatitis B.

Corticosteroids

These are manmade (synthetic) drugs that resemble certain hormones produced naturally by the human body. They work by reducing production of substances that cause inflammation in the body. Corticosteroids are very potent and can provide rapid relief for arthritis pain. However, they have serious side effects and therefore should be used for short periods only. Long-term use of corticosteroids should be reserved only for very serious cases and conducted under strict medical supervision. Common side effects of these drugs include weight gain, muscle weakness, osteoporosis (weakening of the bones), mood swings, blurred vision, glaucoma, and diabetes.

Nonsteroidal Anti-inflammatory Drugs

NSAIDs work by blocking COX enzymes, which are responsible for producing prostaglandins, chemicals produced by the human body that cause pain and inflammation. By blocking COX enzymes, NSAIDs reduce the levels of prostaglandin in the body, thereby reducing pain and inflammation. These drugs have many side effects that range from problems of the gastrointestinal tract, such as nausea, vomiting, heartburn, and diarrhea, to more severe conditions, such as an increased risk of heart attacks and strokes.

DEBATE ABOUT PRESCRIPTION VERSUS OVER-THE-COUNTER MEDICATIONS

Benefits of Treatment with Prescription Medications for Arthritis

Arthritis treatment[2] using prescription medications benefits the patient in two ways. First, medications such as analgesics and NSAIDs provide quick relief from the pain, stiffness, and inflammation that accompany arthritis. Corticosteroids also provide fast relief from severe pain and are normally used if the patient is not responding to analgesics or NSAIDs. The second line of therapy, involving DMARDs and biological treatments, works to arrest the progression of the disease and prevent permanent damage to the joints. A combination of both types of medication, along with other forms of therapy, such as proper diet, exercise, and self-care, can help the patient remain healthy and active.

Drawbacks of Prescription Treatment for Arthritis

While prescription treatments for arthritis provide much-needed relief from painful symptoms, it is important to be aware of the risks associated with them. Most arthritis medications have side effects that may range from mild skin irritation to heart attack. For example, strong analgesics such as tramadol or codeine provide pain relief but may cause nausea, confusion, or delirium. NSAIDs reduce pain and inflammation but may also attack the digestive system, causing stomach upset, ulcers, and even gastrointestinal bleeding. Corticosteroids provide quick relief but have a number of side effects ranging from weight gain to increased blood pressure and osteoporosis. DMARDs block the progression of the disease but come with side effects such as mouth ulcers, diarrhea, hair loss, skin rashes, and liver problems. Prescription biological drugs also have many side effects, usually including skin reactions, nausea, fever, and headache.

The side effects really depend on the drug used, the dosage, and the frequency of administration, as well as the arthritis patient's response to the drug. Even simple over-the-counter (OTC) drugs may have potentially dangerous side effects. Also, certain drugs taken in combination dramatically increase the risks of side effects. According to peer-reviewed research,[3] two common arthritis drugs, alendronate and naproxen, increase the risk of stomach ulcers when taken together. Also, if a patient is on medication for more than one disease, mixing medicines may case dangerous side effects. It is therefore very important that all drugs be taken only as prescribed after due consultation with the doctor.

Over-the-Counter and Prescription Medications

Pharmacological treatment for arthritis includes both OTC and prescription medications. OTC medications do not require a prescription and can be bought off the shelf. Prescription medicines require a doctor's prescription and can be bought only in pharmacies. Prescription medicines are meant only for the person to whom they are prescribed and should never be shared. OTC drugs are generally used for minor pains and are not as strong as prescription medicines. Examples include pain-relieving creams and sprays, as well as pain-relieving drugs such as aspirin. Prescription drugs, on the other hand, are used for the treatment of major arthritis pains and inflammation and are prescribed by the doctor depending on the severity of the condition. NSAIDs, corticosteroids, and DMARDs are prescription drugs.

Arthritis patients may choose OTC or prescription drugs, but even in case of OTC medication, it is still advisable to consult the doctor for two reasons: (1) many OTC drugs have side effects, and it is important for the patient to be aware of risks and benefits associated with each, and (2) while OTC drugs relieve symptoms such as pain and inflammation, they do not stop the progression of the disease. Medical consultation is therefore necessary to take a long-term view of the ailment and provide the necessary medical care before it progresses to an advanced stage.

DISEASE-MODIFYING ANTIRHEUMATIC DRUGS (PRESCRIPTION ONLY)

Some DMARDs used for the treatment of arthritis include the following:[4]

- Methotrexate: Methotraxate is a prescription drug used for the treatment of cancer and arthritis. The mechanism of its action against arthritis is not yet fully understood, but it seems to alter immunity. Its side effects include dizziness, drowsiness, nausea, vomiting, sore throat, mouth sores, diarrhea, and mild stomach pain. More serious side effects include liver problems, lung infection, and tumors.
- Sulfasalazine: Sulfasalazine is a prescription drug that reduces pain and inflammation and also prevents joint damage. The mechanism of its action is not yet clearly understood. The side effects of sulfasalazine include nausea, vomiting, loss of appetite, mild stomach upset, and skin rashes. In some cases, sulfasalazine has been found to cause abnormalities in liver function, lowered white blood cell count, and kidney failure.
- Hydroxychloroquine: Hydroxychloroquine is an antimalarial drug also used for the treatment of lupus and rheumatoid arthritis. Although its mechanism remains unclear, it is thought to act on the immune system. Side effects of hydroxychloroquine include skin rashes, nausea, indigestion, headache, and mild hair loss. In very rare cases, it may cause damage to the retina; hence, it should be used only as prescribed by a physician.
- Leflunomide: Leflunomide works by suppressing the immune cells, which cause swelling and inflammation of the joints. The usual side effects include diarrhea, headache, nausea, and rashes. Since it suppresses the immune cells, leflunomide can increase the risk of infection. In rare cases, it can also cause liver damage.
- Gold salts: Gold salts are prescription drugs containing gold and are used for the treatment of arthritis. They are believed to block the release of a substance called HMGB1 from the nucleus of body cells.[5] HMGB1 affects the immune system and causes inflammation. Common side effects of gold salts are nausea, diarrhea, skin rashes, loss of appetite, and mouth sores. More serious side effects include kidney damage and decreased while blood cell and platelet counts.
- Azathioprine: Like other DMARDs, azathioprine works by suppressing the immune system, though the exact mechanism of its action is not known. Side effects include nausea, vomiting, and loss of appetite. It is also listed as a carcinogen and may cause lymphoma and skin cancer in rare cases.
- Cyclosporine: Much like azathioprine, cyclosporine works by blocking the production of a chemical called cytokine, thereby suppressing the immune system. Its side effects include nausea, vomiting, tremors, headache, body pain, and increased hair growth. Serious side effects include kidney damage, liver toxicity, high blood pressure, and increased risk of cancer.

BIOLOGICAL RESPONSE MODIFIERS[6] OR BIOLOGIC DMARDS
(PRESCRIPTION ONLY)

Some BRMs or biologic DMARDs used for the treatment of arthritis include the following:

- Etanercept: Etanercept is an injectable prescription drug that works by blocking a substance called tumor necrosis factor alpha (TNF-M), which causes pain and inflammation. Common side effects include headache, dizziness, and skin and throat irritation. Since this drug works by suppressing the immune system, etanercept increases the arthritis patient's susceptibility to infections. In rare cases, it may also cause serious conditions such as low white/red blood cell count and heart problems.
- Adalimumab: Adalimumab is another injectable prescription drug that works by blocking the action of TNF-M. Its side effects include headache, rashes, stomach upset, and skin irritation. Like other TNF-blocking drugs, adalimumab also suppresses the immune system and increases the risk of infection. It may also increase the risk of cancer. However, a connection between adalimumab and the risk of cancer has yet to be conclusively established.
- Infliximab: Infliximab also works by blocking TNF-M. Common side effects of infliximab include cough, rashes, nausea, vomiting, headache, stomach pain, urinary and respiratory infections, and allergic reactions. As with other TNF blockers, infliximab also increases the risk of infection. It may also lower the blood cell count and, in rare cases, cause liver and heart problems.
- Certolizmab pegol: Certolizmab pegol is another injectable prescription drug that blocks TNF and thereby reduces pain and inflammation. Side effects include sore throat, fever, cough, and skin irritation at the injection site. It also increases the risk of infection and may cause or aggravate conditions such as tuberculosis, sepsis (blood infection), lowering of blood cell count, and heart conditions.
- Golimumab: Golimumab is an injectable TNF blocker. As with similar medications, its side effects include irritation at the injection site, sore throat, respiratory tract infection, and fever. It may also lower blood cell count and increase the risk of cancer.
- Anakinra: Anakinra works by blocking the effects of a protein called interleukin-1, a substance responsible for causing pain and inflammation. The side effects of anakinra are skin irritation at the injection site, nausea, stomach upset, and allergic reactions, such as sore throat, cough, and itching. Anakinra can also increase the risk of infection and, in the form of a side effect, worsen serious conditions such as tuberculosis.[7]

- Abatacept: Abatacept is an injectable prescription immunosuppressant. It works by blocking the action of T lymphocytes, which cause the symptoms of arthritis. Common side effects are dizziness, headache, nausea, rash, shortness of breath, and allergic reactions, such as swelling of the face, tongue, lips, and throat. Serious side effects may include severe infections or even cancer.
- Rituximab: Rituximab is a prescription drug that works by destroying the immune system's B cells, which cause the symptoms of arthritis. Most common side effects include fever and chills that appear the first time the drug is administered but lessen over subsequent doses. Other side effects include nausea, headache, itching, and a runny nose. Rituximab may also cause serious side effects such as low blood pressure, irregular heartbeat, and heart attack, as well as serious skin conditions that include Stevens-Johnson syndrome.
- Tocilizumab: Tocilizumab is an injectable prescription drug that works by blocking interleukin-6, which causes pain and inflammation. Its side effects include headache, irritation at the injection site, and stomach pain. It may also cause, in the form of a side effect, serious infection, such as tuberculosis, blood infections, reduced blood cell count, and severe allergic reactions.

GLUCORTICOIDS[8] (PRESCRIPTION ONLY)

Some glucorticoids used for the treatment of arthritis include the following:

- Prednisolone: Prednisolone is a prescription medicine that is very similar to glucocorticoid, a substance produced naturally by the human body. Much like glucocorticoids, prednisolone also acts to suppress an overactive immune system in arthritis patients, thereby reducing pain, swelling, and inflammation. Side effects include headache, muscle weakness, fluid retention, weight gain, and increased susceptibility to infection. Other serious side effects may include high blood pressure, peptic ulcer, aggravation of diabetes, glaucoma, cataract, and psychological effects such as irritability, depression, and mood swings.
- Prednisone: Prednisone is another prescription drug[9] that suppresses the immune system of the body and reduces pain and inflammation. Side effects include muscle weakness, fluid retention, headache, glaucoma, cataracts, thinning of the body, bruising, growth of facial hair, euphoria, depression, and mood swings.
- Cortisone acetate: Cortisone acetate is a prescription immunosuppressant. Like other glucocorticoids, its side effects include weight gain, high blood

pressure, low potassium, vision problems, headache, nausea, and mood changes.

- Betamethasone: Betamethasone is a prescription glucocorticoid that is available as a cream, ointment, or lotion and used to treat itching and inflammation of the skin. Side effects are burning, irritation, itching, and dryness of the skin, but these symptoms disappear as the body gets used to the medication.
- Dexamethasone: Dexamethasone is a very potent glucocorticoid used as an immunosuppressant. Like other glucocorticoids, it is used to treat a variety of diseases, including cancer. Prolonged use can cause serious side effects, such as cataract and bone thinning. Common side effects include increased appetite, weight gain, muscle weakness, increased blood sugar, insomnia, irritability, and mood swings.
- Hydrocortisone: Yet another prescription-only glucocorticoid, hydrocortisone works by suppressing the immune system and exhibits similar side effects to other glucocorticoids, including weight gain, muscle weakness, glaucoma, cataract, high blood pressure, and mood swings.
- Methylprednisolone: This is a prescription-only immunosuppressive drug used to treat a variety of conditions. Like other glucocorticoids, its side effects range from weight gain, fluid retention, vision problems, and mood swings to serious conditions such as high blood pressure, glaucoma, and peptic ulcers.

NONSTEROIDAL ANTI-INFLAMMATORY DRUGS[10] (PRESCRIPTION OR OTC)

Some NSAIDs used for the treatment of arthritis include the following:

- Aspirin: Aspirin is an OTC drug used as an analgesic to relieve minor aches and pains associated with arthritis. It works by blocking the production of prostaglandins, substances that cause pain and fever. The most common side effects of aspirin are heartburn, stomach pains, nausea, and vomiting. In some cases, it may cause allergic reactions, such as hives and rashes.
- Choline and magnesium solicylates: Available by prescription, these reduce the level of prostaglandins, chemicals that cause pain and inflammation. Common side effects are heartburn, nausea, vomiting, abdominal pain, stomach ulcers, and hearing loss. In rare cases, they may also increase the risk of heart attack and stroke, especially in people who already have high blood pressure or other heart conditions. They sometimes also cause stomach or intestinal bleeding.

- Diclofenac potassium: Diclofenac potassium is generally a prescription-only drug, although it is also available over the counter in some countries. It also works by reducing the levels of prostaglandins in the body through COX inhibition. Its side effects include nausea, heartburn, stomach upset, chest pain, shortness of breath, and slurred speech. It may also cause serious allergic reactions, high blood pressure, bleeding of the digestive tract, and liver and heart problems.
- Diclofenac sodium: Diclofenac sodium is a prescription drug that is also available over the counter in some countries. It works by reducing the levels of prostaglandins. Side effects include heartburn, nausea, constipation, diarrhea, headache, dizziness, and drowsiness. It may also cause stomach and intestinal ulcers as well as cardiovascular conditions such as heart attacks.
- Naproxen: Naproxen works as a COX inhibitor, thereby reducing the levels of prostaglandins in the body. It is a prescription drug in most countries, although it is also available as an OTC drug in the United States. As with other NSAIDs, the most common side effects of naproxen include nausea, heartburn, constipation, diarrhea, stomach pain, and shortness of breath. It may also cause serious side effects, such as stomach ulcers and intestinal bleeding, heart problems, and liver damage.
- Naproxen sodium: Naproxen sodium is an analgesic drug available over the counter. Like other NSAIDs, it is a COX inhibitor and reduces the levels of prostaglandins, which cause inflammation. As with other NSAIDs, side effects include heartburn, constipation, nausea, stomach pain, dizziness, cardiovascular problems, and liver damage.
- Sodium salicylate: Sodium salicylate is an NSAID available over the counter. It is usually prescribed as an alternative for patients allergic to aspirin. Its side effects are similar to those of other NSAIDs and include nausea, vomiting, gastric irritation, ulceration, and gastrointestinal bleeding.
- Magnesium salicylate: Magnesium salicylate is available over the counter and works by reducing the substances in the body that cause inflammation. Its side effects are similar to other NSAIDs and include stomach upset, nausea, heartburn, weight gain, and hearing changes. Like other NSAIDs, it might cause stomach and intestinal bleeding. It also increases the risk of heart attack.
- Diflunisal: Diflunisal is a prescription drug, and like some other NSAIDs, it acts by reducing the production of prostaglandins. Its side effects are also similar to those of other NSAIDs and include problems of the gastrointestinal system, including nausea, gas, stomach upset, ulcers, gastrointestinal bleeding, and liver problems.
- Etodolac: Etodolac is another prescription NSAID that lowers the levels of prostaglandins in the body, thereby reducing pain and inflammation. It

exhibits common side effects associated with other NSAIDs, including constipation, diarrhea, vomiting, headache, ringing in the ears, and serious conditions such as heart, kidney, and liver problems.

- Fenoprofen calcium: Fenoprofen calcium is a prescription drug, and like other NSAIDs, it works by reducing the production of prostaglandins in the body. Side effects are similar to those of other NSAIDs and include nausea, vomiting, indigestion, dizziness, drowsiness, and headache. Serious side effects include heart problems, gastrointestinal bleeding, and impaired kidney function.
- Flurbiprofen: Another prescription NSAID, flurbiprofen works as a COX inhibitor and is used to treat pain and inflammation. Its side effects range from headache, nausea, stomach upset, dizziness, and insomnia to serious conditions such as gastrointestinal bleeding and cardiovascular, vision, kidney, and liver problems.
- Ibuprofen: Ibuprofen is available both over the counter and by prescription and works by suppressing prostaglandins. The most common side effects of ibuprofen are stomach pain, nausea, and heartburn. Like other NSAIDs, ibuprofen may cause more serious side effects, such as gastrointestinal bleeding, liver and kidney problems, and cardiovascular problems including heart attack and stroke.
- Indomethacin: Indomethacin is a prescription NSAID that works as a COX inhibitor and reduces the production of prostaglandins in the body. Its side effects include indigestion, dizziness, nausea, and vomiting, as well as serious conditions such as gastrointestinal bleeding, liver and kidney problems, and cardiovascular problems including heart attack and stroke.
- Ketoprofen: Ketoprofen is a prescription drug that reduces the production of prostaglandins in the body. Its side effects are similar to those of other NSAIDs and include nausea, stomach pain, vomiting, diarrhea, and other serious conditions such as peptic ulcer, gastrointestinal bleeding, kidney and liver problems, and heart attack and stroke.
- Mobidin: Mobidin is an OTC drug used to treat mild to moderate joint pain related to arthritis. Like other NSAIDs, mobidin works by blocking chemicals in the body that cause pain and inflammation. Its side effects include liver, kidney, and cardiovascular problems and gastrointestinal bleeding, in addition to milder conditions such as nausea, heartburn, stomach upset, and dizziness.
- Mecofenamate sodium: This OTC drug works by reducing the levels of prostaglandins in the body. Its side effects include gastrointestinal problems such as nausea, vomiting, diarrhea, gas, and heartburn. Serious side effects include gastrointestinal bleeding, liver damage, and cardiovascular problems.

- Mefenamic acid: Mefenamic acid is a prescription drug that works by reducing the levels of prostaglandins in the body. Common side effects include nausea, heartburn, stomach upset, dizziness, drowsiness, and headache. Serious side effects range from high blood pressure, heart attack, and stroke to liver problems and gastrointestinal bleeding.
- Meloxicam: Meloxicam is yet another prescription NSAID that reduces prostaglandins in the body. As with other NSAIDs, its common side effects are related to the gastrointestinal tract and include nausea, vomiting, diarrhea, and abdominal pain. Serious side effects include ulcers, gastrointestinal bleeding, kidney problems, liver damage, heart attack, and stroke.
- Nabumetone: Nabumetone is a prescription drug that provides relief from pain and inflammation by reducing the levels of prostaglandins in the body. Common side effects include nausea, constipation, and abdominal pain. Serious side effects include gastrointestinal bleeding, kidney impairment, and liver problems.
- Oxaprozin: Oxaprozin is a prescription drug; like other NSAIDs, it works by reducing the levels of prostaglandins in the body. Its side effects are similar to those of other NSAIDs and range from nausea, abdominal pain, diarrhea, and headache to more serious conditions such as gastrointestinal bleeding, cardiovascular problems, kidney impairment, and liver damage.
- Piroxicam: Piroxicam is a prescription drug and works by reducing prostaglandins. The most common side effects include nausea, constipation, abdominal pain, dizziness, and drowsiness, while more serious side effects include gastrointestinal bleeding, kidney impairment, and heart attack.
- Rofecoxib: Rofecoxib is a prescription NSAID that has been voluntarily withdrawn from the market after studies indicated that it caused an increased risk of serious cardiovascular problems, including heart attack and stroke.
- Salsalate: This prescription drug blocks the production of prostaglandin in the body. As with other NSAIDs, the side effects range from nausea, abdominal pain, diarrhea, and gastritis to more serious conditions, such as gastrointestinal bleeding, cardiovascular problems, kidney impairment, and liver damage.
- Sulindac: Sulindac is another prescription drug that works by reducing the level of prostaglandin in the body. Side effects range from diarrhea, abdominal pain, and heartburn to ulcers, gastrointestinal bleeding, heart attack, stroke, kidney problems, and liver damage.
- Tolmetin sodium: Tolmetin sodium is a prescription drug that, like other NSAIDs, works by blocking chemicals in the body that cause pain and inflammation. Side effects include problems of the digestive tract and serious conditions such as heart attack, stroke, and stomach ulcers.

- Valdecoxib: Valdecoxib[11] is a COX-inhibiting NSAID that has been withdrawn from the market due to a high risk of heart attack, stroke, and serious (sometimes fatal) skin reactions.

STAYING ON THE DEFENSIVE

Taking Side Effects of Pharmacological Drugs Seriously

All medicines for arthritis, whether prescription or OTC, have side effects that may range from mild to serious, and sometimes fatal, conditions. While all drugs are thoroughly tested for possible side effects before being marketed, it is difficult to predict the side effects that may arise from long-term usage. Furthermore, side effects may vary from patient to patient and may affect different parts of the body. Seemingly mild side effects may sometimes indicate a major complication. Therefore, it is important to be aware of all possible risks associated with the medication prescribed. It is equally advisable to discuss these with the doctor to make sure any adverse effects are monitored and appropriate corrective actions are taken.

Prescription Adherence

In case of long-term health problems such as arthritis, it is important to follow the prescription and take the medication strictly as directed by the doctor. This is known as prescription, or medication, adherence. Lack of prescription adherence results in improper treatment of the disease, leading to further complications. Taking medication irregularly or in the wrong dosage may also lead to other serious, potentially fatal, health conditions such as kidney impairment, liver damage, or cardiovascular problems.[12]

Chapter Seventeen

Natural Arthritis Treatments and Surgery

Many pharmacological medications are available to treat arthritis, but most come with a medley of side effects. Although conventional medication provides relief from the symptoms of arthritis and slows its progression, there is still no cure for the condition. Alternative and natural treatments[1] for arthritis are therefore becoming increasingly popular among arthritis sufferers. The term *alternative treatment* refers to natural methods of healing various diseases. Natural treatments have been used since ancient times, and in contrast to conventional medicine, natural treatment is based on the belief that health problems are caused by a combination of factors affecting not just the body but also the mind. While conventional medicines focus on treating symptoms using drugs, natural therapies work from the belief that the body can heal itself naturally and that treatment should focus on physical, mental, and emotional factors, rather than the symptoms of the disease, to achieve a complete cure.

OVERVIEW

Benefits

Natural treatments for arthritis do not involve the use of chemicals and hormones. Herbal cures are derived from plants and contain natural ingredients that do not cause chemical or hormonal changes in the body. They are therefore relatively free of side effects. Prescription drugs, on the other hand, contain chemicals that may cause dangerous and sometimes fatal side effects. For instance, Vioxx, a drug used widely for the treatment of arthritis, was withdrawn from the market in 2004 after a study showed that it drastically increased the risk of heart attack and stroke. According to a news report,[2] the Food and Drug Administration estimated that this drug caused over twenty-seven thousand deaths between 1999 and 2003. Such risks can be avoided through the use of natural remedies.

Drawbacks

It should be noted that natural treatments are not scientifically tested, as there have been no large-scale scientific or clinical trials or studies to prove their effectiveness. Although most forms of natural treatment are believed to be free of side effects, some natural herbs do carry some risks. For example, Asian ginseng lowers blood sugar and therefore may not be suitable for diabetes patients.[3] While going for alternative remedies, one should therefore educate oneself about the effectiveness and risks of the treatment and discuss these with a health-care professional to avoid any adverse effects.

HYALURONIC ACID

Introduction

Hyaluronic acid is a substance produced naturally in the human body and found in all tissues and body fluids, particularly the fluids in the eyes and joints.[4] It is a major component of the synovial fluid that reduces friction in the joints of the body. Hyaluronic acid helps in delivering nutrients and removing toxins from cells that do not have a blood supply, such as those in the cartilage. It also lubricates the joints. Without hyaluronic acid, the joints would become brittle. Hyaluronic acid is therefore injected into the joints to lubricate and cushion them, thereby reducing the pain and inflammation associated with arthritis. Hyaluronic acid also binds with water to increase water retention in body tissue. It locks moisture into cells, thus reducing wrinkles and lines and helping to preserve a youthful appearance. It is therefore used as a filler in plastic surgery and in making cosmetic products such as moisturizers. It is also used in eye surgeries such as corneal transplants and cataract operations to help replace natural eye fluids that may be lost during surgery.

Hyaluronic acid was previously extracted from rooster combs. It can now also be produced in the laboratory through the action of bacteria on plant products. In both cases, the final product is natural hyaluronic acid and not a synthetic chemical substitute. Since it is a natural product and contains only natural ingredients, it is classified as a natural treatment and does not fall into the pharmacological category, even though it can be used only if prescribed by a doctor. The US Food and Drug Administration classifies hyaluronic acid as a medical device and not a drug. Medical devices are products that affect the structure or function of the body but do not do so through chemical action. Hyaluronic acid (1) affects either the volume or shape of body parts, as in cosmetic surgery, or (2) relieves pain via lubrication when injected into the joints for arthritis treatment. Hence it is considered a device and not a drug.

Mechanism of Action

Hyaluronic acid is injected into the cavity around joints to increase the viscosity of the joint fluids, thereby lubricating and cushioning the joints. This improves joint movement and reduces pain and inflammation. This process is known as viscosupplementation. Studies[5] have been conducted on the efficacy of hyaluronic acid in the treatment of arthritis. Some of these experiments have indicated that there is no major benefit of hyaluronic acid, while others have found that it is indeed effective in reducing pain and improving joint function. In the absence of conclusive evidence, hyaluronic acid is normally used as a last resort when all other forms of treatment have failed to show results. It is most effective in patients suffering from mild to moderate arthritis and may not be as effective in older people or those in an advanced stage of the disease. While hyaluronic acid does exhibit some side effects, these are generally mild. Side effects may include bruising, redness, swelling, pain, and itching at the site of the injection. When taken in combination with some other products such as vitamin E supplements and nonsteroidal anti-inflammatory drugs, it may increase the risk of bruising and bleeding. It may also cause acne and necrosis, the death of living tissue.

PHYSICAL APPROACHES

Many forms of natural therapy are used to treat arthritis. Many of these have been used for centuries and have produced results even when conventional methods of treatment have failed. Some of the most commonly used natural therapies are as follows.

Hot Compress

Applying a hot compress[6] to any part of the body dilates the blood vessels, increasing blood circulation, and relaxes the muscles, thereby stimulating the body's natural healing forces. It is also found to alter the body's sensation of pain and has an analgesic effect. As with all other natural remedies, one should be careful while applying hot compresses. Heat should not be applied to a joint that is already hot and inflamed or to an open wound. The temperature should not be unbearably high, and the compress should not be applied for more than twenty to thirty minutes at a stretch. Otherwise, it may cause stiffness and soreness of muscles as well as skin burns.

Cold Compress

Like heat, cold also stimulates the body's natural healing action. Cold compresses restrict the blood vessels, decreasing circulation, and thereby reduces inflammation and numbs the sensation of pain. Like hot compresses, cold compresses should not be used for more than twenty minutes at a time. Nor should cold compresses be used if the arthritis patient has a medical condition that effects circulation, such as scleroderma or lupus.

Relaxation Remedies

Natural healing concentrates not only on the physical body of the patient but on his or her mental well-being as well. Natural remedies are based on the belief that any ailment is a problem not only of the body but also of the mind and that mental factors such as positive emotions and stress release play a major role in their cure. In the case of arthritis, several relaxation techniques are used to reduce anxiety, depression, and stress levels and reinforce positive thinking, which is in turn believed to reduce the physical symptoms of the disease.[7]

The following are some common examples of these mind and body relaxation techniques.[8]

- Yoga: The ancient practice of yoga, which involves gentle stretching movements, increases flexibility of the joints and eases pain and stiffness. Yogic meditation techniques relax the mind and provide stress relief and improved mental health.
- Tai chi: This ancient Chinese form of mind-body exercise also combines slow and gentle body movements, breathing techniques, and meditation. Some studies show that regular practice of tai chi increases flexibility and improves balance.
- Deep breathing: Most people take short, shallow breaths when stressed. This reduces the intake of oxygen and has a negative effect on the body. Deep-breathing exercises involve taking deep, slow breaths, which reduces stress and improves the overall functioning of the body.
- Progressive muscle relaxation: This form of relaxation therapy involves focusing on areas of the body that feel tense and consciously relaxing them while breathing deeply. This relaxes the muscles of the entire body and contributes to stress release.
- Meditation: Meditation is found to lower heart rates, blood pressure, and overall stress levels. It improves the mental health of the patient, which in

turn has a very positive impact on the body. Many arthritis patients say that they have benefitted from the positive effects of meditation.

- Spiritual belief and prayer: When faced with life's problems, many people find solace in spirituality and prayer. Such beliefs can often be a powerful tool in dealing not just with disease and illness but indeed with any of life's challenges. Many studies suggest that when patients believe they will get better, chances are that their condition will improve. Prayer therefore can serve as a very powerful healing tool in arthritis cases by engendering positive thinking and hope.

More on Relaxation Remedies

While it is difficult to obtain scientific evidence of the efficacy of relaxation techniques, many studies show that these are indeed effective in improving the physical and mental well-being of the patient. Whether these techniques really work or merely create a placebo effect is debatable. Regardless, if they provide relief and improve the patient's condition, they are well worth practicing.

Magnotherapy

Magnotherapy involves applying a magnetic field to the body, which is believed to increase blood circulation and thus the supply of oxygen to various body parts, such as the joints.[9] This also improves the supply of nutrients to, and helps to detoxify, the affected areas of the body, thereby reducing pain and inflammation. Magnets affect saline solutions, and since blood is a saline solution, it is possible that magnets have some impact on the blood flow. However, this has yet to be proven conclusively. Magnotherapy products include magnetic bracelets, pads, and insoles. They are considered free of side effects, but people using pacemakers, insulin pumps, or similar devices and epilepsy patients should not use them without first consulting a doctor.

Massage Therapy

Massage therapy is another form of natural treatment that has been practiced since ancient times.[10] It involves rubbing and pressing the body and has been found to be effective in reducing stress levels as well as in providing relief from pain and stiffness in arthritic joints. Although it is not clear how massage therapy works, it is possible that massaging the body releases certain chemicals that block pain, reduce stiffness, and provide a feeling of relaxation. Studies indicate that massage therapy lowers blood pressure and heart rates. Massage therapy also reduces anxiety and stress levels. This form of natural therapy has few side effects if completed by a trained therapist, although some precautions need to be taken. Massage should not be done on areas with fractures, weakened bones, blood clots, wounds, or skin infections. Generally, the risk of negative effects is very low.

Creation of a Supportive Environment

Arthritis can have a devastating impact on the patient's life. Patients may find themselves unable to participate in the activities of their choice and, as a result, may suffer from anxiety and depression. In such cases, it is important to provide the patient with a supportive and helpful social environment. Friends and family should avoid making the patient feeling left out of social activities, and the patient should be encouraged to continue participating in social and leisure activities of choice.

Traveling

Traveling provides a break from the daily routine and takes one's mind off day-to-day problems.[11] New sights and experiences and contact with new places and cultures have a great stress-relieving effect. Travel is therefore highly recommended whether a person is healthy or suffering from any ailment, not only arthritis.

Problems and Solutions

Traveling may be a difficult proposition. Arthritis patients may find it difficult to stand in long lines at the airport or other places, and doing so may cause a flare-up. Changes in weather may also increase pain and inflammation. Arthritis patients should therefore plan a trip and its itinerary carefully. For instance, if the patient suffers from increased pain in cold weather, the trip should be planned for the summer, and the destination should also be chosen with the climate in mind. The itinerary should be planned so that long waiting at airports or train stations can be avoided and the patient is able to rest between legs of the trip. The arthritis patient should pack all medication that may be required for the duration of the trip. With simple precautions such as these, there is no reason why arthritis patients should not be able to enjoy the pleasures of travel.

ROLE OF NUTRITION IN ARTHRITIS

Proper nutrition is important for everyone, and for arthritis patients healthy eating habits are very important. Some food types are found to be very effective in controlling arthritis, while others seem to aggravate the symptoms. For instance, certain minerals and vitamins, such as calcium, magnesium, vitamins C and D, and folic acid, are essential for healthy joints. A diet rich in these nutrients can therefore help combat the disease. Fruits, vegetables, and nuts contain antioxidants, which reduce inflammation. A diet rich in fiber is also found to be effective in combating inflammation. Thus it is important for the patient to follow a balanced diet that provides the required nutrients and helps in keeping the ailment under control. In addition, certain dietary supplements are also believed to be beneficial for arthritis. Some commonly used supplements for arthritis include the following:

- Glucosamine: Glucosamine is a substance that makes up the cartilage present between the joints.[12] Glucosamine supplements are prescribed for arthritis patients in the belief they help in the formation of new cartilage. Their effectiveness has yet to be proven conclusively. Glucosamine supplements are relatively free of side effects, although they may sometimes cause heartburn, nausea, gas, constipation, or diarrhea. Diabetes patients and pregnant women should take glucosamine under medical supervision or approval.
- Chondroitin: Similar, to a certain extent, to glucosamine, chondroitin is a building block of cartilage. Chondroitin supplements are believed to help repair and build new cartilage. The side effects of chondroitin include constipation, diarrhea, heartburn, and nausea.
- Fish oil: Fish oil supplements contain omega-3 fatty acids, which are effective in reducing inflammation. Omega-3 fatty acids work by suppressing chemicals such as COX enzymes, tumor necrosis factor, and interleukin-1, which cause inflammation. Its side effects may include nausea, indigestion, and a fishy aftertaste. It may also increase the chances of internal bleeding, such as gastrointestinal bleeding and hemorrhagic stroke.
- Borage oil: Borage oil contains omega-6 fatty acids that suppress chemicals responsible for inflammation, thereby providing relief from the symptoms of arthritis. Side effects include indigestion, nausea, and headache. Borage oil may also contain traces of a substance called pyrrolizidine alkaloids (PAs), which may be toxic to the liver. One should therefore use only those preparations that are marked PA free.
- Devil's claw: Devil's claw is an herb used for the treatment of arthritis. It appears to work as a COX-2 inhibitor, meaning it suppresses the cyclooxygenase enzymes responsible for causing inflammation. Common side effects include mild gastrointestinal problems. Devil's claw may lower sugar levels and affect one's heartbeat and blood pressure.
- Evening primrose: Evening primrose supplements contain omega-6 fatty acids and are believed to act as an immunosuppressant, thereby reducing inflammation. Side effects include mild indigestion problems such as nausea and stomach upset. These supplements may increase the risk of bleed-

ing and seizures and should be avoided by arthritis patients suffering from bleeding disorders, epilepsy, or schizophrenia.

- Ginkgo: This supplement is extracted from the ginkgo biloba tree and believed to improve blood circulation and reduce pain, in addition to acting as an antioxidant. Side effects include stomach upset, dizziness, and headache. People suffering from epilepsy, seizures, and schizophrenia and those taking any blood-thinning medicines should avoid ginkgo supplements.
- Flaxseed oil: Flaxseed oil contains omega-3 and omega-6 fatty acids, which are believed to help reduce inflammation. Side effects include stomach upset and diarrhea. It also increases the risk of bleeding, hence should be avoided by those with bleeding disorders or scheduled for surgery.
- Indian frankincense: This plant extract is used to treat arthritis. It may have anti-inflammatory properties although there is not enough clinical evidence to support this claim. Side effects include nausea, diarrhea, abdominal pain, and skin rashes.
- Bromelain supplements: Bromelain is an enzyme found in pineapples. These supplements are found to have analgesic and anti-inflammatory properties. Side effects include indigestion, nausea, diarrhea, and vomiting. Possible allergic reactions include breathing problems, rashes, and hives. Bromelain may increase the risk of bleeding.
- Vitamins: Vitamins C, D, and E have been found to be very beneficial to bones and joints. Vitamin C helps in the formation of collagen, a substance that provides strength and structure to bones and joints. In addition, vitamin C also acts as an antioxidant. Vitamin D helps in the absorption of calcium, which is necessary for strong and healthy bones and teeth. Vitamin D deficiency leads to less calcium being absorbed by the bones, which may result in weak and brittle bones, making a person prone to fractures. Vitamin E is an antioxidant that reduces the number of free radicals in the arthritis patient's body, which are known to harm the bones and joints. Vitamin E also suppresses prostaglandins, which are responsible for causing joint pain. This vitamin also helps in the production of cartilage and prevents cartilage breakdown, thereby helping to maintain healthy joints. Arthritis patients should therefore include foods rich in these vitamins in their daily diet.
- S-adenosyl methionine supplements (SAM-e): This is a substance produced naturally by the human body. An artificially synthesized form of SAM-e is used as a dietary supplement to treat joint pains. It is believed to increase the production of chondrocytes, substances that make cartilage. SAM-e is relatively safe, although it may cause side effects such as nausea, diarrhea, headache, and skin rashes. People suffering from bipolar

disorder or other psychiatric conditions should use SAM-e under medical supervision.

- Methylsulfonylmethane: Methylsulfonylmethane is a natural sulfur compound found in all living things. It is marketed as a dietary supplement for a variety of diseases, including arthritis, and is believed to have an anti-inflammatory and analgesic effect. It appears to be relatively free of side effects, although some side effects, such as nausea, diarrhea, headache, itching, and allergies, have been reported.
- Curcumin and turmeric: Curcumin and turmeric are plant products widely used as food spices. They exhibit anti-inflammatory properties and are believed to suppress the chemicals in the body that cause inflammation. They are generally considered safe, although high doses may cause nausea or diarrhea.
- Valerian: Valerian is widely used as a natural remedy for insomnia and anxiety. It is also believed to have a pain-reducing effect. It appears to be beneficial in treating sleep-related problems in arthritis patients. Valerian is considered safe for short-term use, although some side effects, such as headache, uneasiness, excitability, and insomnia, have been reported.
- Cat's claw: This vine has been used for centuries to treat arthritis and inflammation. It is an antioxidant and exhibits anti-inflammatory properties. Side effects include headache, dizziness, and vomiting, though cat's claw is generally considered safe. It may also lower blood pressure.

Foods Great for Arthritis

Several foods are found to be beneficial in controlling arthritis, and patients can benefit from incorporating them into their daily diet:

- Fatty fish, such as salmon and sardines, is a great choice for arthritis sufferers. Fish contains omega-3 fatty acids, which help fight inflammation. Fish also contains vitamin D, which strengthens bones.
- Avocados have high amounts of fatty acids as well as antioxidant properties. Avocados also help in cartilage repair and are therefore very beneficial for arthritis.
- Soybean products contain isoflavones, which are helpful in maintaining strong and healthy bones. Soy items are also rich in omega-3 fatty acids, vitamin E, and calcium and are therefore very helpful in relieving the arthritis symptoms discussed in chapter 5.
- Whole grains such as brown rice, barley, and whole wheat are rich in fiber and help fight inflammation. They are also helpful in controlling body weight.
- Bell peppers and citrus fruits are rich in vitamin C, which helps in the production of collagen and also acts as an antioxidant.

• Green leafy vegetables contain antioxidants, fiber, and omega fatty acids and are therefore very beneficial for arthritis patients.

In addition to the above, nuts, strawberries, olive oil, and green tea are also found to be good for arthritis.

ROLE OF SURGERY IN ARTHRITIS

Arthritis surgery is usually performed to treat severe cases that have not responded to other treatments. Surgery improves the flexibility of a joint and can also improve the alignment of misshapen joints, providing greater ease of movement. All surgeries have associated risks, and arthritis surgery is no exception. Any medical condition such as high blood pressure or diabetes must be under control at the time of surgery. Otherwise, complications might occur. Surgery also carries risk of infection and blood clots. Recovery from surgery is a slow and tedious process, and the patient must follow the doctor's advice to the letter to avoid any postsurgical complications and allow for a full recovery.

Surgical Options for Arthritis

Various types of surgery[13] are used to treat arthritis. While the subject of arthritis and surgery has been covered in detail in chapter 17, the following list does include some additional options available today:

• Arthrodesis: This involves fusing two bones forming a joint. The resultant fused joint cannot be moved and therefore loses flexibility but is no longer painful. This type of surgery is usually done on ankles, wrists, fingers, or thumbs.
• Arthroscopy: In this type of procedure, a thin instrument called an arthroscope is inserted into the joint through the skin. The arthroscope can be connected to a camera and allows the surgeon to see into the joint, assess how much it is affected, and determine suitable treatment. This type of surgery is usually done on knees and shoulders.
• Osteotomy: This surgery involves cutting and repositioning the bone to correct deformities and improve joint alignment. It is usually done on the knees and hips.
• Resection: Resection removes all or part of a bone. This type of surgery is usually done when a damaged joint makes movements very difficult. It is usually done for the joints in the foot and sometimes for the wrist, thumb, or elbow.
• Synovectomy: This involves removal of the synovium, or the tissue lining the joints. This is usually done for rheumatoid arthritis and reduces pain

and prevents joint damage. The effects of this form of surgery are not permanent as the synovium can regrow and the symptoms may reappear.

- Arthroplasty, or joint replacement: In this type of surgery, the damaged bone or joint tissue is removed and replaced with metal or plastic parts. Replacement can be of the entire joint (total arthroplasty) or a part of the joint (hemiarthroplasty). Arthroplasty is done for the knees, hips, shoulders, elbows, fingers, toes, ankles, and spine.

SIDE EFFECTS AND PATIENT ADHERENCE

While natural supplements are believed to be free of side effects, many do have some associated risks. Similarly, while surgery provides relief from the painful symptoms of arthritis, all surgical procedures entail inherent risks, for instance of infection or complications, and a long and slow recovery period. It is therefore very important that the arthritis patient is aware of the risks associated with both natural treatments and surgery and takes the required steps to prevent harmful side effects.

Chapter Eighteen

Addressing the Mental Aspects

Mental disorders are disturbances in the individual's psychological patterns that potentially have a strong bearing on thought processes and emotions. Such disorders are normally attached to distress and disability and may result in sensory or mental impairment strong enough to have a significantly adverse effect on a person's life. The effect of these disorders ranges from imperceptible to causing severe chronic disability.[1]

INTRODUCTION

Beginnings

Long ignored or deemed insignificant, mental health problems have gained a great degree of understanding and recognition from the general public over the past few decades. More disturbing is the predominance of mental illnesses among the general populace, irrespective of the prevalence of arthritis in the world today. The World Health Organization has discovered that an alarmingly high percentage (more than one-third) of people present in most countries have reported symptoms indicative of one or more of the common known mental illnesses.[2] This high figure holds true for the United States, where an estimated one in four Americans is diagnosed with a mental illness every year.[3] Even more surprisingly, this figure is relatively low, though it does not take into account substance disorders, which are recognized worldwide as a mental disorder.[4] The percentage of people actually suffering from mental disorders in the United States in a given year is roughly 32 percent, which amounts to about 75 million people (including those who have arthritis).[5] Mental disorders are slightly more common in women, with around 34 percent of all adult women meeting the criteria for diagnosis of one or more mental disorders, in contrast to almost 30 percent of all men.[6] Moreover, mental disorders are becoming a huge concern as they have been deemed the foremost cause of disability in the United States among the fifteen to forty-four age group. It is also worthwhile to note that roughly 45 percent of individuals with a mental disorder exhibit symptoms that meet the criteria for more than one disorder.[7]

Significance

Studies have determined that lifetime prevalence rates for any mental disorder go as high as roughly 60 percent.[8] This effectively means that more than one in every two Americans suffers from one form or another of mental disorder. This high prevalence of mental illnesses supplicates the link between possible mitigating factors of an arthritis patient's mental suffering. Furthermore, the implications of mental disorders must be considered when approaching arthritis holistically. These disorders are common among arthritis patients undergoing personal hardship. Dismay and stress are natural, especially when these hardships stretch over a long period or are intense. This holds particularly true in medical cases due to the stress and anxiety that often accompany a medical problem. It therefore comes as no surprise that individuals suffering from long-standing chronic illnesses also find themselves falling into the grips of one or more mental disorders. This can be a large problem as mental disorders can aggravate the situation.

HAPPINESS AT LARGE

An integral point made by researchers is that prolonged stress and anxiety hamper the ability of immune cells to respond to hormonal signals, which in turns results in promotion of a disease by inflammation.[9] These findings were supported by a separate study revealing that individuals with a positive outlook on life who experience little stress tend to have longer and healthier lives than people suffering from anxiety, depression, and a general lack of enjoyment of daily activities.[10] Detailed study and lab experiments involving both animals and humans have demonstrated a strong link between stress and poor health. Stress is found to have a direct correlation with a tendency toward heart disease, a weaker immune system, and a shorter life span. Negative mood states have also been consistently shown to be associated with slower healing and poorer immune response.[11]

More than the absence of negative emotions and their side effects is important here, however. Positive emotions and mental states have positive effects on physical health. Even though research is ongoing, the results achieved so far are substantial and significant. A detailed twenty-year study of over six thousand men and women aged twenty-five to seventy-four showed that emotional vitality (enthusiasm, hopefulness, engagement in life, and the ability to deal with stressors) had a distinct and measurable protective effect against coronary heart disease. [12] The researchers discovered that optimism reduces the chances of coronary heart disease by half. Similar studies have pointed toward happiness and optimism as boosting the immunity system and preventing disease. [13]

Having Arthritis and Staying Happy

Negative emotions can have strong negative impacts on the arthritis sufferers' abilities, responsibilities, and relationships, as well as how the patient looks at him- or herself. It is therefore very important for an individual to remain happy. This is primarily because being happy promotes stronger resilience in the individual's immune cells, ensuring that arthritis patients do not suffer from more diseases or illnesses. Furthermore, being happy permits arthritis sufferers to have a fresher outlook on life, and instead of succumbing to isolation, individuals lead a more involved existence. Happier individuals are usually more active in their daily lives, and this activity ensures constant exercising of muscles and thus prevents worsening of their condition. Happiness is a good safeguard against becoming a recluse and is therefore essential to maintaining strong and productive relationships over time. It is important to not cave in to negative emotions as they pave the way for a loss of optimism and hope. It is important for arthritis patients to remain happy to combat a potential sharp increase in frustration levels due to immobility and fatigue. These frustrations can be very destructive as an individual may take them out on loved ones, thereby straining relationships, or experience bursts of anger that hamper day-to-day life.

Sustaining Happiness as an Arthritis Patient

Staying happy is a lot easier said than done. How does an arthritis patient escape the daily nightmare that surrounds him or her? How does one shut out the harsh reality of everyday life and manage to maintain a positive outlook despite a plethora of reasons to feel despair? A lot of effort—both physical and mental—is indeed required, but as demonstrated above, sustaining happiness is essential for those combating arthritis. The most obvious solution is to turn to medication, as a number of available drugs help numb feelings of emotional pain and give arthritis patients a sense of elation. Studies show that these "happy pills" block pain signals to the brain. However, these pills do have a number of side effects and may not be the ideal solution. [14]

Perhaps the most important step arthritis patients can take to sustain happiness is remaining active. Keeping occupied prevents negative thoughts from entering one's head. Moreover, regularly exercising and keeping busy instills a sense that the individual's arthritis is not that bad. The sense of control this provides give patients confidence that they can win the battle with arthritis and thus enables a more positive outlook. [15]

SPECIFIC MENTAL OUTCOMES OF ARTHRITIS

Behavioral Problems

Upon first being diagnosed with arthritis, individuals at first often exhibit a high degree of shock. They seem numb to whatever medical staff tell them, and it may take them a while to come to terms with the diagnosis. Confusion is rampant in arthritis patients, especially the newly diagnosed. They are often not fully informed about the exact implications of their illness and at times exaggerate the condition in their minds, which leads to mental manifestations discussed shortly. An arthritis sufferer might fear the physical pain that they will experience, the medication they will have to take, and the effect on their personal, professional, and family lives, as well as the lives of those around them. Often overwhelming fear gives way to a host of mental illnesses. Arthritis patients exhibit a high degree of anxiety as they dwell on how the chronic illness will impact their lives. People exhibiting high degrees of anxiety often suffer from frequent panic attacks as they despair over their situation.

Depression and Arthritis

A cause of great concern is the high prevalence of mental disorders in arthritis patients. According to a 2012 report, a massive percentage of all arthritis patients suffer from depression. [16] Experts discovered that if pain resulted in a loss of mobility, the risk of depression was significantly larger. This trend was also common when the illness was seen to hamper an individual's social activities. Figures were significant for people with rheumatoid arthritis and osteoarthritis (37 and 33 percent, respectively). [17] Only half of these arthritis patients had sought treatment from mental health experts during the previous year. [18]

The connection between depression and arthritis has many layers. First, individuals experience a varying degree of pain due to both the type of arthritis and differences in pain thresholds. This pain may reach a level at which individuals become depressed because they no longer see it getting better and assume it will only get worse with time. Other physical side effects such as fatigue have also been strongly linked to depression. Depression may result in feelings of being alone in one's suffering, and this isolation can aggravate the individual's mental suffering. A patient may begin to feel hopelessness and despair, especially if things seem to worsen over time.

If an arthritis patient begins to suffer symptoms of depression, it is advisable to contact a mental health specialist at the earliest opportunity. In order to address this problem, one should first gain as much knowledge as possible to eliminate fear of the unknown. Furthermore, one should embrace the challenge of adopting a new lifestyle. This challenge need not be a bad thing and can be an exciting opportunity to explore new hobbies instead of dwelling on those one can no longer pursue. Instead of shutting themselves out, arthritis sufferers should ask for help whenever necessary, as healthy communication is beneficial to overcoming depression. It is also important to keep as active and busy as possible because staying occupied and living life a day at a time helps avoid dwelling too much on the future.[19]

Sadness and Arthritis

Sadness is a more normal and common trait in people with arthritis. Sadness is a natural feeling that accompanies loss, and unlike depression, it is not accompanied by a severe feeling of hopelessness and a decline in one's general level of interest or ability to experience pleasure. Sadness, however, can lead to depression if not properly addressed, so arthritis sufferers should ensure they are accepting of their ailment and adopt a positive outlook so that the bout of sadness may pass and they can be happy.[20]

Anxiety and Arthritis

Anxiety among individuals suffering from arthritis is even more alarmingly prevalent. A high figure—about 30 percent—reported symptoms of anxiety, with almost 85 percent of all people suffering from depression also suffering from anxiety.[21] Individuals normally experience anxiety when they start thinking about the effect arthritis may have on their lives. The level of anxiety tends to vary from individual to individual, but people suffering from anxiety tend to feel uneasy and unable to relax. They start worrying about everything from how their arthritis is causing them pain to how it will impact their jobs and the lives of family members. In extreme cases anxiety can manifest as panic attacks. In order to address anxiety disorders, arthritis patients should immediately contact counselors regarding relaxation techniques. Furthermore, they should try meeting any negative feelings head-on. Individuals should focus on lifestyle changes and how they can use physical activity and improvised exercises to tackle the challenges they face, as this will help mitigate the triggers of anxiety.[22] Patients can also turn to medication to help relax and attend stress-management programs.

Agitation and Arthritis

Agitation is a symptom also reported to go hand in hand with rheumatoid arthritis. Recent studies indicate that this correlation is not as strong as one would believe, with only about 200 in nearly 135,000 arthritis patients exhibiting agitation, according to one study.[23] It must be noted, however, that instances of individuals suffering from both conditions increase sharply with age as more than half of those two hundred were older than sixty. One must take note of the fact that two-thirds of individuals suffering from both afflictions are female.[24]

MENTAL STRESS AND ARTHRITIS

Stress Caused by Therapy

The arthritis sufferer should be wary of the mental disorders caused by therapy itself. Most of this stems from a fear of the unknown, a growing sense of hopelessness, and the need to take various medicines. In order to address the mental stress caused by therapy, patients must try to maintain healthy communication with their medical staff. They should try to obtain as much knowledge as they can about their condition so as not to imagine it is worse than it actually is. Furthermore, they should look positively at their medications as tools for their betterment rather than as evidence of their plight because a positive approach is vital in ensuring that they do not feel undue stress during their therapy.

Stress Caused by Long-term Treatment

Long-term arthritis treatment can result in individuals losing hope and developing depression and negative sentiments. Individuals diagnosed with arthritis should let go of their denial and accept that they will not be able to lead the lives they did before the diagnosis. They should instead restructure and redefine their lives with new activities and hobbies to keep themselves busy. It is also important to maintain to a social life. Arthritis patients should look to establish strong ties with others suffering from similar afflictions so that they do not feel isolated and can turn to someone they can relate to. It is important to not lose hope, and despair can be avoided by remaining as physically and socially active as possible so that patients always feel a semblance of control over their lives.[25]

Stress Caused by Symptoms

In order to combat the stress caused by the various symptoms of arthritis, patients should ensure that they take a proactive and positive approach to facing the numerous challenges the disease presents. They should first and foremost exercise regularly, within the bounds allowed by their ailment, to ensure that they remain active and do not feel that arthritis is getting the better of them. Furthermore, relaxation techniques such as breathing exercises and meditation should be employed to shift focus from arthritic symptoms and keep the mind from dwelling on problems. People with arthritis should get as much sleep and rest as needed because rest is vital to conserve energy. Contemplation is vital to isolate and identify various stressors, which can then be eliminated by developing a clearheaded and positive approach.

Chapter Nineteen

Exercises for Arthritis

Exercise has been touted over and over as vital to arthritis patients' staying healthy and fit. Still, the fact bears repeating to emphasize the importance of exercise, especially since those who are not ill can be complacent and stay sedentary until they get sick. Aside from decreased body fat and accompanying weight loss, other positive benefits of exercise include lowered risk of contracting diabetes, osteoporosis, cancers of the colon and breast, depression, dementia, and cardiovascular disease.

INTRODUCTION TO EXERCISES FOR ARTHRITIS

Exercise Even When in Good Health

Exercise helps improve (1) the range of motion in muscles and joints, (2) how the body breaks down food and fat to build substances that are crucial to the body, and (3) the delivery of oxygen through the blood to all parts of the body, resulting in increased endurance and a greater sense of well-being.

How Exercise Is Helpful for Virtually Any Disorder

When done right, exercise always provides positive effects to patients of any condition or disease, not just arthritis. Exercise itself may not cure or slow the disease, but the so-called happy hormones generated bring about a positive attitude and help minimize pain. In addition, the habits of focus, discipline, and multitasking cultivated by regular exercise help improve quality of life. Since exercise reduces the patient's chances of developing additional health problems and complications, it might help prolong life. A 2005 study that tracked more than three hundred patients with rheumatoid arthritis for a

239

period of two years found that a high-intensity weight-bearing program resulted in a significant decrease in the loss of bone-mineral density in participants' hips.[1] This means that proper exercise helps the arthritic patient fight weakening of the hips.

On the Intensity of Exercise

It might be self-evident, but it bears repeating that different types of exercise suit different types of people in different walks of life. The young may get away with sudden, intense physical exertion, but older people need longer warm-up and cooling-down exercises to gently bring up the heart rate prior to exercising and slowly bring down the blood pressure after activity. A youthful body is more energetic and more resilient to impact sports and sudden rises in heart rate and blood pressure, which may be why some athletes start young and retire early. That said, people in their fifties need not worry that it's too late to start exercising. A study done on men who started exercising between the ages of fifty and sixty showed that mortality rates for that age group were the same as for those who have been exercising their whole adult lives.[2]

When investigating how exercise affects men and women, studies vary in their results. In a study that searched for a link between gender, exercise intensity, and anxiety, men reported lower anxiety after performing low-intensity exercise and were more anxious after medium- to high-intensity exercise.[3] Women reported no change in anxiety levels. In another study that tracked the release of growth hormone in young adults with different levels of exercise intensity, women had higher secretions of growth hormone compared to men as the intensity of the exercise was increased.[4]

Results from Exercise as Compared to Age

Given that the body of an older patient is not as resilient as that of a younger one, exercise affects people differently. The human body starts to decline as it ages, with (1) weakening of bones, (2) degradation of joints, (3) loss of brain and muscle cells, (4) slower metabolism, and (5) deteriorating sense of balance. It is therefore imperative to exercise to slow the decline of the body and to prevent illnesses. Slower metabolism and hormonal changes make it difficult for the elderly to lose weight compared to the young. Older people are also not as active as younger people, which may be due to existing pain or illness or fear of injury.

CENTRALITY OF EXERCISE

A Reasonable Level of Exercise Is Central to Managing Arthritis

It is only natural for an arthritis patient to avoid exercising when in pain. Knowledge that the pain is sometimes caused by degenerated cartilage in the joints has given rise to the idea that exercise worsens arthritis—that much like a rope wears down and ultimately breaks when pushed and pulled consistently, so the cartilage wears down due to the pushing and pulling that happens when a person exercises. One study proved, however, that runners did not contract arthritis of the hip or knee more often than nonrunners.[5] Other experiments involving sixty-year-old men suffering from arthritis who were divided into three groups—those who were given health education, those who had weight training, and those who did aerobic exercise—showed that those who underwent weight training and aerobic exercise had improved disability scores after three months.[6] Even better, those in the aerobic exercise group had less knee pain. Other researchers found a connection between age and the vagus nerve function of the heart: vagus nerves worked better during exercise in those who had regular fitness regimens than in those who were sedentary.[7]

Graded exercise programs, where exercising starts out slowly and gradually increases in intensity over time, are effective and safe for patients with arthritis of the knees or hips.[8] When the body is jolted by extensive exercise caused by overaggression, symptoms and pain may worsen. Joints and muscles need motion in order to remain healthy. Arthritic joints and surrounding tissue stiffen due to prolonged inactivity and a sedentary lifestyle. Even if exercising may not slow or stop the progression of arthritis, it still carries enough benefits for arthritis patients to continue exercising. One reason is that arthritis patients who exercise note that they feel less pain and disability, according to experiments on arthritis patients who performed muscle-strengthening exercises and walking.[9] Exercising releases hormones called endorphins, which act as natural painkillers. Active arthritis patients can keep performing chores and stay independent longer than patients who are inactive. This may motivate patients to continue exercising.

Drawbacks of Overexercising

Exercise has to be done regularly to keep the body fit and maintain exercise's positive effects. Even elite athletes lose as much as half of their aerobic training capacity after a three-month break in training.[10] Those who are highly motivated in the beginning, however, frequently strain themselves by performing inappropriate exercises or exerting themselves too much, too soon, and too often. In some instances people become addicted to exercise and do not allow their bodies to rest. Clinical research suggests that overexercising causes more harm than good.[11] Aside from the inevitable muscle soreness and possible injuries, effects include depression, irritability, disturbed sleeping patterns, and loss of appetite. Worse, the immune system can be compromised due to fatigue caused by overtraining, leading to increased susceptibility to diseases, allergies, and infections. Women athletes who subject themselves to this regimen sometimes lose their menstrual function. Other athletes have lost bone density, which weakens the bones.[12]

BEST EXERCISES FOR JOINTS

Joints must be moved daily so that they are kept mobile. Exercises appropriate for arthritis sufferers ease joint pain and stiffness, improve joint flexibility and mobility, and strengthen surrounding muscles and tissues so that the joints have more support and stability. Moreover, regularly moving the joints aids the movement of nutrients to and waste products from the cartilage, the pliant material that cushions the ends of the bones and prevents them from rubbing against each other. The patient must be alert and self-aware when exercising. Pushing on despite muscle soreness and pain might be dangerous, for the patient will be prone to injury. Thirty minutes of exercise a minimum of three times a week is already valuable to the body. When needed, interspersing short periods of rest between sets of exercise is key. Three ten-minute walks are just as effective as a single thirty-minute walk. The patient must heed the warnings of the body and, when it is tired, let it rest. When the joints become inflamed or red or pain lasts for an hour or more after exercising, the patient must stop and report this to the doctor or physical therapist so that the exercise plan can be changed. If the patient is new to exercise, a trainer or instructor is necessary to make sure that the form is correct and the back is not strained.

Walking

Walking is by many standards the easiest exercise to do: it entails neither gym fees nor training. Walking assists with improving joint flexibility and endurance. After warming up, the arthritis patient can start by walking on a level plain. Hilly or steeply inclined plains or stairs will put extreme stress on the knees. Another form of exercise that will improve the quality of joints is walking in a pool or on the beach. The water provides a bit of resistance to the legs and body, but buoyancy makes the exercise gentle on the knees and hips. Exercising in warm water is most therapeutic for the affected areas. Patients need not know how to swim to engage in pool walking, but if the water is too deep for their liking, they can exercise in shallow areas. The usual depth is waist- or shoulder-deep water. Deeper water increases the difficulty level of the workout. For additional safety, exercising near a bar that can be gripped to avoid slipping is best. Another way to prevent falls is to wear rubber-soled footwear or aqua shoes with cushioning support for the legs, knees, and back. Aqua shoes are lightweight and dry quickly. Socks are unnecessary and disadvantageous because wet socks are heavy. A flotation or buoyancy belt might be useful to keep the body upright in shoulder-level water. To increase the intensity of the exercise, lifting the knees higher while walking backward and forward will aid immensely.

Swimming and Other Water Exercises

Hydrotherapy is a popular form of treatment for arthritis patients. It is also called water aerobics or aquatic exercise. These exercises can be performed in a pool, the common venue for water aerobics classes, or in a hot tub or spa at home, the size of which will determine the kind of movements the patient can make. When getting into the water, the patient must relax and allow the water to soothe the body. When ready, the patient can then slowly perform stretching, strengthening, or aerobic exercises. For patients who know how to swim, swimming is an effective way to exercise most parts of the body because the water makes it an almost nonimpact exercise. Patients would do well to experiment with different swimming styles until they settle on the one they are most comfortable with. As a general rule, the breaststroke is not suitable for those with arthritis in the hips or knees due to the required knee bending.

Stretching

Stretching exercises help the joints and muscles stay limber and the body flexible. A sedentary lifestyle with prolonged sitting and standing worsens joint and limb stiffness and deformities. Stretching exercises done in the morning are a good pick-me-up to revitalize the body in preparation for a new day. For all stretching exercises, extending the body enough to feel the stretch is recommended. The body must not be pushed too hard, and exercise must stop once pain or inflammation results from the workout. Raising the arms over the head, holding for a bit, then bringing the hands down is an easy exercise to get the blood moving more in the arms. For tight shoulders due to sleeping in one position for too long, rolling the shoulders up and down or making windmills with the arms will help them relax. To ease neck stiffness, it is advisable to turn the head to the left and hold for five seconds, turn the head to the right and hold for five seconds, turn the chin up and hold for five seconds, then turn the chin down and hold for five seconds. Rotating the head clockwise and counterclockwise also mitigates stiffness. A stretching exercise that engages the hips is to put the hands on the hips, bending at the waist to the left and holding for five seconds, straightening up, bending at the waist to the right and holding for five seconds, and straightening up.

Targeted stretching of the joints of the extremities can alleviate pain and rigidity in the fingers, toes, wrists, and ankles. These exercises can be done sitting down. One can open the hand and spread the fingers as far apart as possible, as though forming a star; hold for five seconds, then relax. Folding the thumb and each finger one at a time to form a fist, then unfolding each one at a time, like a blossoming flower, enhances the ability of each to move independently. Folding the hand to the wrist then straightening, as well as flexing then relaxing the foot, may remind the arthritis patient of an Egyptian dance move. Giving nicknames to exercises and movements might help the patient remember them so that building the habit of exercise becomes much easier.

Bicycle Riding

Patients who are fit can by all means ride their bicycles outdoors to enjoy the scenery and fresh air. Since mountain biking may be too stressful on the knees due to the rugged terrain, which forces the legs to push harder, biking recreationally on smooth, flat roads is best so that the body is not jarred and the knees do not have to absorb the effects of going over bumps. If outdoor biking is too tough on the patient, stationary and recumbent bicycles are a good alternative. This way, when feeling pain, the patient can stop any time to rest without worrying about timing, balance, or the possibility of a fall. Stationary and reclining bikes use the legs to pedal but keep weight off the knees and hips because the individual is seated. Another advantage is that the resistance can be tweaked to suit the capability and strength of the patient.

Strength-Training Exercises

Two types of strengthening exercises, isometric and isotonic, are added to the exercise plan depending on the severity of patient's condition and the type of arthritis. Isometric exercises do not require joint movements; only the muscles are used. These exercises are the best choice for patients who are unable to move their joints fully without feeling pain. A great upper-body isometric exercise is the handclasp: the patient clasps his or her hands, palms facing and pushing together to create pressure. Exercising the quadriceps muscles that surround the knees through isometric contractions will help patients with arthritis of the knees. Isometric quadriceps contractions are quite easy to do. The patient only needs to lie down on his or her back and work the quadriceps by trying to straighten the legs in the air. Isometric exercises are also recommended for those with arthritis of the neck. The patient places one palm against the back of the head, then the head presses into the palm while the palm resists, holding for five seconds. Succeeding sets are done by moving the palm to the forehead, then each palm to one side of the head above the ear for five counts on each side, then both palms to the cheeks.

Isotonic exercises entail joint movement. For example, the patient sits in a chair and raises the leg to knee level, then lowers it and repeats. In this exercise, the weight of the body and gravity create resistance. The patient can also try squeezing a tennis ball slowly and repeat as often as possible. This engages the joints of the fingers as long as the patient doesn't squeeze too hard. Other isotonic exercises are the partial chair squat and the leg press. The leg press is normally done using an exercise machine on which the legs push a weight away from the body. In a partial chair squat, a seated patient stands up, stretches the arms in front, then bends the knees slowly. This helps with the knee and hip endurance. Small free weights weighing one or two pounds can be used during exercises to turn the regimen up a notch. Exercise machines and elastic bands are also used.

Strengthening exercises can be done every day by a person suffering from arthritis. Consistent exercise brings reliable results and the full benefits of physical activity. The patient must make sure that breathing and movements are coordinated. There is no need to be extremely fast or to pick up heavy weights immediately. The body must ease into the exercise and maintain a smooth and steady rhythm. Bouncing movements and jerky motions should be avoided.

Chapter Twenty

Approaching Arthritis at Home

Home is obviously where the arthritis patient stays and lives. All the members of the household come together, interact, and rest, enjoying the camaraderie and happiness of being together. Medical disorders can rob one of a lot of that joy. Learning to live with arthritis can be tough. Leading a normal life is difficult, and family ties become strained because one family member has been stricken by the condition. People with arthritis become sensitive to their surroundings at home and dependent on the people around them.

SIGNIFICANCE

Family members at home can start to lose their finer feelings and, instead of helping their sibling, parent, or grandparent, exact emotional tolls. This happens when one does not have a full understanding of how to approach arthritis specifically at home. A condition such as arthritis targets the musculoskeletal system of the body. Arthritis affects all people, including men, women, and even children. This condition leads to pain and inflammation, accompanied by soreness and bruising in some cases, which may make it difficult for the patient to move around at home. More than 345 million people worldwide suffer from arthritis, and of these, 40 million are from the United States and include 225,000 children.[1] Arthritis in children can be treated if detected early, and despite being diagnosed with arthritis, children can expect to live a normal and full life. The reasons for arthritis are unknown, and so preventing occurrence of the condition, at home or in any other environment, is not possible.[2]

The movement of the arms and legs depends on the mobility of the joints for tasks ranging from taking a shower to going to bed. The joints are the places where the limbs meet, such as the ankles, wrists, hips, and knees. The bones are protected by the cartilage, which is flexible but deteriorates and becomes rigid after the onset of the disease. The synovial membrane covers the gaps between the two limbs, and synovial fluid provides lubrication. When arthritis sets in, these joints are affected.

Importance of Full Support

Arthritis must be monitored continuously. Infectious arthritis is caused by a bacterium, virus, or fungus, so this form of the condition definitely requires the full involvement of parents. The danger is that it can enter the bloodstream and infect other joints as well. Since arthritis is chronic and degenerative in nature, patients suffer increasing amounts of pain when performing sedentary activities, such as watching television. In some instances, patients respond to treatment. Combinations of legitimately prescribed drugs can help.

Arthritic Children at Home

Children diagnosed with juvenile arthritis (chapter 9) should attend school, take part in extracurricular activities, and socialize within and outside the family as normally as possible. There is a chance of recovery even if the child spends most of his or her time at home, and unless there is extensive damage, a normal routine is recommended. It is further recommended that the child engage in independent activities, such as going for a drive or working in part-time jobs. Children who have arthritis or live with an arthritis sufferer should maintain a positive attitude. Parents or guardians living at home should respond in a positive fashion. Physical activities of all kinds help. The therapist may use splints to help bind the joint so that any damage is avoided. Splints help avoid tightening of joints and deformities. Most people already suffering from one form of arthritis or another are susceptible to infectious or septic arthritis. Juvenile rheumatoid arthritis (JRA) is the arthritis present in children. Of the three types of arthritis present in children, systemic JRA is the least prevalent but most destructive. Pauciarticular JRA is least destructive, and the child will have pain in at most four joints. The third type of arthritis is polyarticular JRA, which affects more than four joints. This type of disease will get progressively worse as time goes on. If diagnosed early and treated properly, the child will grow up to be a healthy person as long as he does not spend all of his time at home. Emotional stress is greater among children suffering from arthritis. Their social lives are disrupted, and they must depend on others even for help with small things, such as carrying their books through the kitchen to the patio and climbing the stairs.[3]

Emotions of Arthritic Children at Home

One should avoid making life stressful for arthritis patients. Children especially find the going tough, and so care should be extended in the form of social-welfare counseling and physiotherapy. Social involvement should be maintained at all times. The best therapy includes full involvement of the child's friends and neighbors. Making the child participate in social activities like games and cultural events such as festivals is a good morale booster. One should ensure that the child is never overstressed. When interacting with the child, remember to behave in a normal fashion. Learning about the disease and its stages from the doctors treating the patient and the physiotherapist will help you put your social interaction with the patient on a sound footing.

TREATING ARTHRITIS AT HOME[4]

Children at Home and Arthritis Medication

Treatment deals with relieving symptoms and protecting the body from further damage. Proper medication in children with arthritis is necessary to see that there is no further spread of the disease. Medicines are used to fight infections since they are the most dangerous form of the spread of the disease. The rate of metabolism is controlled so that there is minimum spread of the disease, the action of drugs is maximized, and there is no resultant degeneration.

Alternative Methods at Home

Acupuncture

While this approach may not be permitted (legally or socially) at home, it is important to know how it works if the opportunity to perform it at home surfaces. Acupuncture therapy uses needles to relieve pain. The medians along the body are identified, and the flow of energy is redistributed. This kind of treatment relieves pain, but whether it will help the patient with arthritis is debatable. Sometimes the doctor may recommend this method to relieve pain when permissible at home.

Massage

While easily done at home, massage therapy should be performed by an expert experienced with arthritis patients. Massage will reduce the stress-producing chemicals and stimulate muscles and hormones. It thus improves sleep and metabolic activity.

Diet

Proper diet is vital for the arthritis patient. Food should be low in saturated fats, and more whole grains, fruits, and nuts should be added. Avoid oily and salty foods, which can increase inflammation of the joints.

Exercises at Home

This is best for growing children. Even elderly patients can benefit from this. Movement improves muscle tone and reduces tension accumulated in the body.

Yoga and Meditation

These bring calmness and help relieve stress. Tensions in the body are automatically reduced. Joining meditation groups will give the patient an additional sense of sharing and belonging. This helps in the healing process.

Conventional Treatment of Arthritis at Home

Treatments use emerging drugs. When comparing injected and oral disease-modifying antirheumatic drugs (DMARDs) and corticosteroids, there is no appreciable difference in the trials conducted using oral DMARDs such as methotrexate, leflunomide, and sulfasalazine. There is some evidence, although not much, of increased clinical response rates to combination therapies using methotrexate and biological DMARDs.[5] Recognizing the symptoms is the first step to treating the disease. Common arthritis symptoms suffered at home include joint pains, which can present either shortly or long after the use of nonarthritis medication. There may be persistent pain or just tenderness, and the joint itself may be sore. Sometimes the joint may be stiff or sore after some period of inactivity. Lumps may form around the joint in the case of osteoarthritis. Most joints in the body, including those of the hands, hips, spine, and knees, are susceptible to infection. The advantage of being at home when drug-related side effects happen is that the arthritis patient can find a place to rest right away.[6]

Conventional treatment at home includes salicylates and nonsteroidal anti-inflammatory drugs (NSAIDs). Common NSAIDs given are naprosyn and tolmetin. At times ibuprofen (approved for small children) is also given. The dosage is based on the patient's body weight. These NSAIDs should be taken with food as they have a tendency to cause severe gastrointestinal disturbances. If the disease is very severe, then surgery is performed. Treatment is done through the use of corticosteroids and disease-modifying agents such as injectable gold, methotrexate, and sulfasalazine.[7]

Treatment, whether at home or elsewhere, helps with the control of symptoms, prevention of damage to joints, and maintenance of normal body function. DMARDs are used as a second line of treatment in cases where there is no response to NSAIDs. Among DMARDs, methotrexate and leflunomide are very common. The most recently developed medicines, the biologics, are anti–tumor necrosis factor agents (etanercept, abatacept, infliximab, and tocilizumab).

Infants at Home

Infants get arthritis from medical disorders that are mostly genetic in nature. Through early diagnosis and prompt treatment, many processes are aborted. The infant's skeleton in its initial phases has good potential for adaptation.[8] Since infants are unable to express their discomfort or illness verbally, one should be on the lookout for symptoms of arthritis such as high temperatures (102 or 103 degrees Fahrenheit or higher), development of reddish marks on the body, and restlessness. Infections and the use of certain drugs can also cause onset of the condition.

Once the child is identified as having the disease, treatment should begin immediately. Elimination of other diseases with similar symptoms is also necessary. Many children are fully cured, and there is no more manifestation of the disease in their adult lives. Regular consultation among the infant's pediatrician and other health professionals is essential. In this manner it is possible to communicate any progress in the treatment of the disease. Any change in the patient's condition will also be conveyed to the doctor, who will have the advice of experts.

Toddlers at Home

For effective treatment of arthritis in toddlers, one relies on evaluation of orthopedic and genetic conditions as well as physical findings. Radiographs and biopsies help determine the scope and nature of treatment to be followed. The symptoms of JRA are very distinct. The patient will develop high fever, often in the range of 103 degrees Fahrenheit or more, and a skin rash will keep appearing and disappearing. Treatment usually consists of NSAIDs and DMARDs if necessary. The combination of drugs such as methotrexate with NSAIDs, the first line of medicines, seems to produce better results. Systemic JRA encompasses nearly 10 percent of all known cases of childhood arthritis.[9] The peak onset period is between one and five years. The likelihood of occurrence is equal for both male and female toddlers, and it may be polyarthritis or oligoarthritis. Systemic JRA is characterized by persistent intermittent fever with one or two daily temperature spikes greater than 101 degrees Fahrenheit. Transient, nonpruritic rash is seen on the trunk. Other multisystemic clinical involvement may include the following:

- Pericarditis
- Hepatosplenomegaly
- Acute phase reactants
- Leukocytosis
- Growth delay
- Anemia
- Diffuse lymphadenopathy
- Pleuritis
- Osteoporosis or osteopenia

Use of DMARDs or conventional therapy using NSAIDs is recommended for the toddler, who remains largely at home. Tests have shown methotrexate to have a superior effect among nonbiological DMARDs. Even when the action mechanisms differed (anakinra, etanercept, and adalimumab) and comparators varied, there was reduced risk of flare-ups. NSAIDs may be used in conjunction with intra-articular corticosteroids. These drugs may be used with or without methotrexate mostly for treating toddlers with JRA. Randomized discontinuation trials have suggested that continued use of drugs help reduce the possibility of flare-ups.[10]

Schoolchildren at Home

The incidence of JRA is greater in females than in males and usually occurs after age eight. Growth retardation is predominant with early closure present in the epiphyseal plates; the onset of swelling is gradual, with stiffness involving the cervical spine and the hips. More than five joints are involved in the initial six months itself. Polyarticular JRA is chronic and erosive. The prognosis is worst when the disease is unremitting. There may be no occurrence of uveitis but formation of subcutaneous nodules. It is best that schoolchildren with arthritis maintain their regular activities and take part in all school functions. They should not be given the opportunity to feel left out, because a decrease in morale may affect the healing process. For children who need an attendant, one should choose only those who are well qualified to deal with any emergencies that may arise.

Use of infliximab on a long-term basis with methotrexate for treating JRA is well tolerated. Many patients in one study did not feel any improvement in their physical condition and stopped using infliximab. This drug is safe and effective. In polyarticular JRA, the treatment is similar to that described above. A combination of NSAIDs and DMARDs is used. DMARDs are used only when NSAIDs are ineffectual. The drugs should be taken only with food.

Adolescents at Home

Arthritis is caused by rheumatic diseases, dermatomyositis, rheumatic fever, or other vasculitic syndromes.[11] Malignancies and infections can also cause arthritis. Identifying the disease early is essential for effective treatment of the patient. Treatment, as described above, consists of combination drug therapy, which is found to be more effective. When the disease is identified early, chances of the patient's complete recovery and continuation of a healthy life are good. In all cases, the patient should follow treatment up with physical therapy. Splints may be used when the pediatrician feels that damage to the joint is imminent. Otherwise, the child should do what other children are doing and follow the same routines. This will improve the child's mental attitude, and he or she will discover that togetherness gives a lot of strength. Encouragement from parents and school friends is helpful to the effectiveness of the treatment. Strict adherence to diet and regular administration of medicines is necessary.

ROLE OF FAMILY MEMBERS

Initial Approaches

The physiotherapist should educate family members about necessary exercises and dietary regulations. Keeping the child in good physical health, from the family members' perspective, involves regular exercises, outward social mobility, and proper diet. Since the disease is progressive and the body is growing, it is necessary to inhibit the disease without affecting the metabolic progress of the healing process. This is done through a series of exercises designed to help the arthritis patient live a normal life. It is important to keep the physiotherapist informed about the progress of the arthritis sufferer. In cases where the patient is in need of an attendant, or if the disease is severe, a social worker should be consulted and possibly asked to meet with family members at home. This will help in orienting the patient better.

Family Relationships at Home

A person suffering the symptoms of arthritis at home must endure the rigor of living with the pain and difficulty of ordinary day-to-day activities. Understanding this will help family members develop strong bonds with the patient. If there are still some difficulties, one should ask for help from a physiotherapist or psychologist, who will have seen a lot of situations the patient is likely to encounter and be able to provide valuable advice. It is necessary for family members to be emotionally and psychologically bonded to the arthritis sufferer when home at all times. Sometimes the child may become confused or disoriented; being there for him or her is the main thing. Once the child has the confidence that family is there, he or she will begin to grow in confidence.

It is a good idea to involve the patient in various tasks or chores around the house. This will boost his or her morale and also help make the atmosphere of the house lively and cheerful. Doing things for the other members of the family will raise enthusiasm and encourage the patient, especially an arthritic child, to do a lot more than he or she normally does. Naturally, one should be careful to see that the child only does what is within the limits of what the doctor has advised. Family members who have a strong relationship with the arthritic child will more willingly arrange get-togethers, but one should be careful not to overstress the child. By increasing the child's social interaction, close family members give him or her a chance to build stronger bonds with friends and neighbors.

ATMOSPHERE AT HOME

Discussions

Family members must find time to discuss whether there are other ways of helping the patient. Sharing chores will help ease the burden. They should provide opportunities for the patient to be socially active and let the latter get in touch with other children who have arthritis so that they can share experiences and understand how others cope with the disease. While discussions regarding the seriousness of the disease are to be avoided in the house or in front of the patient, it is necessary for family members to have a complete understanding of the condition. Talking to the physician or other health-care professionals regularly will help. Family members who discuss arthritis-related matters should talk to the patient and try to understand his or her point of view. This will not only help maintain a comfortable atmosphere but also help the patient express difficulties more clearly.

Direct Factors

Nature of the Disorder

Of the three types that affect the child, systemic JRA is the most serious. Therefore, it is important for people at home to know the living environment of the JRA patient. Degeneration of the joints occurs rapidly, and as time goes on, the patient suffers more. Patients suffering from this kind of disease need to be accompanied by an attendant, especially if the disease is advanced, as it is dangerous to leave them unattended. Pauciarticular JRA does not cause much pain, and symptoms, when they manifest, are minimal. Such patients can be allowed out alone and encouraged to do things independently. Patients with polyarticular disease will have to consult doctors and physiotherapists regarding what they can do and the extent of involvement they are expected to have. Depending on the seriousness of the disease, the doctors will advise them as to whether they can remain without an escort and should participate in games and sports.

Type of Treatment

Pauciarticular JRA requires a lot of physiotherapy. The body's skeletal system is growing and can easily repair itself. One should be careful not to hurt the joints through excessive movements. Medicines should be taken regularly and as prescribed. Social activities and games are required for children in the formative stages of growth. Social interactions also help improve the mental strength and confidence of the child.

Dietary Factors

Foods need not always be cooked separately for arthritic people. They can eat what the family eats but should continue to take supplements prescribed by the doctor. These will improve the chances of the body's recovering through its own repair mechanisms. Many medicines need to be taken with food because of the reaction they cause in the gastrointestinal system.

Indirect Factors

Economic Stability

The financial status of the household will affect the mental well-being and psychological attitude of the child with arthritis. If there is any stress, the child will develop an attitude that may not help in the recovery process. In the event this happens, a psychologist could be consulted and a clear-cut solution found before the child's treatment begins. Psychological evaluation of the child will help doctors and parents determine the nature of the support the child requires. Having too much comfort also may reduce the child's desire to take the initiative, which may impede the growth factor. One should make sure that the child's enthusiasm is always on the rise.

Social Interaction

Encourage the child to take part in get-togethers and celebrations. More than ordinary children, those with JRA need to keep their spirits up. Taking part in functions will encourage them to strengthen social interactions with their neighbors and friends.

Community Functions

Many community functions such as festivals and religious ceremonies will help arthritis patients maintain strong a mental attitude.

Arthritis-Related Stress at Home

Arthritis as a condition is not always well understood in social circles. When people see others moving slowly or waiting, they tend to assign different meanings to these behaviors. An arthritis patient becomes the target of gossip, which can lead to unpleasant situations. People living with the arthritis sufferer should be understanding, cope with the situation, and make family life pleasant. If the patient is a child, one way is to invite other children affected by arthritis to the house. This will help everyone in the family understand and appreciate how other children are living with the condition. Some camps tell one everything about the disease and how to cope with situations that may emerge. Regular discussions among family members keep everyone's spirits high. Some family members may feel shy about expressing their feelings about situations they have been through. Talking will likely eliminate misunderstandings and increase confidence levels.

Chapter Twenty-One

Finding Motivation

Motivation is essential to an individual's personal life simply because it provides the energy and confidence to move. With motivation, it is easy to attain goals and accomplish tasks because the determination to achieve is present. Motivation is also essential in the arthritis patient's workplace because it can generate productivity.[1] Motivation also ensures higher-quality performance and initiative.[2]

POSITIVITY AND MOTIVATION

People experiencing arthritis may refuse to work out regularly, as the exercise itself requires great effort and they fear pain or further harm to an already fragile joint. Arthritis sufferers might also feel let down and try to isolate themselves due to low self-esteem and anxiety. When they are elderly and have accepted that arthritis is largely part of aging, they may be reluctant to do something about the problem. Refusal or reluctance to exercise is also brought on by physical barriers, such as difficulty walking, grasping, standing, bending, and lifting heavy objects.[3] According to a 2006 study, nearly 40 percent of people with arthritis do no exercise, while the remainder either perform strengthening exercises or other exercises of a serious or moderate nature.[4] The motivation of people with arthritis to exercise is vital, as exercise can lessen episodes and the pain itself. People who exercise also have a more positive attitude about their own health and being wholesome.

ROADBLOCKS

Pain Factors

It is not always easy to fortify oneself against the pitfalls of arthritis; thus arthritis patients may inadvertently barricade themselves against achieving motivation. The first thing to consider for a person with arthritis is the pain he or she is dealing with, which can impede motivation. The patient might feel discouraged by the physical pain or fear breaking a bone or exacerbating pain. Finding the motivation to fight the pain will help families, caregivers, and people suffering with arthritis. An active person who regularly exercises can tolerate and adapt to pain, thereby improving mobility. Patients who do not exercise regularly comment on the pain and feel that they are physically unable to cope, which discourages them from even trying to work out.[5]

Lifestyle

A busy life can also make finding motivation difficult for arthritis patients. There is so much stress that overall health, as well as the drive to exercise, may be put aside. There are so many things to do in a twenty-four hour period, and fatigue is inevitable, so there is not much time for exercise. Free time might be allotted to finishing other tasks, resulting in (1) cramming, (2) lack of rest or sleep, and (3) diminished energy levels. Occupational stress in arthritis patients can be triggered by deadlines, extensive work hours, heavy workloads, workplace bullying, and "toxic" environments.[6] Getting fit and fighting arthritis might be the lowest priority for these patients. Workplace stress can also be accompanied by emotional stress due to anxiety about meeting deadlines, getting along with coworkers or bosses, and fatigue. This is again connected with depression, which is known to decrease motivation. Patients need the motivation not only to confront arthritis but also to work hard and achieve certain goals.

Deprivation

According to a major report from 2010,[7] around 8 percent of people between the ages of eighteen and forty-four have reported doctor-diagnosed arthritis, while approximately 30 percent of people age forty-five to sixty-four have noted doctor-diagnosed arthritis. Of persons sixty-five and older, 50 percent have doctor-diagnosed arthritis. Arthritis occurs mostly in senior citizens, and "ageism" at times interferes with motivation. Ageism is defined as stereotyping of and discrimination against the elderly because of their age.[8] Age bias can fall into the positive or negative category. "Positive" in this case refers to a more generous and kind attitude toward the elderly, while "negative" basically refers to identifying the old as sick, mentally deficient, or weak. Because of this, senior citizens encounter psychological and physical deprivations, such as the following:[9]

- Mandatory early retirement or being phased out (replaced) by younger employees
- Difficulty with public transportation, especially on busy days
- Limited supportive education, which makes it difficult to overcome various technological barriers
- Denial of access to elder employees to education programs
- Devalued contributions
- Vast limitations on freedom and life choices
- Lack choices and privileges
- Discrimination in decision making

Some people are kinder to the elderly because of the negative view of the latter that is apparently engraved into society. No matter what, negativity should never hinder elderly arthritis patients looking for motivation, as they should remain active despite their aging bodies. Good health is their human right. Legal rights such as those rendered by the Age Discrimination in Employment Act of 1967[10] protect older Americans from discrimination on the job, as long as they fit the job description and can do the work properly. The act also gives seniors the right to receive pensions in old age after retirement. Lack of motivation can be expected, despite this legislation, as seniors may not only be suffering from arthritis; they may have other disorders such as depression and anxiety, coupled with possible expectations of death.

Relationships and Difficulty Finding Motivation

Disruptive relations with caregivers and family members are another potential roadblock. Disruptive relations are associated with prolonged depression, which can decrease motivation and increase a tendency to relapse.[11] Family intervention plays a noteworthy role in the treatment and recovery process, and negative interactions with family and friends pose a great risk for (1) physiological malfunctioning, (2) depression, (3) mood and anxiety disorders, (4) cancer,[12] (5) diabetes,[13] (6) coronary heart disease,[14] (7) stroke,[15] and (8) death.[16] In some cases family and friends may not believe the patient is sick, and medical attention might not be sought immediately. This might prolong or complicate the illness. Unsupportiveness not only leads to physical limitations and other maladies but can arise from too much help, such that the patient does not find the motivation to recover and depends on family and friends instead. In that regard, overly optimistic comments, not pushing the patient to be more independent, and overprotectiveness are somewhat unsupportive.[17] Essential motivation soon weakens as arthritis patients feel help-less and believe that loved ones cannot support them in the long run.

HOW TO GET MOTIVATED AS AN ARTHRITIS PATIENT

Healthy Approaches

A lifestyle involving regular physical activity and a healthy diet is essential in enhancing both physical and mental health and can play an important role in maintaining the motivation to fight arthritis. Physical activity can keep the muscles surrounding the affected joints strong, decreasing bone loss and controlling joint swelling and pain. It also enhances stamina and energy by improving sleep and reducing fatigue. According to studies, a combination of modest weight loss and moderate exercise leads to better overall improve-ment in pain and mobility for overweight or obese arthritis patients.[18] As arthritis keeps sufferers from moving freely to the optimal extent, it is likely that they will become overweight or obese. A healthy lifestyle can promote weight loss and long-term weight management.[19] Such a lifestyle can also reduce the risk of heart disease, diabetes, high blood pressure, colon and breast cancer, and premature death.[20] Healthy individuals are reported to save money as they make less frequent trips to the doctor or hospital, pay less for prescription drugs, and are at less risk for surprise medical expenses.[21] Studies prove that people who lack financial problems find motivation with more ease. Healthy lifestyle is also psychologically beneficial[22] as it can (1) decrease symptoms of depression, such as the feeling that life is not worth-while, (2) boost the overall level of spirit, (3) remove anxiety factors such as restlessness and tension, (4) help alleviate malaise, and (5) improve sleep. Motivation has given people suffering with arthritis a positive attitude and a more active social life.

Self-esteem Approach

Another way to get motivated is by retaining and boosting self-esteem, which is said to be an actual human need. Psychologist Abraham Maslow included self-esteem in the hierarchy of needs. He also argued that there are two forms of esteem: outer and inner. The outer form pertains to the combination of personal self-respect and respect from others.[23] Related topics include whether arthritis patients have self-confidence or value themselves. Self-esteem can do the following for arthritis sufferers and their caregivers:[24]

- Set the difference between success and failure
- Affect thinking, resulting in a positive or negative outlook
- Affect confidence

- Give value to the self
- Enable the right attitude to succeed
- Promote happiness

Self-confidence is important as it gives a person the determination to do things and might affect self-esteem. Valuing one's self and actions can boost one's morale. Self-esteem is important for ill patients such that a healthy outcome depends on coping strategies and self-esteem. The help of family and peers lessens stress and the inability to adjust easily to situations and environments, decreasing the chance of suicide.[25]

Optimism versus Pessimism

Thoughts and emotions strongly affect motivation. When the mind of the individual suffering from arthritic pain thinks it is capable of exercising for an hour, the individual believes he or she can perform that action. The body then responds by engaging physically in such action. An individual who does not have this belief might not exercise for a full hour. This is an example of how the mind influences a patient's perceptions of and reactions to things in life, which determines how satisfied he or she will be. Emotional intelligence is also achieved by attaining goals and controlling negative thoughts and emotions. If negative thoughts and thinking habits are left unmanaged, pessimism will control the life of an arthritis patient who would otherwise try to find motivation.[26] One study showed that negative thinking is associated with unhealthy patterns of physiological functioning, while optimism is associated with healthy patterns of physiological functioning of the cardiovascular and immune systems.[27] Optimism boosts the immune system such that there is a decline in sickness. Moreover, arthritis patients and caregivers who are pessimistic about their condition suffer depression and anxiety and soon become less motivated to fix the problem. In the end, the patient's health declines. An optimistic person, however, exhibits a healthy body and mind and is more likely to find enough motivation to ward off illness and exercise frequently.

Second Opinions and Motivation

Half of all Americans do not get a second opinion from doctors. In 30 percent of medical cases, getting a second opinion can alter the treatment plan and even the diagnosis.[28] In some cases previously undiagnosed illnesses are discovered. Second opinions boost the patient's motivation as they provide reassurance that an illness really exists and the diagnosis is correct. Once the arthritis sufferer accepts the diagnosis, motivation will come much easier.

5

Wrap-up

Chapter Twenty-Two

Collective Efforts

A disease or condition such as arthritis should be approached collectively for the reason that severe suffering from a malady cannot be alleviated easily by patients alone or only by the people surrounding them. At this point the patient cannot handle emotional stress well and will need all the support possible.

SIGNIFICANCE AND FOCUS OF COLLECTIVE APPROACHES

Magnitude of the Problem

Another reason for a collective approach to this chronic illness is its high prevalence. In the United States 50 million people have arthritis, and the number is likely to increase in the future, making arthritis a common disability among US residents. Arthritis may influence a patient's lifestyle for a lifetime. Knee arthritis can cause serious pain, and individuals who have had past knee injury or are obese are at increased risk for it. Arthritis can also result in severe financial damage due to hospitalizations and outpatient visits, not to mention lost earnings and other indirect costs. Social support, whether financial or physical (e.g., driving a patient to the clinic), can be very helpful to a patient of any medical condition, not just arthritis. Arthritis is nevertheless a big contributor to multiple chronic conditions and is associated with a decline in life expectancy, such that almost half of arthritis patients also have another underlying illness. Moreover, diabetic and heart disease patients commonly have arthritis.[1] These are some of the reasons to why arthritis should not be ignored and must be approached collectively.

Social Aspects

Social isolation faced by arthritis sufferers is one of the condition's greatest concerns, as these patients often find it difficult to open up to others, including other patients. Social support is very important since the absence of interpersonal relationships affect fatigue and place limitations on the sufferer that can result in dependence.[2] If left to cope alone, the arthritis patient may make poor judgments and take actions that lead to complications or development of another disorder. It is important that a patient seeks dependence and garners strength from surrounding individuals, as well as help from government and arthritis interest groups.

A Word or Two about Focus Groups

Health focus groups, which are initiated by the marketing departments of medical companies, are an excellent way to gather basic qualitative feedback on health-care issues. Multiple individuals are gathered together for a group interview or discussion on a certain topic such as arthritis. This technique is used to investigate the topic more or discover new themes. Focus groups are likely to target people of different age groups. Feedback from physicians and hospital administrators is also valuable.[3]

Problems Solved

An arthritis focus group can be convened to (1) face complex problems, (2) clarify existing issues, (3) quickly dispense opinions, beliefs, and ideas, (4) extract rich and raw information so long as it is accurate, and (5) sustain the need for thinking with others about not only unfamiliar ideas but also known topics for further understanding and development of patients' perspectives on arthritis. When there is a need to scrutinize the points of view of patients or others belonging to a group, ideas can be tested within a focus group to determine practicality.[4] For instance, a focus group about cervical cancer might hold a group discussion and, at the end, come up with the idea that screening for cervical cancer should be incorporated into everyone's life as a formal routine. Participants may not realize that a pap smear plays a big role in early detection of cervical cancer, but fear and fatalism are the dominant reactions to cancer in general. In spite of this, the group might still agree that early detection and diagnosis leads to a better prognosis for cervical cancer sufferers.[5]

Information gathered in arthritis focus groups might include needs, history, concerns, reactions, perceptions, and behavioral issues. These focus groups can also help with the following:

- Learning in advance how the population will react to methods, policies, and services
- Discerning problems, limitations, costs, and benefits
- Setting priorities for everyone, including the facilitator or host
- Attaining a more comprehensive plan
- Stimulating logical thinking about potential solutions, opportunities, and linkages that can identify future or possible impacts of arthritis
- Gathering a more accurate understanding of cultural or social factors that differ from the facilitator's opinion and perception
- Collecting feedback faster, as multiple individuals are available at once
- Gathering public input in less time, with fewer meetings and more focused agendas[6]

Arthritis focus groups are an ideal method for examining the stories, experiences, opinions, beliefs, practices, needs, and concerns of an individual. The groups permit participants to develop questions and frameworks as well as to voice their own needs and concerns in their own words. The groups also allow researchers to access different communication forms used in day-to-day interaction. Being able to access the diverse knowledge and attitudes of participants plays a vital part in the outcome of the discussions.

A FURTHER LOOK INTO FOCUS GROUPS

Advantages

Arthritis focus groups have additional advantages over attempts to address all of one's arthritis-related problems alone. Focus groups are inexpensive and can be flexible in terms of format, types of questions, and desired outcomes. The groups are also relatively easy to assemble as they have to take place within a certain population. Groups are easy to conduct because the interactions are similar to those of day-to-day conversations. Arthritis groups allow participants to confirm their contributions to the group because of the open form of talking and listening. Direct interaction between researchers and participants provides accurate and rich data with the facilitator asking a question and participants brainstorming about ideas and answers. The data is rich and accurate because participants have firsthand experience of the topic and can contribute largely to the knowledge of facilitators and group members. As participants are not required to answer every question, group members are able to build on one another's responses. New professional and personal connections develop as people help each other release ideas via brainstorming. Individuals build confidence in each other by instigating positive verbal and physical responses.

Limitations

While there are advantages, there are also drawbacks in terms of accuracy and quantity. Findings may not be that accurate. A limited number of individuals comprise a single arthritis focus group. This may mean the group represents a larger population but some people's concerns are neglected in meetings due to the small number of participants. Members' ability to handle various roles that people might normally play in society, but which might be absent in self-care, is required. Examples include being nonviolent, friendly, and quiet and coping with outsiders. Arthritis groups also require good facilitation skills. Data compilations might be difficult to analyze scientifically because they are unstructured (relative to clinical investigations) and based on emotions.[7]

Censoring, conflict avoidance, conformance, and other unexpected reactions need to be addressed in light of proper data analysis and might not generate desired results.[8] Moreover, the output can be biased as the arthritis focus group can be influenced by one or two dominant participants in the session, preventing submissive members from airing their opinions and leading them to submit to the dominant members' views. Simply put, not all participants can express their feelings on a sensitive topic due to social and emotional background. The group setting can also influence participants' behavior.[9] This might in turn hinder their emotional outlet, and certain concerns might go unvoiced. The possible dissemination of (inaccurate) scientific theories that would otherwise be clinical facts is a noteworthy limitation of arthritis focus groups. Negativity on the side of the participants, as well as the lack of a guarantee that certain verbiage will remain confidential within the group, are additional limitations.

A TOP-LEVEL AFFAIR

Action Plans

Organizations can add to the collective arthritis efforts by sponsoring tests for optimal methods. An example is using the International Classification of Functioning, Disability, and Health (ICF) core set to gain arthritis patients' perspectives about their illness. A focus group in this case is used to understand the aspects of functioning health that are important to arthritis patients. It can accomplish this using two approaches: the open approach and the ICF-based approach. Of the two, the ICF core set is more appropriate than the open approach[10] and is effective in focus groups. Problems can be easily diffused and acknowledged by testing methods and techniques that can lead to an improving patient pool and better outcomes of arthritis focus groups.

Nonprofit organizations provide medical information, physician referrals, guidebooks such as this volume, brochures, and other resources to give patients in-depth knowledge about arthritis and how to live with it. Aside from publishing magazines,[11] nonprofit entities organize exercise classes, year-round events,[12] and fund-raisers to create awareness.[13] Nonprofit organizations such as the Arthritis Foundation have invested in research about arthritis, generating new ideas for "miracle drugs"[14] and even organizing advocacy summits.[15]

The government needs to take more action to limit the growing number of arthritis cases and prioritize arthritis as a public health issue. The government has acted on arthritis using three national agencies: (1) the Centers for Disease Control (CDC), (2) the Arthritis Foundation, and (3) the Association of State and Territorial Health Officials. These organizations are joining together to come up with a strategy to deal with the public health challenges of arthritis. The collaboration, known as the National Arthritis Action Plan (NAAP), links government agencies, volunteer organizations, academic institutions, interest groups, and associations to work toward the prevention and control of arthritis. The CDC has its own arthritis program with a team of full-time public health experts. The CDC has addressed the leading causes of disability and how to improve quality of life, which in turn has made arthritis a health issue addressed on a national, collective level. While the Arthritis Foundation and CDC have helped with the issue of funding, the NAAP has developed proposals and public health programs on arthritis. A conference titled "Building Partnerships to Address Arthritis" was held by the Arthritis Foundation, which continues to receive numerous proposals for developing health awareness about arthritis and reducing the burden of the condition. This allows for grants in several states (1) to establish and develop arthritis programs, and (2) to build partnerships among national agencies and interested organizations.[16]

Moreover, the CDC has also led in strategic public health effort to promote well-being, prevention of arthritis and other chronic diseases, and balanced health. It partners with state health departments to improve states' ability to monitor the status of arthritis, promote illness control and prevention, and expand interventions by collaborating with existing health-care delivery systems. Collaboration in the line of policy and system changes has also been a priority of the CDC as it is a member and sponsor of the Osteoarthritis Action Alliance, which promotes recommendations about approaching arthritis. The CDC and Arthritis Foundation, through the Osteoarthritis Action Alliance, have reduced the burden of osteoarthritis through strategies that address self-management education, physical activity, prevention of further injury, and management of weight.

It is helpful to apply for Social Security assistance as an arthritis sufferer. If the Social Security Administration denies the initial application, a medical professional such as a doctor can give a statement about the arthritis sufferer's condition for use as evidence at a hearing. [17]

A HELPING HAND

When Influence Matters

It is important for an arthritis sufferer to receive empathy from another patient. Arthritis is an ailment that requires collective sympathy, and patients need someone they can relate to and learn from. At every stage, the patient will have questions and concerns that are difficult to answer or resolve. Support groups in which patients reach out to other arthritis sufferers for collective support are beneficial in giving patients somebody to talk to. Individuals suffering from arthritis can discuss ideas for coping with the general symptoms of the illness. This is better if partnered patients talk weekly so as to share thoughts and insights [18] associated with arthritis. If the patient can feel localized pain, the other patient has likely felt it too. The two can help each other since the latter gives advice and support for the former's pain. This improves patient confidence on both sides.

On Patient-to-Patient Interaction

Arthritis patients can give each other advice about preventing pain from reoccurring and living with the disorder. Patient-to-patient advice can help arthritis sufferers evaluate attitudes developed from personal experiences and recognize growth over the time. Giving off positive vibrations and affirmation increases good vibrations and boosts emotion, not only for the patient being affirmed but also for the one providing the affirmation. Sharing ideas and expectations about treatment might ease making treatment-related decisions. [19] Reaching out to other sufferers can give the arthritis sufferer a positive outlook on the following:

- Bringing in a friend who can serve as an emotional outlet and learning from shared experiences
- Volunteering and helping someone else to enlarge the group so that patients feel they have more reinforcement
- Organizing a get-together with patients for a movie or other indoor activity
- Going out with a friend for lunch or coffee (or perhaps setting up a tea party)
- Letting "buddy patients" meet relatives and meeting theirs
- Playing cards together
- Going for a walk with a friend who also suffers from arthritis

- Setting up a dinner date
- Joining clubs or taking classes that can let the patient experience new surrounding and meet new people
- Keeping a pet together
- Reminding each other of bad habits that need to be corrected and eradicating negativity that may cause loss of hope[20]
- Exercising together
- Attending arthritis events held by nonprofit organizations

The arthritis sufferer gains by building new relationships and meeting new friends. This not only elicits comfort and assurance but also boosts confidence, positivity, and hope. For the sufferer of arthritis or any chronic disorder, life can be very fragile and irritating. Not only do patients have the power to lift the spirits of other patients with shared experience, but also the support of the family and others. This can be very helpful, allowing patients to feel loved and accepted whatever the severity of their arthritis.

Chapter Twenty-Three

Conclusion

For the sake of well-being, it is important for the arthritis sufferer to overestimate how glowing the future will be. Overexpectation of great health not only creates motivation but also affects current happiness and actual health. Females tend to place more importance in anticipated or future health than men, who do not find future health as important.[1] Unless arthritis sufferers can change their behavior to alter future health completely on their own, caregivers or health-care professionals supply patients with information regarding their health, which in turn can add to hope.[2]

IN LIGHT OF HOPE

Hope really happens in the brain since a positive outlook on life can help an individual recover or improve faster—it is often said that disease can be fought in the mind.[3] A simple placebo effect can help arthritis sufferers feel happier as they face pain. The placebo effect refers an idea or material thing that has no medical value in reality but is used to appease or reassure an individual. When a person believes that he or she will have a great health outcome, the body produces endorphins, hormones that reduce feelings of pain, and enkephalins, neurotransmitters involved in pain reception, movement, mood, and behavior. Enkephalins (specifically beta-enkephalin) cause chemical changes in the brain that send a message to the nervous system thought to lessen and block out pain. Endorphins block chemical signals sent to the brain from any part of the nervous system. In the absence of pain, the patient's body is able to exert the energy necessary to recover from an illness. It is also thought that endorphins and enkephalins strengthen the immune system, for if the body is not ill, it is able to fight a life-threatening disease. Negative outcomes of immune response send harmful signals to the body that can prolong an illness and thus lower survival rates. This creates a cycle that can be broken by hope. [4]

Gaining Hope

While hope is an intangible and sometimes elusive concept, an individual suffering from arthritis should still make the effort to find it. Each person has his own way of coping, and each must have the will and determination to find out what best suits his or her well-being. A good way for an arthritis patient to preserve hope is to develop old relationships or build new ones. It might be difficult to reach out due to depression, but ways for arthritis sufferers to open up include the following:

- Speaking about feelings to their caregiver
- Volunteering and helping someone else
- Going out for coffee or lunch with a friend
- Letting a loved one check in regularly
- Getting together with friends for movies or indoor activities
- Getting in touch with an old friend
- Going for a walk with others
- Scheduling a dinner date
- Taking classes or joining clubs
- Taking up sessions with a therapist

Studies confirm that having a pet also strengthens hope: it not only brings companionship but also drives away the patient's bad energy and thus creates positive thinking.

Negative modalities such as (1) all-or-nothing thinking, (2) overgeneralization, (3) emotional reasoning or self-pity, (4) labeling, and (5) mental filters (whereby the patient ignores the positive and focuses on the negative) should be eliminated to make room for hope. Negative thinking can be balanced with the following:

- Thinking of what the arthritis patient wants to say and pondering if he or she should listen to other people's advice
- Getting over mistakes
- Socializing with people who bring good energy or positivity
- Keeping a log of negative thoughts for later review [5]

A fit mind comes with a healthy body, so patients should get in shape, eat healthily, and get enough sleep. As hope comes hand in hand with positivity, positive actions and thinking can develop hope and eradicate mental pain in an arthritis patient.

CONFIDENCE BOOSTERS

Confidence is a big indicator of arthritis sufferers and caregivers future actions. Having poor self-confidence tends to lead to the wrong decisions. Instead of choosing what is best, patients make decisions based on fear. Without confidence, life can be filled with destructive thoughts and may hinder the pursuit of dreams. It is very important to face fear and boost confidence. It is great if one can acknowledge failures, but focusing on successes is more helpful. Sometimes a patient fears exercise because of the pain associated with arthritis. It is more important to focus on the positive points that exercise brings, such as improving one's body. The key is for the arthritis sufferer to anticipate positive outcomes from actions. Likewise, it is important to avoid procrastination, which often results in fear and excessive tension at "the last minute." Exercise, whether for an arthritis patient or someone else, requires a lot of discipline. Voluntarily skipping exercise despite a prescribed regimen because one is not in the mood can become a habit. The more a patient talks himself out of exercise and manufacture excuses, such as things that might go wrong, the more fear can develop. Acting quickly is the best way to fight procrastination.

Confident thinking results in confident action. For example, a person might not know what to do in a tense situation but act as if he does. When building confidence, it is equally important for arthritis patients to put themselves in others' shoes. Like everyone, arthritis patients have fears and desires. Addressing these can help a patient to act properly and displace concern about speaking or acting wrongly. Moreover, maintaining a positive mental attitude rather than focusing on negative feelings can bring out the best in a patient. As depression sinks in with a lack of confidence, self-esteem may decrease, and the arthritis sufferer may feel useless. However, if the patient focuses on the positive side of things, such as thinking that arthritis will not cause harm, that confidence will ultimately bring out the best in the person.

THE PATIENCE FACTOR

Patience is also very important since every person must recognize that things will not necessarily happen as expected or as soon as desired. For instance, a male arthritis patient who wants to get out of the hospital and go home may suffer setbacks and complicate his own situation if he checks out early. In the end, he'll come back to the hospital. If he had more patience, he could have remained under hospital care until he felt better. It may be difficult for patients who have terminal illness, but practicing patience is still important as it can help avoid rash action. By being patient and thinking and relaxing before making a decision and acting, the individual can control his or her emotions and think things thorough rationally. Manifestations of patience also include the following:

- Waiting for an outcome without being anxious, tense, or frustrated
- Letting go of the need for instant gratification
- Displaying tolerance and understanding of others' maturity, coping capabilities, and emotional freedom
- Accepting one's frailty in pursuit of growth
- Tempering enthusiasm and exuberance
- Feeling peaceful and content

Signs of impatience in the arthritis patient can include the following:

- Always feeling dissatisfied
- Easily losing control of just about any situation
- Wasting energy by worrying about how slow things are going instead of focusing on desired changes
- Withdrawing effort prematurely because of slow changes
- Ignoring achievements and focusing on what has not yet been achieved
- Becoming pessimistic
- Burning out quickly
- Getting overwhelmed with large tasks that eventually sap motivation
- Quickly growing intolerant of setbacks and mistakes
- Constantly getting angry

In today's fast-paced world, people expect things to come instantly. Not everyone is willing to wait—period. A lack of patience can alter attitude negatively. Rudeness, anxiety, and bitterness can engulf patients. Caregivers can become aggravated over minor issues. To make matters worse, there is no good outcome with all the hurrying and psychological coercing.[6]

The following indicators can assess the current state of one's patience:

- A personalized definition of patience
- The level of tolerance when a problem arises
- How patient a person is with others' successes
- How patient a person is with his or her own personal growth
- Thoughts about the negative consequences of impatience
- Thoughts about why others react with impatience
- Thoughts about how others reacts to impatience
- Other emotions felt with impatience
- Beliefs hindering acquisition of patience
- New traits required to develop patience

To increase patience, arthritis sufferers and their caregivers must develop a strong life philosophy. It is all about taking life one day at a time and considering each day a gift and a stepping-stone on the path to growth. It takes time, effort, and energy to accept reality while still working to grow. Resistance may come when a person wants to change long-standing beliefs, actions, and habits. Moving on and not dwelling on past mistakes and failures can frame the arthritis sufferer's perspectives and make each day seem like a fresh start. It is also important to break larger goals down into smaller, shorter-term objectives. This can provide a more realistic and singularized goal for the immediate future.

The arthritis patient needs to be systematic when it comes to planning, as this gives rationality to action and removes unnecessary mental clutter. As a result of accepting some flaws, arthritis patients can begin to accept their other imperfections, fragilities, and weaknesses. This is when having too much patience is a negative addition. In any case, one should be aware of the surrounding realities, and those who come into contact with the arthritis sufferer will have suffered their own setbacks, weaknesses, struggles, and issues about their own personal growth and recovery.[7] Arthritis can limit a patient's mobility and cause severe lifestyle restrictions. Even the smallest tasks can become more challenging as symptoms surface. As far as patience is concerned, an important insight is that arthritis does not—and cannot—control the patient's life unless he or she allows it to. Remaining aware of patterns of daily actions can help with managing symptoms patiently. Finally, strong communication is also needed, and a desire to work together can help patients understand their current situation.[8]

THE FAREWELL

A Close Look at the Patient-Caregiver Relationship

Studies show high patient satisfaction when patients share thoughts openly during consultation.[9] A professional relationship with a caregiver in good standing leads to more psychological satisfaction. The long-term effect of the intervention is simply a significant health improvement in the patient.[10] A doctor-patient relationship can be established in various ways to assist doctors in improving their communication with patients, as that has been proven to better the patient's satisfaction and to allow both the arthritis sufferer and the caregiver to express empathy, concern, and humility.[11] Furthermore, malpractice cases against physicians cite poor communication and lack of empathy.[12]

Shared decision-making between the health-care professional and patient has a great influence in drug treatments also. Many patients do not take the treatment prescribed because (1) they do not share the doctor's opinion of the appropriateness of the drug, or (2) they are worried about harmful side effects. To avoid this, ample concordance in a doctor-patient relationship is needed. [13]

Benefits of Seeing a Doctor Regularly

By planning check-ups, the arthritis sufferer will attain a substantial, though not comprehensive, understanding of his or her situation. Medical advances can have a great impact on one's health, and screenings can detect underlying and undiagnosed conditions. It is imperative that a doctor take a complete medical history and family background so as to (1) prevent compounding symptoms, and (2) provide an explanation for a patient's behavior that can lead to self-management of the condition. Diagnosis at an early stage resulting from a visit to the physician's office necessitates a lifestyle change and timely medications to avoid further complications. A patient can save more by having routine screenings and follow-up visits than severe and invasive treatments such as surgery. This is another benefit of seeing a doctor regularly—saving money by spending a little in the present so as to avoid heavy expenses down the road. Also, public health events sponsored by corporate screening programs can allow a patient to see a doctor for a routine check-up either for free or at a discounted rate. [14]

Dangers of Avoidance

People are perhaps cutting back health-care spending due to the worldwide economic recession. Instead of professional medical treatment, alternative home remedies and self-help regimens are being used to "cure" a variety of disorders. According to the Centers for Disease Control, more stress-related health disorders are threatening lives due to the current economic crisis. Arthritis patients need to avoid the consequences of bypassing visits to health-care professionals at the prescribed times. Leaving pain and other feelings unattended may exacerbate the condition and lead to surgical intervention or hospitalization, which may cost more in the long term. One must also see a physician for the basic care a doctor can provide. Arthritis itself needs to be checked, but so do vitals signs, such as blood pressure and sugar. For instance, not all people realize that their blood pressure is rising or that there is a high sugar content in their urine without visiting a health-care professional. Accurate reading of vitals can reveal other disorders that may need further testing or exploration. Certain tests need to be done to detect hypertension, diabetes, and other conditions that can multiply pain and might hinder recovery. Another danger of avoiding a trip to the doctor is that developing symptoms might be overlooked. At the end of the day, the road to approaching arthritis is tricky but manageable, and keeping everything routinely in check benefits both patient and caregiver.

Appendix A

Arthritis-Related Links

www.arthritis-symptom.com
www.arthritis.ca
www.arthritis.org
www.arthritisaustralia.com.au
www.arthritisireland.ie
www.arthritisresearchuk.org
www.cdc.gov/arthritis/basics/rheumatoid.htm
www.emedicinehealth.com/arthritis/article_em.htm
www.everydayhealth.com/arthritis/index.aspx
www.mayoclinic.com/health/arthritis/ds01122
www.medicinenet.com/arthritis/focus.htm
www.netdoctor.co.uk/diseases/facts/arthritis.htm
www.severearthritis.net
www.stoparthritispain.co.uk/arthritissymptoms
www.webmd.com/rheumatoid-arthritis/guide/exercise-and-rheumatoid-arthritis

Appendix B

Research and Training

American College of Rheumatology
2200 Lake Blvd. NE
Atlanta, GA 30319
(404) 633–3777
Fax: (404) 633–1870
www.rheumatology.org

Arizona Arthritis Center
1501 N. Campbell Ave, Rm. 8303
Tucson, AZ 85724
(520) 626–5026
Fax: (520) 626–5018
aac@arthritis.arizona.edu
www.arthritis.arizona.edu

Arthritis and Joint Replacement Center
1500 Owens St.
San Francisco, CA 94158
(415) 353–2808
Fax: (415) 353–2956

Arthritis Center of Nebraska
3901 Pine Lake Rd., Ste. 120
Lincoln, NE 68516
(402) 420–1212
Fax: (402) 328–0961
info@nebraskaarthritis.com
www.nebraskaarthritis.com

Arthritis Community Research and Evaluation Unit
Toronto Western Research Institute
399 Bathurst St.

MP–10th Fl., Ste. 316
Toronto, ON M5T 2S8
Canada
(416) 603–6269
Fax: (416) 603–6288
acreu@uhnres.utoronto.ca
www.acreu.ca

Arthritis Foundation, Heartland Region
9433 Olive Blvd, Ste. 100
St. Louis, MO 63132
(314) 991–9333

Arthritis Research and Therapy
BioMed Central
236 Gray's Inn Rd.
London WC1X 8HB
United Kingdom
+44 (0) 20 3192 2009
Fax: +44 (0) 20 3192 2010
info@arthritis-research.com
www.arthritis-research.com

Barnes-Jewish Hospital
Washington University
1 Barnes-Jewish Hospital Plaza
Saint Louis, MO 63110
(314) 747–3000
www.barnesjewish.org

Brigham and Women's Hospital
75 Francis St.
Boston, MA 02115
(617) 732–5500
www.brighamandwomens.org

Center for Rheumatology
Steffens Scleroderma Clinic
2 Palisades Dr.
Albany, NY 12205
(518) 584–4953
www.steffens-scleroderma.org

Center of Excellence for Arthritis and Rheumatology
1501 Kings Highway
PO Box 33932
Shreveport, LA 71130
(318) 675–5000
www.lsuhscshreveport.edu

Center on Aging Studies
University of Missouri, Kansas City
5215 Rockhill Rd.
Kansas City, MO 64110

(816) 235–1747
Fax: (816) 235–5193
bullc@umkc.edu
www.iml.umkc.edu

Centre for Health Evaluation and Outcome Sciences
1081 Burrard St.
St. Paul's Hospital
Vancouver, BC V6Z 1Y6
Canada
Fax: (604) 806–8210
www.cheos.ubc.ca

Centre for Hip Health and Mobility
2635 Laurel St.
Vancouver, BC V5Z 1M9
Canada
(604) 675–2575
Fax: (604) 675–2576
www.hiphealth.ca

Johns Hopkins Arthritis Center
Wes Linda Mason F. Lord Center Tower
5200 Eastern Ave., Ste. 4100
Baltimore, MD 21224
www.hopkins-arthritis.org

Johns Hopkins Continuing Medical Education Office
Asthma and Allergy Center
5501 Hopkins Bayview Cir., Fl. 1B
Baltimore, MD 21224
(410) 550–8089
Fax: (410) 550–5601
www.hopkins-arthritis.org

Massachusetts General Hospital
55 Fruit St.
Boston, MA 02114
(617) 726–2000
www.massgeneral.org/rheumatology

McCaig Institute for Bone and Joint Health
3330 Hospital Dr. NW
Calgary, AB T2N 4N1
Canada
(403) 220–4554
Fax: (403) 283–7742
www.mccaiginstitute.com

Medical Arts and Research Building
University of Connecticut Health Center
263 Farmington Ave.
Farmington, CT 06030

Missouri Arthritis Rehabilitation Research and Training Center (MARRTC)
1205 University Ave., Ste. 1100
Columbia, MO 65211
(573) 884–1220
Fax: (573) 884–5509
erichardsjo@health.missouri.edu
www.marrtc.org

New England Musculoskeletal Institute
263 Farmington Ave.
Farmington, CT 06030–5352
(800) 535–6232
www.nemsi.uchc.edu

New York–Presbyterian University Hospital of Columbia and Cornell
525 E. 68th St.
New York, NY 10065–4870
(212) 746–5454
www.nyp.org

Northwest Missouri Regional Arthritis Center
802 N. Riverside, Ste. 160
St. Joseph, MO 64507
(800) 443–8858
www.moarthritis.typepad.com

Rheumatic Disease Clinic
4825 Almeda Rd.
Houston, TX 77004
(713) 521–7865
Fax: (713) 521–7856
www.rdch.org

Rheumatology Center at Miller Children's Hospital
2865 Atlantic Ave., Ste. 110
Long Beach, CA 90806
(562) 933–0590
www.millerchildrenshospitallb.org

Rheumatology Center of Princeton
23 Franklin Corner Rd., Ste. 106
Lawrenceville, NJ 08648
(609) 896–2505
www.princetonrheumatology.com

Saint Luke's Hospital
Arthritis Center
4401 Wornall Rd.
Kansas City, MO 64111
(816) 932–2351

Scleroderma, Vasculitis and Myositis Center
535 E. 70th St.
Office 797W, 7W Rheumatology

New York, NY 10021
(212) 774–2123

Scoliosis Research Society
555 E. Wells St., Ste. 1100
Milwaukee, WI 53202
(414) 289–9107
www.srs.org

St. John's Clinic–SGC
Arthritis Center
3231 S. National, Ste. 400
Springfield, MO 65807
(417) 888–6789

A. T. Still University Arthritis Center
800 W. Jefferson St.
Kirksville, MO 63501
(866) 626–2878

Temple University School of Medicine
Section of Rheumatology
3322 N. Broad St.
Philadelphia, PA 19140
(215) 707–0791
Fax: (215) 707–3508
www.temple.edu

University of Alabama Hospital at Birmingham
619 19th St. S.
Birmingham, AL 35249
(205) 934–4011
www.health.uab.edu

University of Colorado Hospital
12401 E. 17th Ave.
Aurora, CO 80045
(720) 848–0000
www.uch.edu

University of Missouri, School of Medicine
1 Hospital Dr.
Columbia, MO 65212
(573) 882–1566
Fax: (573) 884–4808
mumedicine@missouri.edu
www.medicine.missouri.edu

University of Missouri, School of Health Professions
Arthritis Center
1205 University Ave., Ste. 1100
Columbia, MO 65211
(573) 882–8097

University of North Carolina, Chapel Hill
3330 Thurston Building
Chapel Hill, NC 27599
(919) 966–1739
Fax: (919) 966–1739

Appendix C

Arthritis Organizations

Agency for Healthcare Research and Quality
540 Gaither Rd.
Rockville, MD 20850
(301) 427–1364
www.ahrq.gov

American Academy of Orthopedic Surgeons (AAOS)
6300 N. River Rd.
Rosemont, IL 60018
(847) 823–7186
Fax: (847) 823–8125
www.aaos.org

American Behcet's Disease Association
PO Box 869
Smithtown, NY 11787
(800) 723–4238
www.behcets.com

American Chronic Pain Association
PO Box 850
Rocklin, CA 95677
(800) 533–3231
Fax: (916) 632–3208
www.theacpa.org

American College of Rheumatology
1800 Century Pl., Ste. 250
Atlanta, GA 30345
(404) 633–3777
www.rheumatology.org

American Juvenile Arthritis Organization
1330 W. Peachtree St.
Atlanta, GA 30309
(404) 965–7538

American Medical Association
515 N. State St.
Chicago, IL 60654
(800) 621–8335
www.ama-assn.org

American Occupational Therapy Association
4720 Montgomery Ln.
PO Box 31220
Bethesda, MD 20824
(301) 652–2682
Fax: (301) 652–7711
www.aota.org

American Pain Foundation (APF)
201 N. Charles St., Ste. 710
Baltimore, MD 21201
www.painfoundation.org

American Physical Therapy Association
1111 N. Fairfax St.
Alexandria, VA 22314
Fax: (703) 706–8536
www.apta.org

Arthritis Foundation
PO Box 7669
Atlanta, GA 30357
(800) 283–7800
www.arthritis.org

Arthritis National Research Foundation
200 Oceangate, Ste. 830
Long Beach, CA 90802
(800) 588–2873
Fax: (562) 437–6057
www.curearthritis.org

Association of Rheumatology Health Professionals (ARHP)
1800 Century Pl., Ste. 250
Atlanta, GA 30345
(404) 633–3777
www.rheumatology.org

Coalition of State Rheumatology Organizations
1121 Military Cutoff, Ste. 337
Wilmington, NC 28405
(910) 256–9898

Fax: (910) 256–6058
info@csro.info
www.csro.info

Division of Population Health
Centers for Disease Control and Prevention
1600 Clifton Rd.
Atlanta, GA 30333
(800) 232–4636
www.cdc.gov

Ehlers-Danlos National Foundation
3200 Wilshire Blvd.
Ste. 1601, South Tower
Los Angeles, CA 90010
(213) 368 –3800
Fax: (213) 427–0057
www.ednf.org

International Scleroderma Network
7455 France Ave. S., Ste. 266
Edina, MN 55435
(800) 564–7099
www.sclero.org

International Still's Disease Foundation
1123 S. Kimbrel Ave.
Panama City, FL 32404
(850) 871–6656
Fax: (850) 871–6656
www.stillsdisease.org

Lupus Foundation of America
2000 L St. NW
Washington, DC 20036
(800) 558–0121
www.lupus.org

Lyme Disease Foundation
PO Box 332
Tolland, CT 06084
(860) 870–0070
Fax: (860) 870–0080
www.lyme.org

National Council on the Aging
1901 L St. NW, 4th Fl.
Washington, DC 20036
(202) 479–1200
www.ncoa.org

National Fibromyalgia Association
2121 S. Towne Centre, Ste. 300,
Anaheim, CA 92806

(714) 921–0150
www.fmaware.org

National Institute of Arthritis and Musculoskeletal and Skin Diseases
1 AMS Cir.
Bethesda, MD 20892
(301) 495–4484
Fax: (301) 480–2814
www.niams.nih.gov

National Marfan Foundation
22 Manhasset Ave.
Port Washington, NY 11050
(800) 862–7326
Fax: (516) 883–8040
www.marfan.org

National Organization of Rheumatology Managers (NORM)
1121 Military Cutoff, Ste. 337
Wilmington, NC 28405
(910) 520–0515
Fax: (910) 254–1091
www.normgroup.org

National Osteoporosis Foundation
1150 17th St. NW, Ste. 850
Washington, DC 20036
(800) 231–4222
Fax: (202) 223–2237
www.nof.org

National Psoriasis Foundation
6600 SW 92nd Ave., Ste. 300
Portland, OR 97223
(503) 244–7404
www.psoriasis.org

Paget Foundation
120 Wall St., Ste. 1602
New York, NY 10005
(212) 509–5335
Fax: (212) 509–8492

Rheumatology Associates and Osteoporosis Center
8902 N. Meridian St., Ste. 210
Indianapolis, IN 46260
(317) 844–6444
Fax: (317) 848–6605
www.indyrheumatology.com

Scleroderma Foundation
300 Rosewood Dr., Ste. 105
Danvers, MA 01923
(978) 463–5843

www.scleroderma.org

Scoliosis Association
PO Box 811705
Boca Raton, FL 33481
(561) 994–4435
www.scoliosis-assoc.org

Sjogren's Foundation
6707 Democracy Blvd.
Bethesda, MD 20817
(800) 475–6473
Fax: (301) 530–4415
www.sjogrens.org

Spondylitis Association of America
PO Box 5872
Sherman Oaks, CA 91413
(818) 892–1616
www.spondylitis.org

Appendix D

Nationally Recognized Arthritis Clinics

A. T. Still University
Arthritis Center
800 W. Jefferson St.
Kirksville, MO 63501
(866) 626–2878

Arthritis and Joint Replacement Center
1500 Owens St.
San Francisco, CA 94158
(415) 353–2808
Fax: (415) 353–2956

Arthritis Foundation, Heartland Region
9433 Olive Blvd, Ste. 100
St. Louis, MO 63132
(314) 991–9333

Barbara Volcker Center for Women and Rheumatic Diseases
Hospital for Special Surgery
535 E. 70th St., 8th Fl., Rm. 848H
New York, NY 10021
(212) 774–2291
Fax: (212) 774–2374
volckerctr@hss.edu

Barnes-Jewish Hospital
Washington University
1 Barnes-Jewish Hospital Plaza
Saint Louis, MO 63110
(314) 747–3000
www.barnesjewish.org

Center for Rheumatology
Steffens Scleroderma Clinic
2 Palisades Dr.
Albany, NY 12205
(518) 584–4953
www.steffens-scleroderma.org

Centre for Hip Health and Mobility
7/F, 2635 Laurel St.
Robert H. N. Ho Research Centre
Vancouver, BC V5Z 1M9
Canada
(604) 675–2575
Fax: (604) 675–2576
www.hiphealth.ca

Children's Hospital of Pittsburgh of UPMC
4401 Penn Ave.
Pittsburgh, PA 15224
(412) 692–5325
www.chp.edu

Columbia University
Division of Rheumatology
161 Fort Washington Ave., 2nd Fl.
New York, NY 10032
(212) 305–4308
Fax: (212) 342–6835
www.rheumatologyatcolumbia.org

Johns Hopkins Arthritis Center
Wes Linda Mason F. Lord Center Tower
5200 Eastern Ave., Ste. 4100
Baltimore, MD 21224
www.hopkins-arthritis.org

Johns Hopkins Continuing Medical Education Office
5501 Hopkins Bayview Cir., Fl. 1B
Baltimore, MD 21224
(410) 550–8089
Fax: (410) 550–5601
www.hopkins-arthritis.org

Mayo Clinic
13400 E. Shea Blvd.
Scottsdale, AZ 85259
(480) 301–8000
www.mayoclinic.com

McCaig Institute for Bone and Joint Health
3330 Hospital Dr. NW
Calgary, AB T2N 4N1
Canada

(403) 220–4554
Fax: (403) 283–7742
www.mccaiginstitute.com

Missouri Arthritis Rehabilitation Research and Training Center
1205 University Ave., Ste. 1100
Columbia, MO 65211
(573) 884–1220
Fax: (573) 884–5509
erichardsjo@health.missouri.edu
www.marrtc.org

National Center for Farmworker Health (NCFH)
1770 FM 967
Buda, TX 78610
(800) 531–5120
Fax: (512) 312–2600
info@ncfh.org
www.ncfh.org

New England Musculoskeletal Institute
263 Farmington Ave.
Farmington, CT 06030
(800) 535–6232
www.nemsi.uchc.edu

New Mexico Arthritis Center
4901 Lang NE, Ste. 305
Albuquerque, NM 87109
(505) 822–1309
Fax: (505)822–1393

New York–Presbyterian University Hospital of Columbia and Cornell
525 E. 68th St.
New York, NY 10065
(212) 746–5454
www.nyp.org

Northwest Missouri Regional Arthritis Center
802 N. Riverside, Ste. 160
St. Joseph, MO 64507
(800) 443–8858
www.moarthritis.typepad.com

Ohio State University Hospital
370 W. 9th Ave.
Columbus, OH 43210
(614) 293–8000
www.osumedcenter.edu

Rheumatic Disease Clinic
4825 Almeda Rd.
Houston, TX 77004
(713) 521–7865

Fax: (713) 521–7856
www.rdch.org

Rheumatology Associates
8144 Walnut Hill Ln., Ste. 800
Dallas, TX 75231
(214) 540–0700
Fax: (214) 540–0701
www.arthdocs.com

Rheumatology Center at Miller Children's Hospital
2865 Atlantic Ave., Ste. 110
Long Beach, CA 90806
(562) 933–0590
www.millerchildrenshospitallb.org

Rheumatology Center of Princeton
23 Franklin Corner Rd., Ste. 106
Lawrenceville, NJ 08648
(609) 896–2505
www.princetonrheumatology.com

Saint Francis Medical Center
Arthritis Center
150 S. Mount Auburn Rd.
Cape Girardeau, MO 63703
(888) 216–3293

Saint Louis University
221 N. Grand Blvd.
St. Louis, MO 63103
(314) 977–2500
www.slu.edu

Saint Luke's Hospital
Arthritis Center
4401 Wornall Rd.
Kansas City, MO 64111
(816) 932–2351

Scleroderma, Vasculitis and Myositis Center
Rheumatology Office
535 E. 70th St.
New York, NY 10021
(212) 774–2123

St. John's Clinic–SGC
Arthritis Center
3231 S. National, Ste. 400
Springfield, MO 65807
(417) 888–6789

Texas Rheumatology Center
16659 Southwest Fwy.

Bldg. 2, Ste. 235
Sugar Land, TX 77479
(281) 980–2717
Fax: (281) 265–3806
www.angelamccainmd.com

UCLA Health System
Peter Morton Medical Building
200 UCLA Medical Plaza, Ste. 365-B
Los Angeles, CA 90095
(310) 825–2448
Fax: (310) 794–6553
www.rheumatology.ucla.edu

University of Missouri, School of Medicine
1 Hospital Dr.
Columbia, MO 65212
(573) 882–1566
Fax: (573) 884–4808
mumedicine@missouri.edu
www.medicine.missouri.edu

University of Missouri, School of Health Professions
Arthritis Center
1205 University Ave., Ste. 1100
Columbia, MO 65211
(573) 882–8097

Appendix E

For Further Reading

Aesoph, Laurie M. *How to Eat Away Arthritis: Gain Relief from the Pain and Discomfort of Arthritis through Nature's Remedies*. 2nd ed. Upper Saddle River, NJ: Prentice Hall, 1996.

Airola, Paavo. *There Is a Cure for Arthritis*. Upper Saddle River, NJ: Prentice Hall Press, 1988.

Bales, Peter. *Osteoarthritis: Preventing and Healing without Drugs*. New York: Prometheus Books, 2008.

Berkley, George E. *Arthritis without Aspirin: Effective New Ways to Control Arthritic Pain*. Upper Saddle River, NJ: Prentice Hall, 1982.

Carr, Rachel. *Arthritis: Relief beyond Drugs*. New York: HarperCollins, 1984.

Challem, Jack. *The Inflammation Syndrome: The Complete Nutritional Program to Prevent and Reverse Heart Disease, Arthritis, Diabetes, Allergies, and Asthma*. Hoboken, NJ: John Wiley and Sons, 2003.

D'Adamo, Peter J., and Catherine Whitney. *Arthritis: Fight It with the Blood Type Diet*. Eat Right 4 Your Type Library. New York: G. P. Putnam's Sons, 2004.

Darlington, Gail. *Diet and Arthritis*. London: Random House, 1999.

Delgado, J. L. *The Buena Salud Guide to Arthritis and Your Life*. New York: HarperCollins, 2012.

Dore, Robin K. *Arthritis: Your Comprehensive Guide to Pain Management, Medication, Diet, Exercise, Surgery and Physical Therapies*. New York: DK Publishing, 2009.

Fife, Bruce. *The New Arthritis Cure: Eliminate Arthritis and Fibromyalgia Pain Permanently*. Colorado Springs, CO: Piccadilly Books, 2009.

Firestein, Gary S., Gabriel S. Panayi, and Frank A. Wollheim. *Rheumatoid Arthritis*. 2nd ed. New York: Oxford University Press, 2006.

Fishman, Loren, and Ellen Saltonstall. *Yoga for Arthritis: The Complete Guide*. New York: W. W. Norton and Company, 2008.

Fox, Barry, Nadine Taylor, Jinoos Yazdany, and Dr. Sarah Brewer. *Arthritis for Dummies*. 2nd ed. Indianapolis: Wiley, 2011.

Fries, James F. *Arthritis: A Take Care of Yourself Health Guide*. New York: Perseus Books, 1999.

Hills, Margaret. *Treating Arthritis Diet Book*. London: Sheldon Press, 2001.

Hozack, William J., Javav Parvizi, and Benjamin Bender. *Surgical Treatment of Hip Arthritis: Reconstruction, Replacement, and Revision*. Philadelphia: Saunders, 2009.

Kantrowitz, Fred G. *Taking Control of Arthritis*. New York: HarperCollins, 1991.

Klippel, John H., ed. *Primer on the Rheumatic Diseases*. 13th ed. New York: Springer, 2007.

Koehn, Cheryl, Taysha Palmer, and John Esdaile. *Rheumatoid Arthritis: Plan to Win.* New York: Oxford University Press, 2002.

Konshin, Victor. *Beating Gout: A Sufferer's Guide to Living Pain Free.* 2nd ed. Williamsville, NY: Ayerware Publishing, 2009.

Lawrence, Ronald, and Martin Zucker. *Preventing Arthritis: A Holistic Approach to Life without Pain.* New York: Berkley Trade, 2002.

Lee, Thomas F. *Conquering Rheumatoid Arthritis.* Amherst, NY: Prometheus Books, 2001.

Leong, Amye, and Joseph Layden. *Get a Grip: A Take-Charge Approach to Living with Arthritis.* New York: Penguin Group, 2002.

Lewis, Faye Cashatt. *All Out against Arthritis.* Upper Saddle River, NJ: Prentice Hall, 1973.

McNeil, M. E. A. *The First Year: Rheumatoid Arthritis: An Essential Guide for the Newly Diagnosed.* New York: Da Capo Press, 2005.

Mosher, Dianne, Howard Stein, and Gunnar Kraag. *Living Well with Arthritis: A Sourcebook for Understanding and Managing Your Arthritis.* Toronto: Penguin Canada, 2007.

Nelson, Miriam E., Kristin Baker, Lawrence Lindner, and Ronenn Roubenoff. *Strong Women and Men Beat Arthritis.* New York: G. P. Putnam's Sons, 2003.

Rothfeld, Glenn S., and Suzanne LeVert. *Natural Medicine for Arthritis: The Best Alternative Methods for Relieving Pain and Stiffness: From Food and Herbs to Acupuncture and Homeopathy.* Emmaus, PA: Rodale Books, 1996.

Sharma, Leena, and Francis Berenbaum. *Osteoarthritis: A Companion to Rheumatology.* New York: Elsevier Health Sciences, 2007.

Shlotzhauer, Tammi L., and James L. McGuire. *Living with Rheumatoid Arthritis.* A Johns Hopkins Press Health Book. 2nd ed. Baltimore: Johns Hopkins University Press, 2003.

Shomon, Mary J. *Living Well with Autoimmune Disease: What Your Doctor Doesn't Tell You . . . that You Need to Know.* New York: HarperCollins, 2002.

Sobel, D., and A. C. Klein. *Arthritis, What Exercises Work: Breakthrough Relief for the Rest of Your Life, Even After Drugs and Surgery Have Failed.* New York: St. Martin's Press, 1995.

Szer, Llona S., Yukiko Kimura, and Peter N. Malleson. *Arthritis in Children and Adolescents: Juvenile Idiopathic Arthritis.* New York: Oxford University Press, 2006.

Theodosakis, Jason, and Sheila Buff. *The Arthritis Cure, Revised and Updated: The Medical Miracle that Can Halt, Reverse, and May Even Cure Osteoarthritis.* 2nd ed. New York: St. Martin's Press, 2004.

Glossary

AAOS. American Academy of Orthopedic Surgeons.

Abatacept. Injectable prescription immunosuppressant medication that specifically blocks the function of T cells.

Adalimumab. Injectable prescription immunosuppresant medication that blocks the function of TNF, which causes pain and inflammation.

Adverse effects. See *side effects*.

Anakinra. Prescription drug that blocks the effects of the protein interleukin-1 to suppress pain and inflammation.

Analgesic. A pain-relieving medication.

Antibodies. See *immunoglobulin*.

Antigens. Protein peptides that may exist on the surface of certain cells.

Arthritis urethritica. See *reactive arthritis*.

Arthritis. Term that literally means "joint inflammation." The condition affects joints, bones, muscles, and nearby soft tissues to a certain degree. The two major forms of this condition are osteoarthritis and rheumatoid arthritis.

Arthrodesis. Surgical fusion of the joint; considered a final-resort surgery for arthritis.

Arthrology. Study of the anatomy, physiology, and dysfunction of the joints.

Arthroplasty. Surgical replacement of a joint with a prosthesis.

Arthrotomy. Surgical intervention that drains fluid inside a joint through an incision.

Autoimmune disease. Disease caused by the body's autoimmune response.

Autoimmune response. Immune response directed against the body's own cells.

Azathioprine. Prescription immunosuppresant drug that blocks the function of cytokine; still classified as a DMARD and also as a carcinogen.

B cell. Type of lymphocyte that is mainly responsible for tagging foreign pathogens for identification by killer T cells.

Bacteremic infection. Infection caused by bacteria.

Bacteria. Single-celled organisms that are capable of living inside and outside the body.

Bacterial arthritis. See *septic arthritis*.

Biological response modifiers. Substances that are naturally produced by the body in small amounts to fight infection and disease.

Bipedal. Land animal that is capable of moving around using two limbs.

Bone marrow. Semisolid substance located inside the compact bone that is responsible for producing blood cells.

BRM. Biological response modifier.

Bursitis. Inflammation of one or more bursae, the small sacs of synovial fluid that serve to cushion the bones, muscles, tendons, and joints.

C-reactive proteins. Proteins found in the bloodstream that can activate the complement system. The presence of elevated C-reactive proteins indicates an inflammatory disease.

CBC. Complete blood count.

CD4+. Type of glycoprotein that serves as an HIV receptor.

Certolizmab pegol. Injectable prescription immunosuppresant medication that blocks the function of TNF, which causes pain and inflammation.

Chronic disease. Long-lasting or recurring disease.

Clinical assessment. Systemic evaluation of a patient's condition based on his or her medical history and the results of physical and laboratory examinations; used to develop the patient's diagnosis, prognosis, and treatment.

Complete blood count. A diagnostic exam that can measure the levels of different blood cells and components found in a certain amount of blood.

Computed tomography scan. Diagnostic imaging technique that uses X-rays in conjunction with computers to produce clear cross-sectional images.

Connective tissue. Diverse tissue type that includes most of the body's tissues, excluding muscles, nerves, and epithelial tissue, which makes up the glands and all outer and inner linings of the body.

Corticosteroid. Chemical substance that mimics cortisol in the body to limit inflammation and suppress immune system activity.

COX enzyme. Enzyme responsible for producing prostaglandin.

Cross-reactivity. Thought to be responsible for autoimmune conditions such as reactive arthritis; characterized by inflammation of parts of the body due to an infection located elsewhere in the body.

CRP. C-reactive protein.

CT scan. Computed tomography scan.

Cyclosporine. Prescription immunosuppresant drug that blocks the function of cytokine; still classified as a DMARD.

DEXA. Dual-energy X-ray absorptiometry.

Disease. Pathological condition that causes a deviation from the normal structure or physiology of an organism.

Disease-modifying antirheumatic drugs. Medications used to treat arthritis even though their specific mechanism of action is still unknown.

Disseminated gonococcal infection. Process that spreads gonococcal infections systemically throughout the various body systems.

Dizygotic. Developed from individual fertilized ova.

DMARD. Disease-modifying antirheumatic drug.

Endocarditis. Inflammation of the endocardium, or the inner lining of the heart.

Enteropathic arthritis. An inflammatory joint disease triggered by inflammatory gastrointestinal diseases.

Enzyme. A substance that serves as a biochemical catalyst and functions to speed up chemical or metabolic reactions.

ESR. Erythrocyte sedimentation rate.

Estrogen. Hormone, produced by the ovaries, with many uses, including the protection of bones from calcium loss.

Etanercept. An injectable prescription immunosuppresant medication that blocks the function of TNF, which causes pain and inflammation.

Eunuch. Male individual intentionally castrated early in life. This early castration causes a deviation from normal hormonal secretions and may in turn cause physiological deviations from the normal male human body.

Fever response. The resetting and increasing of the body's temperature in response to the detection of toxins in the body system.

Fibromyalgia. Condition that causes fatigue, pain, and tenderness in various parts of the body, including muscles, tendons, and ligaments.

Fungi. Plantlike multicelled organism that takes nutrition from other living organisms, such as plants and animals.

Glucocorticoids. Corticosteroids specifically involved in the metabolism of carbohydrates.

Gold salts. Prescription immunosuppresant drug that contains gold; still classified as a DMARD.

Golimumab. Injectable prescription immunosuppresant medication that blocks the function of TNF, which causes pain and inflammation.

Gonococcal arthritis. The most prevalent form of septic arthritis in the United States. The causative organism behind this form of arthritis is the Gram-negative diplococcus *Neisseria gonorrhoeae*, which is most likely spread systemically due to disseminated gonococcal infection.

Gout. Recurrent form of arthritis mostly attributed to the buildup of uric acid crystals in the joints.

Gram stain. Diagnostic exam named after Danish doctor Hans Christian Gram, who created the test to identify and differentiate Gram-positive bacteria, which have peptidoglycan in their outer layers, from Gram-negative bacteria by staining the peptidoglycan-containing bacteria a bluish color.

Health-care delivery system. Organized system composed of people, institutions, and re-sources that aims to deliver health-care services in response to the health-care needs of its target population.

Helper T cells. T cells that instruct B cells to create specific antibodies based on the antigens received from macrophages that have digested a specific pathogen.

Histamine. Chemical responsible for activation of the inflammatory response.

HLA-B27. Gene that commonly occurs in the DNA of Caucasian populations and makes them more susceptible to reactive arthritis than individuals from other races.

Hydroxychloroquine. Type of DMARD that alters the immune system. This was originally an antimalarial medication.

Immunoglobulin. Chemical compounds that bind to antigens on the outer layers of foreign pathogens for identification and destruction by T cells.

Immunosuppressant medications. Medications used to reduce oversensitivity or exaggerated reactions of the immune system.

Immunoturbidimetry. Immunologic technique used for scanning for specific antigens (foreign substances).

Infectious arthritis. See *septic arthritis*.

Inflammatory response. The immune system's response to infection; characterized by pain, redness, heat, and swelling.

Infliximab. Injectable prescription immunosuppresant medication that blocks the function of TNF, which causes pain and inflammation.

Interferon. A chemical protein that binds to healthy cells to protect them from invading viruses.

Interleukins. Chemicals that serve as the immune system's neurotransmitters.

Internists. Physicians who specialize in internal medicine, which is concerned with various multisystem conditions.

Iritis. Inflammation of the eye, specifically the iris.

ISMH. International Society of Medical Hydrology.

Juvenile rheumatoid arthritis. Inflammatory joint disorder that affects young children and teenagers.

Leflunomide. Medication that can suppress immune cells responsible for joint inflammation; still classified as a DMARD.

Leukocytes. Cells responsible for the body's specific immune response. They can be further classified as eosinophils, macrophages, or lymphocytes.

Lupus erythematosus. Inflammatory autoimmune disease that affects the skin, joints, and some organs.

Lymphocytes. Leukocytes responsible for identifying and destroying specific pathogens. They can be further subdivided into B cells, NK cells, and T cells.

Macrophages. A phagocytic type of leukocyte.

Magnetic resonance imaging. A diagnostic procedure used in radiology to create 2-D or 3-D images of internal body structures by exposing the body to a magnetic field.

Magnotherapy. Arthritis treatment involving the use of magnetic fields on the body.

Menopause. Natural, permanent loss of the ovaries' ability to secrete ova and hormones, resulting in hormone-related physiological changes such as the cessation of menses.

Metacarpophalangeal joints. Ball-and-socket joints located between the metacarpals and the phalanges.

Methotraxate. Immunity-altering prescription drug used to treat cancer and arthritis; classified as a DMARD.

Monozygotic. Developed from a single fertilized ovum.

MRI. Magnetic resonance imaging.

Neutrophils. Phagocytic type of leukocyte.

Nonsteroidal anti-inflammatory drugs. Anti-inflammatory drugs that do not contain corticosteroids. They work by blocking the COX enzymes responsible for producing prostaglandin.

NSAIDs. Nonsteroidal anti-inflammatory drugs.

Oligoarthritis. A form of arthritis that affects only a few joints.

Orthopedic surgeons. Surgeons who specialize in surgical interventions for the musculoskeletal system.

Osteoarthritis. Disease encompassing a group of mechanical abnormalities that result in a degenerative joint disease.

Osteomyelitic condition. A medical condition involving the infection and subsequent inflammation of the bone and bone marrow.

Over-the-counter (OTC) medications. Medications that can be purchased without a prescription.

Pathogen. Organism that causes disease; usually a microorganism that can be classified as a bacterium, mycobacterium, fungus, parasite, or virus.

Podagra. Gout affecting the big toe.

Primary prevention. The promotion of health through provision of protective measures against specific health problems to healthy individuals or groups. This includes assessment of health risks, immunization, and health education on the prevention of disease.

Protozoa. Single-celled organisms that live in and are spread through water.

Psoriatic arthritis. Inflammatory joint disease triggered by the skin disease called psoriasis.

Purulent. See *suppurative.*

Pyrogen. Chemical responsible for the fever response.

Quadrupedal. Capable of moving around using four limbs.

Quaternary prevention. Prevention of unnecessary medical intervention if avoidable.

Reactive arthritis. Form of arthritis that results from the body's faulty systemic autoimmune response to an infection inside the body that is not located on the arthritic joint, which may result in polyarthritis.

Reiter's syndrome. Former terminology used to refer to reactive arthritis; named for German physician Hans Conrad Julius Reiter. The term was later dropped in favor of the current terminology due to his Nazi connections. See *reactive arthritis.*

Rheumatic diseases. See *rheumatism.*

Rheumatism. Medical problems targeting the joints and connective tissues.

Rheumatoid arthritis. An autoimmune disease that results in a system-wide inflammatory disorder characterized by swollen and inelastic synovial joints.

Rheumatoid factor. Antibody directed against the body's own tissues that is regarded to be the significant culprit behind rheumatoid arthritis. It is known to specifically react against immunoglobulin G (IgG).

Rheumatologists. Physicians who specialize in the nonsurgical management of arthritic diseases.

Rheumatology. Medical subspecialty focusing on the prevention, diagnosis, and treatment of rheumatic diseases.

Risk factors. Factors that predispose an individual or group to a specific illness.

Rituximab. A prescription immunosuppressant medication used to treat autoimmune disorders.

Scleroderma. Thickening and hardening of the skin.

Secondary prevention. The alleviation of health problems associated with disease through early identification of those problems and subsequent early treatment of disease. Measures include disease screening, medications, and reactive lifestyle changes.

Sepsis. Refers to systemic compromise due to the spread of infection.

Septic arthritis. A form of arthritis that results from direct infection of the joint(s).

Side effects. Undesired or harmful effects resulting from medications or other medical interventions.

Signs. Objective manifestations of an underlying health problem.

Spondyloarthropathies. Inflammatory diseases of the spinal column.

Sulfasalazine. Medication used in arthritis to control inflammation and pain; classified as a DMARD.

Suppurative arthritis. See *septic arthritis.*

Surgical debridement. The surgical removal of dead tissue to allow for better healing.

Symptoms. Subjective manifestations of an underlying health problem.

Synovectomy. Removal of the synovium.

Synovial fluid. Viscous lubricating fluid found inside the cavities of joints.

T cells. The type of lymphocyte mainly responsible for identification and destruction of pathogens.

Tertiary prevention. The restoration of health through rehabilitation or the alleviation of complications related to terminal disease. Measures include medication, rehabilitation, and lifestyle changes.

TNF. Tumor necrosis factor.

Tocilizumab. Prescription drug that blocks the effects of the protein interleukin-6 to suppress pain and inflammation.

Treatment modalities. Methods of treatment.

Uveitis. Inflammation of the uvea of the eye.

Venereal arthritis. See *reactive arthritis*.

Viruses. Multicelled organisms that invade and reproduce inside other microbial organisms.

WBC. White blood cell.

White blood cells. See *leukocytes*.

X-ray. Diagnostic imaging technique that uses electromagnetic radiation.

Z-thumb. Metacarpophalangeal deformity with a square appearance.

Notes

PREFACE

1. Joint Commission Resources Inc., *Joint Commission Guide to Patient and Family Education* (Oakbrook Terrace, IL: Joint Commission on Accreditation of Healthcare Organization, 2003), 154.

2. W. Shiel, "Arthritis," Emedicine, accessed July 27, 2012, www.emedicinehealth.com/arthritis.

3. C. Doak, "Teaching Patients with Low Literacy Skills," Harvard School of Public Health, 1996, accessed July 24, 2012, http://www.hsph.harvard.edu/healthliteracy/resources/doak-book.

4. F. London, *No Time to Teach: The Essence of Patient and Family Education for Health Care Providers* (Atlanta: Pritchett & Hull, 2009); S. H. Rankin, K. Stallings, and F. London, *Patient Education in Health and Illness*, 5th ed. (Philadelphia: Lippincott Williams & Wilkins, 2005).

5. National Alliance for Caregiving, AARP, *Caregiving in the U.S.* (Bethesda, MD: National Alliance for Caregiving, AARP, 2004).

6. P. S. Arno, "Well-being of Caregivers: The Economic Issues of Caregiving: Data from 1987/1988 National Survey of Families and Households," in *New Caregiving Research Symposium, American Association of Geriatric Psychiatry Annual Meeting*, ed. T. McRae (Orlando, FL: American Association of Geriatric Psychiatry, 2002).

7. H. Brus, M.A. van de Laar, E. Taal, J. J. Rasker, and O. Wiegman, "Effects of Patient Education on Compliance with Basic Treatment Regimens and Health in Recent Onset Active Rheumatoid Arthritis," *Annals of the Rheumatic Diseases* 57, no. 3 (1998): 146–51.

8. H. Brus, van de Laar, Taal, Rasker, and Wiegman, "Effects of Patient Education."

9. J. M. Hootman, C. G. Helmick, and T. J. Brady, "A Public Health Approach to Addressing Arthritis in Older Adults: The Most Common Cause of Disability," *American Journal of Public Health* 102, no. 3 (2012): 426–33.

10. Alliance for Excellent Education, "Healthier and Wealthier: Decreasing Health Care Costs by Increasing Educational Attainment," November 2006, accessed August 2, 2012, www.all4ed.org.

11. T. Sells, "Prevention Is Most Cost-effective Health Strategy, Says CDC Director," Scripps Interactive Newspapers Group, July 16, 2010, accessed August 2, 2012, http://www.commercialappeal.com/news/2010/jul/16/ailing-health-care.

12. J. L. Longe, *The Gale Encyclopedia of Medicine* (Belmont, CA: Gale Group, 2011).

13. C. A. Shourt, C. S. Crowson, S. E. Gabriel, and E. L. Matteson, "Orthopedic Surgery among Patients with Rheumatoid Arthritis 1980-2007: A Population-Based Study Focused on Surgery Rates, Sex, and Mortality," *Journal of Rheumatology* 39, no. 3 (2012): 491–95; G. A. Kelley, K. S. Kelley, J. M. Hootman, and D. L. Jones," Effects of Community-Deliverable Exercise on Pain and Physical Function in Adults with Arthritis and Other Rheumatic Diseases: A Meta-analysis," *Arthritis Care & Research* 63, no. 1 (2011): 79–93.

1. INTRODUCTION TO RHEUMATISM

1. M. Stein and G. Taylor, *The Encyclopedia of Arthritis* (New York: Facts on File, 2004), ix.

2. American College of Rheumatology, "History of the ACR," accessed April 25, 2012, www.rheumatology.org/about/leadership/75th_anniversary.asp.

3. G. Henkel, "Reflections on a Diamond Celebration," *Rheumatologist*, accessed April 25, 2012, www.the-rheumatologist.org.

4. J. Harrison, K. Kulkarni, M. Baguneid, and B. Prendergast, *Oxford Handbook of Key Clinical Evidence* (London: Oxford University Press, 2009), 490.

5. G. Pasero and P. Marson, "Hippocrates and Rheumatology," *Clinical and Experimental Rheumatology* 22 (2004): 687.

6. Pasero and Marson, "Hippocrates and Rheumatology," 687.

7. A. Feigenbaum, "A Description of Behçet's Syndrome in the Hippocratic Third Book of Endemic Disease," *British Journal of Ophthalmology* 40 (1956): 355–56.

8. Feigenbaum, "A Description of Behçet's Syndrome," 357.

9. Pasero and Marson, "Hippocrates and Rheumatology," 688.

10. Pasero and Marson, "Hippocrates and Rheumatology," 688.

11. Pasero and Marson, "Hippocrates and Rheumatology," 688–89.

12. J. R. Coxe, trans., "Section V: On Diseases," in *The Writings of Hippocrates and Galen*, ed. J. R. Coxe (Philadelphia: Lindsay and Blakiston, 1846).

13. W. W. Buchanan and W. F. Kean, "Rheumatoid Arthritis: Beyond the Lymphocyte," *Journal of Rheumatology* 28, no. 4 (2001): 691–93.

14. D. Garrison and M. Hast, "De Humani Corporis Fabrica," Northwestern University, accessed July 23, 2012, www.vesalius.northwestern.edu.

15. W. Harvey, *De Motu Cordis* (Frankfurt: n.p., 1628).

16. K. B. Kansupada and J. W. Sassani, "Sushruta: The Father of Indian Surgery and Ophthalmology," *Documenta Ophthalmologica* 93, no. 1–2 (1997): 159–67.

17. D. M. Dunlop, "The General Principles of Avicenna's 'Canon of Medicine,'" *Medical History* 12, no. 4 (1968): 418–21.

18. P. Lutz, *The Rise of Experimental Biology: An Illustrated History* (New York: Humana Press, 2002), 60.

19. I. B. Syed, "Islamic Medicine: 1000 Years Ahead of Its Time," *Journal of the International Society for the History of Islamic Medicine* 2 (2002): 8.

20. M. H. Pillinger, P. Rosenthal, and A. M. Abeles, "Hyperuricemia and Gout: New Insights into Pathogenesis and Treatment," *Bulletin of the NYU Hospital for Joint Diseases* 65, no. 3 (2007): 215.

21. S. Schwartz, "A Disease of Distinction," accessed June 4, 2012, www.stephanaschwartz.com/PDF/disease_of_distinction.pdf.

22. G. Nuki and P. A. Simkin, "A Concise History of Gout and Hyperuricemia and Their Treatment," *Arthritis Research and Therapy* 8 (suppl. 1) (2006). Published online ahead of print.

23. P. Shulten, J. Thomas, M. Miller, M. Smith, and M. Ahern, "The Role of Diet in the Management of Gout: A Comparison of Knowledge and Attitudes to Current Evidence," *Journal of Human Nutrition and Diet* 22, no. 1 (2009): 3–11.

24. C. Dubow, "The Disease of Kings," *Forbes*, accessed May 10 2012, www.forbes.com; M. Scholtens, "The Glorification of Gout in 16th- to 18th-Century Literature," *Canadian Medical Association Journal* 179, no. 8 (2008): 804.

25. Dubow, "The Disease of Kings."

26. Scholtens, "The Glorification of Gout," 804.

27. Schwartz, "A Disease of Distinction."

28. Roy Porter, "Gout: Framing and Fantasizing Disease," *Bulletin of the History of Medicine* 68 (1994): 5.

29. Nuki and Simkin, "A Concise History of Gout."

30. Scholtens, "The Glorification of Gout," 804.

31. P. Marson, "*Gout and the Spider* by Jean de la Fontaine (1621–1695), or the Metamorphoses of a Rheumatologic Tale," *Reumatismo* 54, no. 4 (2002): 379.

32. L. F. Wright, R. P. Saylor, and F. A. Cecere, "Occult Lead Intoxication in Patients with Gout and Kidney Disease," *Journal of Rheumatology* 11, no. 4 (1984): 517–20.

33. Dubow, "The Disease of Kings."

34. G. Parker, *Philip II: Library of the World Biography* (London: Hutchinson, 1978), 191–92.

35. Scholtens, "The Glorification of Gout," 804.

36. L. D. Kritzman, *The Fabulous Imagination: On Montaigne's Essays* (New York: Columbia University Press, 2009), 240.

37. Scholtens, "The Glorification of Gout," 805.

38. Dubow, "The Disease of Kings."

39. G. Low, "Thomas Sydenham: The English Hippocrates," *Australian and New Zealand Journal of Surgery* 69, no. 4 (1999): 258–62.

40. Harrison, Kulkarni, Baguneid, and Prendergast, *Oxford Handbook*, 490.

41. T. Sydenham, *A Treatise of the Gout and Dropsy* (rpt.; Philadelphia: College of Physicians, 1963), 193.

42. Pillinger, Rosenthal, and Abeles, "Hyperuricemia and Gout," 215.

43. Nuki and Simkin, "A Concise History of Gout."

44. Schwartz, "A Disease of Distinction."

45. Nuki and Simkin, "A Concise History of Gout."

46. Harrison, Kulkarni, Baguneid, and Prendergast, *Oxford Handbook*, 490.

47. A. B. Garrod, "Observations on Certain Pathological Conditions of the Blood and Urine in Gout, Rheumatism and Bright's Disease," Medico-Chirurgial Society of Edinburgh 31 (1848): 83–97.

48. A. B. Garrod, The Nature and Treatment of Gout and Rheumatic Gout (London: Walton and Maberly, 1859).

49. D. J. McCarty and J. L. Hollander, "Identification of Urate Crystals in Gouty Synovial Fluid," *Annals of Internal Medicine* 54 (1961): 452–60.

50. H. Amer, A. Swan, and P. Dieppe, "The Utilization of Synovial Fluid Analysis in the UK," *Rheumatology* 40, no. 9 (2001): 1060–63.

51. Harrison, Kulkarni, Baguneid, and Prendergast, *Oxford Handbook*, 490.

52. Stein and Taylor, *The Encyclopedia of Arthritis*, 342.

2. UNDERSTANDING BONE AND JOINT HEALTH

1. P. H. White and R. W. Chang, "Public Health and Arthritis: A Growing Imperative," in *Primer on the Rheumatic Diseases*, ed. J. H. Klippel, J. H. Stone, L. J. Crofford, and P. H. White (New York: Springer, 2008), 1.

2. White and Chang, "Public Health and Arthritis," 2.

3. J. Kluger, *Splendid Solution: Jonas Salk and the Conquest of Polio* (New York: Putnam, 2005), 384.

4. White and Chang, "Public Health and Arthritis," 2–3.

5. C. M. Ripsin, H. Kang, and R. J. Urban, "Management of Blood Glucose in Type 2 Diabetes Mellitus," *American Family Physician* 79, no. 1 (2009): 29–36.

6. B. Williams, N. R. Poulter, M. J. Brown, M. Davis, G. T. McInnes, J. F. Potter, P. S. Sever, and S. McG-Thom, "Guidelines for Management of Hypertension: Report of the Fourth Working Party of the British Hypertension Society, 2004-BHS IV," *Journal of Human Hypertension* 18, no. 3 (2004): 139–85.

7. White and Chang, "Public Health and Arthritis," 3.

8. White and Chang, "Public Health and Arthritis," 3.

9. T. Kuehlein, D. Sghedoni, G. Visentin, J. Gérvas, and M. Jamoule, "Quaternary Prevention: A Task of the General Practitioner," *Primary Care* 10, no. 18 (2010): 350–54

10. B. J. Turnock, *Public Health: What It Is and How It Works*. Burlington, MA: Jones and Bartlett Publishers, 2011.

11. J. P. Bunker, H. S. Frazier, and F. Mosteller, "Improving Health: Measuring Effects of Medical Care," *Milbank Quarterly* 72, no. 2 (1994): 225–58.

12. Turnock, *Public Health*, 23.

13. Centers for Disease Control and Prevention, "Ten Great Public Health Achievements—United States, 1900–1999," *Morbidity and Mortality Weekly Report* 48, no. 12 (1999): 241–43; Turnock, *Public Health*, 24.

14. E. Tognotti, "The Eradication of Smallpox, a Success Story for Modern Medicine and Public Health: What Lessons for the Future?," *Journal of Infection in Developing Countries* 4, no. 5 (2010): 264.

15. Turnock, *Public Health*, 23.

16. US Department of Health, Education and Welfare, *Smoking and Health: Report of the Advisory Committee to the Surgeon General of the Public Health Service* (Washington, DC: Office of the Surgeon General, 1964).

17. F. G. O'Connor, J. P. Kugler, and R. G. Oriscello, "Sudden Death in Young Athletes: Screening for the Needle in a Haystack," *American Family Physician* 57, no. 11 (1998): 2763–70.

18. M. J. Thun, L. M. Hannan, L. L. Adams-Campbell, P. Boffetta, J. E. Buring, D. Feskanich, D. Flanders, S. H. Jee, K. Katanoda, L. N. Kolonel, I.-M. Lee, T. Marugame, J. R. Palmer, E. Riboli, T. Sobue, E. Avila-Tang, L. R. Wilkens, and J. M. Samet, "Lung Cancer Occurrence in Never-Smokers: An Analysis of 13 Cohorts and 22 Cancer Registry Studies," *Public Library of Science Medicine* 5, no. 9 (2008): e185.

19. American Academy of Orthopaedic Surgeons (AAOS), *The Burden of Musculoskeletal Diseases in the United States: Prevalence, Societal and Economic Cost* (Rosemont, IL: AAOS, 2008).

20. Anthony D. Woolf and Bruce Pfleger, "Burden of Major Musculoskeletal Conditions," *Bulletin of the World Health Organization* 81, no. 9 (2003): 646.

21. Woolf and Pfleger, "Burden of Major Musculoskeletal Conditions," 653.

22. Bone and Joint Decade's Musculoskeletal Portal, "Key Goals," accessed May 10, 2012, www.boneandjointdecade.org.

23. W. G. Gilliar, "Musculoskeletal Component," *Foundation of Osteopathic Medicine*, ed. Anthony Chila, American Osteopathic Association (New York: Lippincott, Williams, and Wilkins, 2010), 326.

24. Gilliar, "Musculoskeletal Component," 323.

25. R. Pattinson, "Volume of World Beer Production," European Beer Guide, accessed July 22, 2012, www.europeanbeerguide.net.

26. G. Nuki and P. A. Simkin, "A Concise History of Gout and Hyperuricemia and Their Treatment," *Arthritis Research and Therapy* 8 (suppl. 1) (2006): 1–5.

27. D. V. Haslam and W. P. James, "Obesity," *Lancet* 366, no. 9492 (2005): 1197–209.

28. Woolf and Pfleger, "Burden of Major Musculoskeletal Conditions," 648.

29. Woolf and Pfleger, "Burden of Major Musculoskeletal Conditions," 652.

30. Woolf and Pfleger, "Burden of Major Musculoskeletal Conditions," 652.

31. Gilliar, "Musculoskeletal Component," 324.

32. B. K. Choi, J. H. Verbeek, W. Wai-San Tam, and J. Y. Jiang, "Exercises for Prevention of Recurrences of Low-Back Pain," *Cochrane Database of Systematic Reviews* 20, no. 1 (2010): CD006555.

33. K. B. Hagen, G. Hilde, G. Jamtvedt, and M. Winnem, "Bed Rest for Acute Low-Back Pain and Sciatica," *Cochrane Database of Systematic Reviews* 18, no. 4 (2004): CD001254; cf. Woolf and Pfleger, "Burden of Major Musculoskeletal Conditions," 653.

34. Woolf and Pfleger, "Burden of Major Musculoskeletal Conditions," 653.

35. Gilliar, "Musculoskeletal Component," 323.

36. Woolf and Pfleger, "Burden of Major Musculoskeletal Conditions," 653.

37. White and Chang, "Public Health and Arthritis," 2–3.

38. L. Keir, B. A. Wise, C. Krebs, and C. Kelley-Armey, *Medical Assisting: Administrative and Clinical Competencies*, 6th ed. (Independence, KY: Cengage Learning, 2007), 392.

39. M. H. Sayler, *The Encyclopedia of the Muscle and Skeletal Systems and Disorders* (New York: Infobase Publishing, 2005), 315.

40. M. A. Liston, "Reading the Bones: Interpreting the Skeletal Evidence for Women's Lives in Ancient Greece," in *A Companion to Women in the Ancient World*, ed. S. L. James and S. Dillon (Hoboken, NJ: John Wiley and Sons, 2012), 127.

41. L. Schienberg, "More Than Skin Deep: The Scientific Search for Sexual Difference," in *The Mind Has No Sex* (Cambridge, MA: Harvard University Press, 1991), 189–213.

42. Schienberg, "More Than Skin Deep," 210.

43. Liston, "Reading the Bones," 128.

44. Liston, "Reading the Bones," 129.

45. H. Schutkowski, "Sex Determination of Infant and Juvenile Skeletons: I. Morphognostic Features," *American Journal of Physical Anthropology* 90, no. 2 (1993): 199–205.

46. Liston, "Reading the Bones," 127.

47. N. K. Lee, H. Sowa, E. Hinoi, M. Ferron, J. D. Ahn, C. Confavreux, R. Dacquin, P. J. Mee, M. D. McKee, D. Y. Jung, Z. Zhang, J. K. Kim, F. Mauvais-Jarvis, P. Ducy, and G. Karsenty, "Endocrine Regulation of Energy Metabolism by the Skeleton," *Cell* 130, no. 3 (2007): 456–69.

48. Shirō Kondō, *Primate Morphophysiology, Locomotor Analyses, and Human Bipedalism* (Tokyo: University of Tokyo Press, 1985).

49. H. M. McHenry, "Human Evolution," in *Evolution: The First Four Billion Years*, eds. M. Ruse and J. Travis (Cambridge, MA: Belknap Press of Harvard University Press, 2009), 263.

50. C. Darwin, *The Descent of Man and Selection in Relation to Sex* (London: Murray, 1871), 52.

51. S. K. Thorpe, R. L. Holder, and R. H. Crompton, "Origin of Human Bipedalism as an Adaptation for Locomotion on Flexible Branches," *Science* 316, no. 5829 (2007): 1328–31.

52. P. Wheeler, "Human Ancestors Walked Tall, Stayed Cool," *Natural History* 102, no. 8 (1993): 65–66.

53. L. Aiello and C. Dean, *An Introduction to Human Evolutionary Anatomy* (Oxford: Elsevier Academic Press, 1990), 246.

54. Weijie Wang, Robin H. Crompton, Tanya S. Carey, Michael M. Günther, Yu Li, Russell Savage, and William I. Sellers, "Comparison of Inverse-Dynamics Musculoskeletal Models of AL 288-1 Australopithecus Afarensis and KNM-WT 15000 Homo Ergaster to Modern Humans, with Implications for the Evolution of Bipedalism," *Journal of Human Evolution* 47, no. 6 (2004): 453–78.

55. Wang, Crompton, Carey, Günther, Li, Savage, and Sellers, "Comparison of Inverse-Dynamics Musculoskeletal Models."

56. Aiello and Dean, *Introduction to Human Evolutionary Anatomy*, 247.

57. K. S. Saladin, *Anatomy and Physiology: The Unity of Form and Function*, 3rd ed. (New York: McGraw-Hill, 2003), 286–87.

58. Aiello and Dean, *Introduction to Human Evolutionary Anatomy*, 483ff.

59. Saladin, *Anatomy and Physiology*, 281.

60. P. S. Bridges, "Prehistoric Arthritis in the Americas," *Annual Review of Anthropology* 21 (1992): 67–91.

61. H. Smith, "Dinosaurs Suffered from Painful Arthritis, Say Scientists," Metro. May 15, 2012, accessed May 16, 2012, www.metro.co.uk/news.

62. S. Gomez, "Crisóstomo Martinez, 1638–1694: The Discoverer of Trabecular Bone," *Endocrine* 17, no. 1 (2002): 3–4.

63. Gordana Vunjak-Novakovic, Nina Tandon, Amandine Godier, Robert Maidhof, Anna Marsano, Timothy P. Martens, and Milica Radisic, "Challenges in Cardiac Tissue Engineering," *Tissue Engineering* 16, no. 2 (2010): 169–87.

64. R. Rubin and D. S. Strayer, *Rubin's Pathology: Clinicopathologic Foundations of Medicine* (New York: Lippincott, Williams, and Wilkins, 2007), 90.

65. M. McKinley and V. O'Loughlin, *Human Anatomy* (New York: McGraw-Hill Companies, 2011), 147.

66. E. N. Marieb, P. B. Wilhelm, and J. Mallat, *Human Anatomy, Media Update* (Upper Saddle River, NJ: Pearson Education, 2011), 125.

67. D. Shier, J. Butler, and R. Lewis, *Hole's Human Anatomy and Physiology* (New York: McGraw-Hill Companies, 2009), 261.

68. Marieb, Wilhelm, and Mallat, *Human Anatomy*, 207.

69. Shier, Butler, and Lewis, *Human Anatomy and Physiology*, 261.

70. Marieb, Wilhelm, and Mallat, *Human Anatomy*, 208.

71. McKinley and O'Loughlin, *Human Anatomy*, 257.

72. McKinley and O'Loughlin, *Human Anatomy*, 257.

73. PhysiologyWeb, "What Is Physiology?," last modified April 9, 2011, accessed June 23, 2012, www.physiologyweb.com/physiology.html.

74. PhysiologyWeb, "What Is Physiology?"

75. T. R. Nichols, "Musculoskeletal Mechanics: A Foundation of Motor Physiology," *Advances in Experimental Medicine and Biology* 508 (2002): 473–79.

76. R. T. Kell, G. Bell, and A. Quinney, "Musculoskeletal Fitness, Health Outcomes and Quality of Life," *Sports Medicine* 31, no. 12 (2001): 863–73.

77. S. Hossain, S. Tada, T. Akaike, and E. H. Chowdhury, "Influences of Electrolytes and Glucose on Formulation of Carbonate Apatite Nanocrystals for Efficient Gene Delivery to Mammalian Cells," *Analytical Biochemistry* 397, no. 2 (2010): 156–61.

78. Salem Communications Corporation, "Phusis," Bible Study Tools, accessed August 6, 2012, www.biblestudytools.com.

79. Bryn Mawr College, "Thinking about Brain Size . . . ," March 7, 2003, accessed May 9, 2012, www.brynmawr.edu.

80. N. M. Varki, E. Strobert, E. J. Dick Jr., K. Benirschke, and A. Varki, "Biomedical Differences between Human and Nonhuman Hominids: Potential Roles for Uniquely Human Aspects of Sialic Acid Biology," *Annual Review of Pathology* 6 (2011): 365–93.

81. American Society for Microbiology, "Microbial Reproduction," accessed June 21, 2012, http://archives.microbeworld.org.

82. J. Lian, J. Gorski, and S. Ott, "Bone Structure and Function," American Society for Bone and Mineral Research, last modified January 16, 2004, accessed August 1, 2012, http://depts.washington.edu/bonebio.

83. K. Kawano, A. Nagano, N. Ochiai, T. Kondo, Y. Mikami, and Y. Tajiri, "Restoration of Elbow Function by Intercostal Nerve Transfer for Obstetrical Paralysis with Co-contraction of the Biceps and the Triceps," *Journal of Hand Surgery* (European volume) 32, no. 4 (2007): 421–26.

84. M. L. Mahowald, "Animal Models of Infectious Arthritis," *Rheumatic Disease Clinics* 12, no. 2 (1986): 403–21.

85. National Center for Biotechnology Information and US National Library of Medicine, "Bone Diseases," last updated January 30, 2012, accessed August 13, 2012, www.nlm.nih.gov.

86. P. A. Gholve, D. M. Scher, S. Khakharia, R. F. Widmann, and D. W. Green, "Osgood Schlatter Syndrome," *Current Opinions in Pediatrics* 19, no. 1 (2007): 44–50.

87. TeachPe.com, "Types of Joint," accessed June 15, 2012, www.teachpe.com/anatomy.

88. H. J. Krzwicki and K. S. Chinn, "Human Body Density and Fat of an Adult Male Population as Measured by Water Displacement," *American Journal of Clinical Nutrition* 20, no. 4 (April 1967): 305–10.

89. J. R. Cameron, J. G. Skofronick, and R. M. Grant, *Physics of the Body*, 2nd ed. (Madison, WI: Medical Physics Publishing, 1999), 96.

90. G. M. Morriss-Kay and A. O. Wilkie, "Growth of the Normal Skull Vault and Its Alteration in Craniosynostosis: Insights from Human Genetics and Experimental Studies," *Journal of Anatomy* 207, no. 5 (2005): 637–53.

91. L. Favors, "Male Vs. Female Skeleton," eHow.com, accessed May 27, 2012, www.ehow.com.

92. L. J. Standley, "The Skeletal System," accessed June 5, 2012, www.drstandley.com.

93. R. Stander, "Athletic Omnibus—Differences between Men and Woman," docstoc.com, December 18, 2009, accessed July 8, 2012, www.docstoc.com.

94. J. M. Soucie, C. Wang, A. Forsyth, S. Funk, M. Denny, K. E. Roach, and D. Boone, "Range of Motion Measurements: Reference Values and a Database for Comparison Studies," *Haemophilia* 17, no. 3 (2001): 500–507.

95. B. Kumar, S. Pai, B. Ray, S. Mishra, and A. K. Pandey, "Radiographic Study of Carrying Angle and Morphometry of Skeletal Elements of Human Elbow," *Romanian Journal of Morphology and Embryology* 51, no. 3 (2010): 521–26; D. W. Golden, J. T. Jhee, S. P. Gilpin, and J. R. Sawyer, "Elbow Range of Motion and Clinical Carrying Angle in a Healthy Pediatric Population," *Journal of Pediatric Orthopaedics B* 16, no. 2 (2007): 144–49.

3. THE REAL MEANING AND HISTORY OF ARTHRITIS

1. J. Cluett, "What Does It Mean to Have Arthritis?," About.com, last updated July 18, 2008, accessed July 23, 2012, www.orthopedics.about.com.

2. J. Beasley, "Osteoarthritis and Rheumatoid Arthritis: Conservative Therapeutic Management," *Journal of Hand Therapy* 25, no. 2 (2012): 163–71.

3. M. Kelly, "De Arthritide Symptomatica of William Muscgrave (1657–1721): His Description of Neuropathic Arthritis," *Bulletin of the History of Medicine* 37 (1963): 372–77.

4. J. U. Scher and S. B. Abramson, "The Microbiome and Rheumatoid Arthritis," *Nature Reviews Rheumatology* 7, no. 10 (2011): 569–78.

5. D. R. Shreeve, "William Roentgen's (1845–1923) Influence: Contrasts and Comparisons," *Journal of Medical Biography* 18, no. 3 (2010): 158–62.

6. H. L. Tidy, *A Synopsis of Medicine* (Cheshire, UK: John Wright and Sons, 1946).

7. F. D. Hart, "History of the Treatment of Rheumatoid Arthritis," *British Medical Journal* 1 (1976): 763–65.

8. H. Kaiser and W. Keitel, "[Guillaume de Baillou (1538–1616)—the Father of 'Rheumatism'?]," *Zeitschrift für Rheumatologie* 65, no. 8 (2006): 743–46.

9. P. S. Hench, E. C. Kendall, C. H. Slocumb, and H. F. Polley, "Adrenocortical Hormone in Arthritis: Preliminary Report," *Annals of the Rheumatic Diseases* 8, no. 2 (1949): 97–104.

10. Farlex, "Arthritis," The Free Dictionary, accessed May 25, 2012, www.thefreedictionary.com/arthritis.

11. Merriam-Webster, "Arthritis," accessed July 2, 2012, www.merriam-webster.com/medical/arthritis.

12. Dictionary.com, "Arthritis," accessed June 25, 2012, www.dictionary.reference.com/browse/arthritis.

13. M. Lefers and the Holmgren Lab, "Arthritis," Northwestern University Department of Molecular Biosciences, accessed May 27, 2012, www.molbiosci.northwestern.edu.

14. New York Times Company, "Medical Condition," About.com, last updated January 30, 2009, accessed June 3, 2012, http://firstaid.about.com/od/glossary.

15. National Center for Biotechnology Information and US National Library of Medicine, "Arthritis, Joint Inflammation," last reviewed February 2, 2012, accessed May 26, 2012, www.ncbi.nlm.nih.gov.

16. Marsh, *The Economic and Social Impact of Emerging Infectious Disease* (Andover, MA: Phillips Healthcare, 2008), 48.

1

17. World Health Organization, "Physical Inactivity a Leading Cause of Disease and Disability, Warns WHO," April 4, 2002, accessed June 9, 2012, www.who.int.

18. Hart, "History of the Treatment of Rheumatoid Arthritis," 763–65.

19. B. Strauss, "Did Dinosaurs Have Arthritis?," About.com, accessed June 23, 2012, www.dinosaurs.about.com.

20. R. Waugh, "Fossil Shows Off that Even the Dinosaurs Suffered Arthritis 150 Million Years Ago," *Daily Mail*, May 15, 2012, updated May 15, 2012, accessed July 19, 2012, www.dailymail.co.uk.

21. P. S. Bridges, "Prehistoric Arthritis in the Americas," *Annual Review of Anthropology* 21 (1992): 67–91.

22. M. A. Ruffer, "Studies in Palaeopathology: Some Recent Researches on Prehistoric Trephining," *Journal of Pathology* 22, no. 1 (1919): 90–104; M. A. Ruffer, "Studies in Palaeopathology in Egypt," *Journal of Pathology* 18, no. 1 (2005): 149–62; M. A. Ruffer, "Study of Abnormalities and Pathology of Ancient Egyptian Teeth," *American Journal of Physical Anthropology* 3 (1920): 335–82.

23. G. D. Storey, "Alfred Baring Garrod (1819–1907)," *Rheumatology* 40, no. 10 (2001): 1189–90.

24. Estate of James J. Braddock, "The Man," accessed July 3, 2012, www.jamesjbraddock.com.

4. ANATOMY AND PATHOLOGY OF ARTHRITIS

1. H. Gray, *Anatomy of the Human Body*, 20th ed. (New York: Churchill Livingstone, 1918), accessed June 13, 2012, www.bartleby.com/107.

2. C. Mazzio, *The Body in Parts: Discourses and Anatomies in Early Modern Europe* (New York: Routledge, 1997).

3. R. Richardson, "A Historical Introduction to Gray's Anatomy," in *Gray's Anatomy: The Anatomical Basis of Clinical Practice*, ed. S. Standring, 39th ed. (electronic) (New York, NY: Churchill Livingstone, 2004).

4. HighBeam Research, "W. Hunter," Encyclopedia.com, 2008, accessed March 20, 2012, www.encyclopedia.com.

5. HighBeam Research, "J. Cruveilhier," Encyclopedia.com, 2008, accessed March 23, 2012, www.encyclopedia.com.

6. W. W. Buchanan, "William Hunter (1718–1783)," *Rheumatology* 42, no. 10 (2003): 1260–61; J. Kobler, *The Reluctant Surgeon: A Biography of John Hunter* (New York: Doubleday, 1960).

7. Demand Media, "Bones of the Human Body," eHow.com, accessed May 23, 2012, www.ehow.com.

8. The Synergy Company, "Healthy Bones Are the Foundation of Wellness," accessed April 28, 2012, www.thesynergycompany.com.

9. A. Epstein, "Believe It or Not, Your Lungs Are Six Weeks Old—and Your Taste Buds Just Ten Days! So How Old Is the Rest of Your Body?," *Daily Mail*, accessed July 2, 2012, www.dailymail.co.uk.

10. D. Gentry Steele and C. A. Bramblett, *The Anatomy and Biology of the Human Skeleton* (College Station: Texas A&M University Press, 1988), 4.

11. J. Z. Ilich and J. E. Kerstetter, "Nutrition in Bone Health Revisited: A Story beyond Calcium," *Journal of the American College of Nutrition* 19, no. 6 (2000): 715–37.

12. K. L. Minaker, "Common Clinical Sequelae of Aging," in Cecil Medicine, ed. L. Goldman and D. Ausiello, 23rd ed. (Philadelphia: Saunders Elsevier, 2007), ch. 23.

13. G. Cooper, "How Your Posture Can Cause (and Affect) Arthritis," Health Central, accessed March 21, 2012, www.healthcentral.com.

14. American Society for Arthritis of the Hand, "Osteoarthritis of the Hand," accessed April 29, 2012, www.assh.org.

15. MedicineNet, "Psoriatic Arthritis," accessed April 30, 2012, www.medicinenet.com.

16. A. Asher, "Arthritis of the Neck—Cervical Spondylosis," About.com, updated January 2, 2012, accessed April 30, 2012, www.backandneck.about.com; Healthy Back Institute, "Less Pain and More Life," accessed May 24, 2012, www.losethebackpain.com.

17. J. Cluett, "Shoulder Arthritis: What Is the Most Common Type of Shoulder Arthritis?," About.com, accessed March 30, 2012, www.orthopedics.about.com.

18. F. J. Jiménez-Balderas and G. Mintz, "Ankylosing Spondylitis: Clinical Course in Women and Men," *Journal of Rheumatology* 20, no. 12 (1993): 2069–72.

19. J. Cluett, "Lumbar Spine Arthritis: Wear and Tear Arthritis of the Lumbar Spine," About.com, accessed March 30, 2012, www.orthopedics.about.com.

20. P. F. Ulrich, "Sacrum (Sacral Region)," Spine-Health, accessed April 27, 2012, www.spine-health.com.

21. J. Cluett, "Hip Arthritis: Information about Hip Arthritis and Available Treatments," About.com, accessed April 1, 2012, www.orthopedics about.com.

22. L. Newell, "How Does Arthritis Affect the Knee?," Livestrong.com, October 2009, accessed April 1, 2012, www.livestrong.com.

23. B. J. Sangeorzan, "Ankle Arthritis," University of Washington Orthopaedics and Sports Medicine, updated December 2009, accessed April 2, 2012, www.orthop.washington.edu.

24. K. Blanchard, "Foot Arthritis Symptoms," Livestrong.com, May 16, 2011, accessed July 11, 2012, www.livestrong.com.

25. W. C. Shiel, "Psoriatic Arthritis," MedicineNet, accessed May 2, 2012, www.medicinenet.com.

26. Royal College of Pathologists of Australia, "What Is Pathology?," accessed April 30, 2012, www.rcpa.edu.au/pathology.htm.

27. C. K. Hurley, "DNA-Based Typing of HLA for Transplantation," in *Handbook of Human Immunology*, ed. M. S. Leffell, A. D. Donnenberg, and N. R. Rose (Boca Raton, LA: CRC Press, 1997), 521–55.

28. P. B. Martens, J. J. Goronzy, D. Schaid, and C. M. Weyand, "Expansion of Unusual CD4+ T Cells in Severe Rheumatoid Arthritis," *Arthritis Rheumatology* 40 (1997): 1106–14.

29. M. Feldman and R. Maini, "TNF Defined as a Therapeutic Target for Rheumatoid Arthritis and Other Autoimmune Diseases," *Nature Medicine* 9, no. 10 (2003): 1245–50.

30. G. Manning, D. B. Whyte, R. Martinez, T. Hunter, and S. Sudarshanam, "The Protein Kinase Complement of the Human Genome," *Science* 298, no. 5600 (2002): 1912–34.

31. A. J. Ridley, H. F. Paterson, C. L. Johnston, D. Diekmann, and A. Hall, "The Small GTP-Binding Protein RAC Regulates Growth Factor-Induced Membrane Ruffling," *Cell* 70 (1992): 401–10.

32. T. Hirano, T. Harada, K. Nakajima, A. Iwamatsu, K. Yasukawa, T. Taga, Y. Watanabe, T. Matsuda, S. Kashiwamura, and K. Koyama, "Complementary DNA for a Novel Human Interleukin (BSF-2) that Induces B Lymphocytes to Produce Immunoglobulin," *Nature* 324, no. 6092 (1986): 73–76.

33. J. Edwards, "Rheumatoid Arthritis and Autoimmunity: A New Approach to Their Cause and How Long Term Cure Might Be Achieved," Centre for Rheumatology, University College, London, accessed June 23, 2012, www.lupus-support.org.uk.

34. P. Bass, "What Are Macrophages?," About.com, accessed April 11, 2012, www.asthma.about.com.

35. A. Wilson, H. T. Yu, L. T. Goodnough, and A. R. Nissenson, "Prevalence and Outcomes of Anemia in Rheumatoid Arthritis: A Systematic Review of the Literature," *American Journal of Medicine* 16 (suppl. 7A) (2004): 50S–57S.

36. C. Eustice, "Can Rheumatoid Arthritis Cause a Low Red Blood Cell Count?," About.com, updated May 29, 2007, accessed April 11, 2012, www.arthritis.about.com.

37. G. J. Silverman and D. A. Carson, "Roles of B Cells in Rheumatoid Arthritis," *Arthritis Research and Therapy* 5 (suppl. 4) (2003): S1–S6.

38. W. Ouyang, J. K. Kolls, and Y. Zheng, "The Biological Functions of T-Helper 17 Cells Effector Cytokines in Inflammation," *Immunity* 28, no. 4 (2008): 453–67.

39. C. Ospelt and S. Gay, "The Role of Resident Synovial Cells in Destructive Arthritis," *Best Practices and Research in Clinical Rheumatology* 22, no. 2 (2008): 239–52.

40. S. Shahrara, Q. Huang, A. M., Mandelin, and R. M. Pope, "TH-17 Cells in Rheumatoid Arthritis," *Arthritis Research and Therapy* 10, no. 4 (2008): 1–7.

41. Steele and Bramblett, *The Anatomy and Biology of the Human Skeleton*, 4.

42. C. Eustice, "Rheumatoid Arthritis—10 Things You Should Know from Diagnosis to Disease Management," About.com, updated April 16, 2012, accessed April 29, 2012, www.arthritis.about.com.

43. A. D. Pearle, R. F. Warren, and S. A. Rodeo, "Basic Science of Articular Cartilage and Osteoarthritis," *Clinics in Sports Medicine* 24, no. 1 (2005): 1–12.

5. CAUSES AND SYMPTOMS OF ARTHRITIS

1. R. B. Rosenbaum and D. P. Ciaverella, "Disorders of Bones, Joints, Ligaments, and Meninges," in Neurology in Clinical Practice, ed. W. G. Bradley, R. B. Daroff, G. M. Fenichel, and J. Jankovic, 5th ed. (Philadelphia: Butterworth-Heinemann, 2008), ch. 77.

2. Computer Posture UK, "Thoracic Outlet Syndrome, Cervical Osteoarthritis and Cervical Spondylosis; General Computer Posture RSI Advice for Employers," accessed June 5, 2012, www.computer-posture.co.uk.

3. J. Cluett, "Does Sports Participation Cause Arthritis?," About.com, accessed April 8, 2012, www.orthopedics.about.com.

4. J. Lee, D. Dunlop, L. Jones-Ehrlich, P. Semanik, J. Song, L. Manheim, and R. W. Chang, "The Public Health Impact of Risk Factors for Physical Inactivity in Adults with Rheumatoid Arthritis," *Arthritis Care and Research* 64, no. 4 (2012): 488–93.

5. K. Goel and L. Pearson, "Obesity Takes Heavy Toll on Knee Arthritis," American Academy of Orthopaedic Surgeons, accessed April 25, 2012, www6.aaos.org/news.

6. H. Buchwald, Y. Avidor, E. Braunwald, M. D. Jensen, W. Pories, K. Fahrbach, and K. Schoelles, "Bariatric Surgery: A Systematic Review and Meta-analysis," *Journal of the American Medical Association* 292, no. 14 (2004): 1724–37.

7. Arthritis Foundation, "Recent Headlines: Rheumatoid Arthritis," June 24, 2008, accessed April 13, 2012, www.arthritis.org.

8. W. L. Haskell, "Health Consequences of Physical Activity: Understanding and Challenges Regarding Dose-Response," *Medicine and Science in Sports and Exercise* 26 (1994): 649–60.

9. Centers for Disease Control and Prevention, "Physical Activity: The Arthritis Pain Reliever," accessed April 26, 2012, www.cdc.gov; K. L. Depkin, "The Effects of Exercise on the Human Bones," eHow.com, accessed April 8 2012, www.ehow.com.

10. National Space Biomedical Research Institute, "Bone Development and Structure," accessed April 25, 2012, www.nsbri.org.

11. A. N. Malaviya, "Can Climbing Stairs Lead to Arthritis?," Doctor NDTV, October, 2007, accessed April 8, 2012, www.doctor.ndtv.com.

12. S. L. Reynolds and J. M. Mcilvane, "The Impact of Obesity and Arthritis on Active Life Expectancy in Older Americans," *Obesity* 17, no. 2 (2009): 363–69.

13. C. Stehling, N. E. Lane, M. C. Nevitt, J. Lynch, C. E. McCulloch, and T. M. Link, "Subjects with Higher Physical Activity Levels Have More Severe Focal Knee Lesions Diagnosed with 3T MRI: Analysis of a Non-symptomatic Cohort of the Osteoarthritis Initiative," *Osteoarthritis Cartilage* 18, no. 6 (2010): 776–86.

14. R. H. Straub, J. R. Kalden, "Stress of Different Types Increases the Proinflammatory Load in Rheumatoid Arthritis," *Arthritis Research and Therapy* 11, no. 3 (2009): 114.

15. N. C. Wright, G. K. Riggs, J. R. Lisse, and Z. Chen, "Self-reported Osteoarthritis, Ethnicity, Body Mass Index, and Other Associated Risk Factors in Postmenopausal Women—Results from the Women's Health Initiative," *Journal of the American Geriatrics Society* 56, no. 9 (2008): 1736–43.

16. P. Carrera-Bastos, M. Fontes-Villalba, J. O'Keefe, S. Lindeberg, and L. Cordain, "The Western Diet and Lifestyle and Diseases of Civilization," *Research Reports in Clinical Cardiology* 2 (2011): 1–21.

17. T. M. Pollard, *Western Diseases: An Evolutionary Perspective* (Cambridge: Cambridge University Press, 2008).

18. T. A. Kutscher, "Barefoot Walking and Living Health Benefits (and 125 Reasons to Go Barefoot)," Barefoot Hikers, accessed April 9, 2012, www.barefootkc.com.

19. K. Alagakrishnan and A. Chopra, "Health and Care of Asian American Elders," Stanford University, accessed April 13, 2012, www.stanford.edu/group/ethnoger/asianindian.html.

20. Hospital for Special Surgery, "Patellofemoral Arthritis in the Knee: An Overview. Interviews with Drs. Boettner, Della Valle, and Shubin Stein about Knee Arthritis, Total Knee Replacement and Patellofemoral Knee Replacement (Partial Knee Replacement)," March 17, 2012, reviewed March 26, 2010, accessed April 13, 2012, www.hss.edu.

21. J. E. Hart, "Air Pollution May Cause Rheumatoid Arthritis: Research Presented during the ACR Annual Scientific Meeting at the McCormick Place Convention Center," American College of Rheumatology, accessed April 28, 2012, www.rheumatology.org.

22. S. Philomena, "Link between Air Pollution and Rheumatoid Arthritis," MedIndia, November 7, 2011, accessed April 23, 2012, www.medindia.net/news.

23. E. V. Hess, "Environmental Chemicals and Autoimmune Disease: Cause and Effect," *Toxicology* 181–82 (2002): 65–70.

24. R. Krulwich, "Cracking the Code of Life," Public Broadcasting System (PBS), April 17, 2001, accessed June 28, 2012.

25. F. C. Arnett and S. Assassi, "Heredity and Arthritis," American College of Rheumatology, 2012, accessed April 14, 2012, www.rheumatology.org.

26. Science Daily, "Identical Twins, Identical Problems: Scientists Discover New Genes Linked to Rheumatoid Arthritis," July 1, 2007, accessed July 12, 2012, www.sciencedaily.com.

27. T. Pincus, "Rheumatoid Arthritis: A Medical Emergency?," *Scandinavian Journal of Rheumatology* 100 (1994): 13.

28. M. Ahern and M. Smith, "Rheumatoid Arthritis," *Medical Journal of Australia* 166 (1997): 93.

29. Ahern and Smith, "Rheumatoid Arthritis," 134.

30. E. Harris, R. Budd, G. Firestein, M. Genovese, J. Sergent, S. Ruddy, and C. Sledge, *Kelley's Textbook of Rheumatology*, 8th ed. (Philadelphia: Saunders Elsevier, 2004), 2:186.

31. Harris, Budd, Firestein, Genovese, Sergent, Ruddy, and Sledge, *Kelley's Textbook of Rheumatology*, 2:1012–53.

32. W. J. Koopman, *Arthritis and Allied Conditions: A Textbook of Rheumatology* (Philadelphia: Lippincott, Williams, and Wilkins, 1997), 145–77.

33. Ahern and Smith, "Rheumatoid Arthritis," 156–61.

34. Pincus, "Rheumatoid Arthritis: A Medical Emergency?," 25–30.

35. Harris, Budd, Firestein, Genovese, Sergent, Ruddy, and Sledge, *Kelley's Textbook of Rheumatology*, 2:562–675.

6. DIAGNOSING ARTHRITIS

1. F. Wolfe, K. Ross, D. J. Hawley, F. K. Roberts, and M. A. Cathey, "The Prognosis of Rheumatoid Arthritis and Undifferentiated Polyarthritis Syndrome in the Clinic: A Study of 1141 Patients," *Journal of Rheumatology* 12 (2005): 133–45.

2. F. Wolfe and D. J. Hawley, "Remission in Rheumatoid Arthritis," *Journal of Rheumatology* 2 (1985): 245.

3. E. Harris, R. Budd, G. Firestein, M. Genovese, J. Sergent, S. Ruddy, and C. Sledge, *Kelley's Textbook of Rheumatology*, 8th ed. (Philadelphia: Saunders Elsevier, 2004), 2:1121–45.

4. Wolfe and Hawley, "Remission in Rheumatoid Arthritis," 250–52.

5. Wolfe, Ross, Hawley, Roberts, and Cathey, "The Prognosis of Rheumatoid Arthritis and Undifferentiated Polyarthritis Syndrome in the Clinic," 162–66.

6. C. Eustice, "What Is Rheumatoid Factor?," About.com, accessed July 22, 2012, www.arthritis.about.com.

7. J. B. Little, "Ionizing Radiation," in *Holland-Frei Cancer Medicine*, ed. R. C. Blast Jr., D. W. Kufe, and R. E. Pollock, 5th ed. (Hamilton, ON: B. C. Decker, 2000).

8. W. J. Koopman, *Arthritis and Allied Conditions: A Textbook of Rheumatology* (Philadelphia: Lippincott, Williams, and Wilkins, 1997), 145–332.

9. Koopman, *Arthritis and Allied Conditions*, 675–722.

10. Wolfe, Ross, Hawley, Roberts, and Cathey, "The Prognosis of Rheumatoid Arthritis and Undifferentiated Polyarthritis Syndrome in the Clinic," *Journal of Rheumatology* 12 (2005): 153.

7. THE ROLES OF VARIOUS TYPES OF PHYSICIANS IN ARTHRITIS

1. A. Santiago, "Career Overview for Family Medicine Physician, or Family Medicine Doctor," About.com, accessed June 16, 2012, www.healthcareers.about.com.

2. Demand Media, "How Does a Family Doctor Spend a Workday?," eHow.com, accessed June 24, 2012, www.ehow.com; R. Lo, "How Does a Medical Doctor Spend a Workday?," eHow.com, accessed June 24, 2012, www.ehow.com.

3. "Arthritis Doctor," Arthritis M.D., accessed July 12, 2012, www.arthritismd.com/arthritis-doctor.html.

4. Agency for Healthcare Research and Policy (AHRQ), "Primary Care Workforce Facts and Stats No. 1: The Number of Practicing Primary Care Physicians in the United States," updated October 2011, accessed May 22, 2012, www.ahrq.gov.

5. AHRQ, "Primary Care Workforce Facts and Stats No. 1."

6. American Dental Education Association, "Family Medicine," September 29, 2010, updated July 25, 2012, www.explorehealthcareers.org.

7. UCSF Medical Center, "Rheumatic Disorders," accessed May 23, 2012, www.ucsfhealth.org.

8. New York Times Company, "Arthritis and Joint Conditions," About.com, accessed May 12, 2012, www.arthritis.about.com.

9. A. K. Poznanski, "Radiological Approaches to Pediatric Joint Disease," *Journal of Rheumatology* 33 (1992): 88.

10. D. Gordon and D. R. Siegfried, "Calling All Rheumatologists," Arthritis Today, accessed May 24, 2012, www.arthritistoday.org.

11. C. L. Deal, R. Hooker, T. Harrington, N. Birnbaum, F. Hogan, E. Bouchery, M. Klei-Gitelman, and W. Barr, "The United States Rheumatology Workforce: Supply and Demand, 2005–2025," *Arthritis and Rheumatism* 56, no. 3 (2007): 722–29.

12. Gordon and Siegfried, "Calling All Rheumatologists."

13. Arthritis Today, "The Downside of Demand," accessed June 14, 2012, www.arthritistoday.org.

14. Poznanski, "Radiological Approaches to Pediatric Joint Disease," 90–93.

15. Poznanski, "Radiological Approaches to Pediatric Joint Disease," 78–86.

16. N. J. Cooper, "Economic Burden of Rheumatoid Arthritis: A Systematic Review," *Rheumatology* 39 (2000): 33.

17. Poznanski, "Radiological Approaches to Pediatric Joint Disease," 81–88.

18. Philip Allen Orthopaedic, "About Orthopaedics," accessed July 2, 2012, www.bonedoctor.com.au.

19. HealthAlliance Hospital, "Orthopedics," accessed July 5, 2012, www.umassmemorial.org.

20. North Jersey Regional Arthritis Center, "Orthopedics," accessed July 5, 2012, www.atlantichealth.org/morristown.

21. Cottage Health System, "Outpatient Surgery," accessed July 21, 2012, www.sbch.org.

22. Cottage Health System, "Outpatient Surgery."

23. Cottage Health System, "Outpatient Surgery."

24. American Academy of Orthopaedic Surgeons (AAOS), "Arthritis: An Overview," accessed July 5, 2012, www.orthoinfo.aaos.org.

25. AAOS, "Arthritis: An Overview."

26. AAOS, "Arthritis: An Overview."

27. AAOS, "Arthritis: An Overview."

28. C. Wilson, "Orthopaedic Surgeon," Arthritis Research UK, accessed July 5, 2012, www.arthritisresearchuk.org.

29. C. Merrill and A. Elixhauser, "Hospital Stays Involving Musculoskeletal Procedure, 1997–2005," Agency for Healthcare Research and Quality, July 2007, accessed May 22, 2012, www.hcup-us.ahrq.gov.

30. Merrill and Elixhauser, "Hospital Stays Involving Musculoskeletal Procedure, 1997–2005."

31. AAOS, "About the AAOS," accessed July 7, 2012, www.aaos.org.

32. AAOS, "AAOS Orthopaedic Surgeon Census," accessed July 7, 2012, www.aaos.org.

33. AAOS, "Orthopaedic Surgeon Quick Facts," accessed July 7, 2012, www.aaos.org.

34. AAOS, "Practice Setting," 2010, accessed July 7, 2012, www.aaos.org.

35. AAOS, "Career in Orthopedics," last reviewed December 2007, accessed July 5, 2012, www.orthoinfo.aaos.org.

36. American Osteopathic Academy of Orthopedics, "Resident American Osteopathic Academy of Orthopedics," accessed June 4, 2012, www.aoao.org.

37. H. Natividad and H. Schmalz, "OPUS 2008: An Orthopaedic Snapshot," AAOS, accessed July 15, 2012, www.aaos.org.

38. AAOS, "Degree of Specialization," 2010, accessed July 7, 2012, www.aaos.org.

39. AAOS, "Specialty Areas," 2010, accessed July 7, 2012, www.aaos.org.

40. AAOS, "Orthopaedic Surgeons: Who Are They and What Do They Do?," accessed July 7, 2012, www6.aaos.org.

41. AAOS, "Orthopaedic Surgeons."

42. Merrill and Elixhauser, "Hospital Stays Involving Musculoskeletal Procedure, 1997–2005."

43. Merrill and Elixhauser, "Hospital Stays Involving Musculoskeletal Procedure, 1997–2005."

44. B. W. Young, "How Many Surgeons in the U.S.?," Orthopedics This Week, January 31, 2011, accessed June 2, 2012, www.ryortho.com.

45. Young , "How Many Surgeons in the U.S.?"

46. Young , "How Many Surgeons in the U.S.?"

47. Merrill and Elixhauser, "Hospital Stays Involving Musculoskeletal Procedure, 1997–2005."

48. International Association of Orthopedic Surgeons, "Welcome to the International Association of Orthopedic Surgeons," accessed July 7, 2012, http://www.iaorthopedics.com.

49. AAOS, "Questions to Ask Your Doctor before Surgery," March 2002, accessed April 23, 2012, www.orthoinfo.aaos.org.

50. Orthopaedic Specialists of North Carolina, "Pre-operative FAQs," accessed July 10, 2012, www.orthonc.com.

51. Orthopaedic Specialists of North Carolina, "Pre-operative FAQs."

52. AAOS, "Questions to Ask Your Doctor before Surgery."

53. AAOS, "Questions to Ask Your Doctor before Surgery."

54. Orthopaedic Specialists of North Carolina, "Pre-operative FAQs."

55. K. Strange, "Patient Education and Physical Therapy after Orthopedic Surgery," May 26, 2011, www.livestrong.com.

8. RHEUMATOID ARTHRITIS

1. N. J. Cooper, "Economic Burden of Rheumatoid Arthritis: A Systematic Review," *Rheumatology* 39 (2000): 28–30.

2. E. Harris, R. Budd, G. Firestein, M. Genovese, J. Sergent, S. Ruddy, and C. Sledge, *Kelley's Textbook of Rheumatology*, 8th ed. (Philadelphia: Saunders Elsevier, 2004), 2:833–43.

3. M. H. Pillinger and R. T. Keenan, "Update on the Management of Hyperuricemia and Gout," *Bulletin of the NYU Hospital for Joint Diseases* 66, no. 3 (2008): 231–39.

4. Centers for Disease Control and Prevention (CDC), "Arthritis-Related Statistics," accessed July 22, 2012, www.cdc.gov.

5. M. C. Hochberg, A. J. Silman, J. S. Smolen, M. E. Weinblatt, and M. H. Weisman, eds., *Rheumatology*, 3rd ed. (New York: Mosby, 2003): 122–23.

6. CDC, "Arthritis-Related Statistics."

7. D. Symmons, C. Mathers, and B. Pfleger, "The Global Burden of Rheumatoid Arthritis in the Year 2000," World Health Organization, accessed April 27, 2012, www.who.int.

8. Mayo Clinic, "Rheumatoid Arthritis," accessed July 23, 2012, www.mayoclinic.com.

9. Mayo Clinic, "Young Women with Rheumatoid Arthritis at More Risk for Broken Bones," accessed July 23, 2012, www.mayoclinic.org.

10. Arthritis Foundation, "The Genetics of Rheumatoid Arthritis," accessed July 20, 2012, www.arthritis.org/genetics-ra.php.

11. D. Mann, "Scientists Search for Rheumatoid Arthritis Genes," WebMD, accessed July 20, 2012, www.webmd.com.

12. S. Raychaudhuri, C. Sandor, E. A. Stahl, J. Freudenberg, H.-S. Lee, X. Jia, L. Alfredsson, L. Padyukov, L. Klareskog, J. Worthington, K. A. Siminovitch, S.-C. Bae, R. M. Plenge, P. K. Gregersen, and P. W. de Bakker, "Five Amino Acids in Three HLA Proteins Explain Most of the Association between MHC and Seropositive Rheumatoid Arthritis," *Nature Genetics* 44, no. 3 (2012): 291–96.

13. D. Mann, "Smoking Raises Rheumatoid Arthritis Risk," MedicineNet, accessed July 20, 2012, www.medicinenet.com.

14. S. Saevarsdottir, S. Wedrén, M. Seddighzadeh, C. Bengtsson, A. Wesley, S. Lindblad, J. Askling, L. Alfredsson, and L. Klareskog, "Patients with Early Rheumatoid Arthritis Who Smoke Are Less Likely to Respond to Treatment with Methotrexate and Tumor Necrosis Factor Inhibitors: Observations from the Epidemiological Investigation of Rheumatoid Arthritis and the Swedish Rheumatology Register Cohorts," *Arthritis and Rheumatism* 63, no. 1 (2011): 26–36.

15. I. Vallbracht, J. Rieber, M. Oppermann, F. Forger, U. Siebert, and K. Helmke, "Diagnostic and Clinical Value of Anti-cyclic Citrullinated Peptide Antibodies Compared with Rheumatoid Factor Isotypes in Rheumatoid Arthritis," *Annals of Rheumatic Disease* 63 (2004): 1079–84.

16. S. Rantapää-Dahlqvist, B. A. W. de Jong, E. Berglin, G. Hallmans, G. Wadell, H. Stenlund, U. Sundin, and W. J. van Venrooij, "Antibodies against Cyclic Citrullinated Peptide and IgA Rheumatoid Factor Predict the Development of Rheumatoid Arthritis," *Arthritis and Rheumatism* 48 (2003): 2741–49.

17. Quest Diagnostics, "Rheumatoid Arthritis Laboratory Markers for Diagnosis and Prognosis," accessed November 28, 2012, www.questdiagnostics.com.

18. J. Vencovský, S. Macháček, L. Šedová, J. Kafková, J. Gatterová, V. Pešáková, and Š. Růžičková, "Autoantibodies Can Be Prognostic Markers of an Erosive Disease in Early Rheumatoid Arthritis," *Annals of Rheumatic Disease* 62 (2003): 427–30.

19. E. Lindqvist, K. Eberhardt, K. Bendtzen, D. Heinegard, and T. Saxne, "Prognostic Laboratory Markers of Joint Damage in Rheumatoid Arthritis," *Annals of Rheumatic Disease* 64 (2005): 196–201.

20. C. Bates, "Arthritis Breakthrough Could Stop Crippling Condition before It Starts," *Daily Mail*, accessed July 20, 2012, www.dailymail.co.uk.

21. Arthritis Research UK, "New Potential Target for Rheumatoid Arthritis," accessed July 20, 2012, www.arthritisresearchuk.org.

22. R. Hirshfeld, "Israeli Medical Breakthroughs Offer Hope to Auto-immune Patients," Israel National News, accessed July 20, 2012, www.israelnationalnews.com.

23. N. Walsh, "IL-6 Blocker Stops RA Joint Damage," Medpage Today, accessed July 20, 2012, www.medpagetoday.com.

24. Walsh, "IL-6 Blocker Stops RA Joint Damage."

25. G. S. Firestein, "Evolving Concept of Rheumatoid Arthritis," *Nature* 423, no. 6937 (2003): 356–61.

26. J. P. Leombruno, T. R. Einarson, and E. C. Keystone, "The Safety of Anti-tumour Necrosis Factor Treatments in Rheumatoid Arthritis: Meta and Exposure-Adjusted Pooled Analyses of Serious Adverse Events," *Annals of Rheumatic Diseases* 68, no. 7 (2009): 36–45.

9. JUVENILE RHEUMATOID ARTHRITIS

1. R. Lagier, "Nosology versus Pathology: Two Approaches to Rheumatic Diseases," *Rheumatology* 40, no. 4 (2001): 467–71.

2. American Academy of Orthopedic Surgeons, "Juvenile Arthritis," last modified December 2010, accessed June 4, 2012, www.orthoinfo.aaos.org.

3. K. Young, "Juvenile Rheumatoid Arthritis and Rheumatoid Arthritis," Rheumatoid Arthritis Warrior, last modified on January 19, 2010, accessed June 4, 2012, www.rawarrior.com.

4. C. Hoffart and D. D. Sherry, "Early Identification of Juvenile Idiopathic Arthritis," *Journal of Musculoskeletal Medicine* 27, no. 2 (2010): 52–56.

5. Hoffart and Sherry, "Early Identification of Juvenile Idiopathic Arthritis," 52–56.

6. WebMD, "Juvenile Idiopathic Arthritis," accessed May 24, 2012, www.emedicinehealth.com.

7. J. Rudis, "Juvenile Rheumatoid Arthritis," New York University (NYU) Longone Medical Center, last reviewed August 12, 2012, last modified September 2011, accessed August 23, 2012, www.pediatrics.med.nyu.edu.

8. J. Pope, reviewer, "Medical History and Physical Examination for Juvenile Idiopathic Arthritis," WebMD, last modified June 11, 2011, accessed April 23, 2012, www.webmd.com.

9. Krames StayWell, "Health Encyclopedia: Juvenile Rheumatoid Arthritis," last modified March 24, 2011, accessed June 1, 2012, www.carefirst.staywellsolutionsonline.com.

10. Autoimmune Technologies, "Areas of Research: Juvenile Rheumatoid Arthritis," accessed August 18, 2012, www.autoimmune.com.

11. National Institute of Arthritis and Musculoskeletal and Skin Diseases (NIAMS), "Juvenile Rheumatoid Arthritis Research Registry," ClinicalTrials.gov, last updated June 5, 2009, accessed July 1, 2012, www.clinicaltrials.gov.

12. NIAMS, "Q&A about Juvenile Rheumatoid Arthritis," last modified September 2011, accessed July 2, 2012, www.niams.nih.gov.

10. OSTEOARTHRITIS

1. G. Slowik, ed., "What Is Osteoarthritis?," ehealthMD, last updated April 23, 2012, accessed April 26, 2012, www.ehealthmd.com.

2. Slowik, "What Is Osteoarthritis?"

3. M. Suszynski, "Understanding Primary and Secondary Osteoarthritis," Everyday Health, last updated March 4, 2009, accessed July 4, 2012, www.everydayhealth.com.

4. M. A. Davis, W. H. Ettinger, J. M. Neuhaus, and K. P. Mallon, "Knee Osteoarthritis and Physical Functioning (Evidence from the NHANES I Epidemiologic Followup Study)," *Journal of Rheumatology* 18, no. 4 (1991): 591–98.

5. R. W. Moskowitz, "The Burden of Osteoarthritis: Clinical and Quality-of-Life Issues," *American Journal of Managed Care* 15 (suppl. 8) (2009): S223–S229.

6. ThirdAge Media, "Osteoarthritis Risk Factors," accessed May 24, 2012, www.thirdage.com.

7. A. Maetzel, M. Mäkelä, G. Hawker, and C. Bombardier, "Osteoarthritis of the Hip and Knee and Mechanical Occupational Exposure—a Systematic Overview of the Evidence," *Journal of Rheumatology* 24, no. 8 (1997): 1599–607.

8. K. Inoue, S. Hukuda, P. Fardellon, Z. Q. Yang, M. Nakai, K. Katayama, T. Ushiyama, Y. Saruhashi, J. Huang, A. Mayeda, I. Catteddu, and C. Obry, "Prevalence of Large-Joint Osteoarthritis in Asian and Caucasian Skeletal Populations," *Rheumatology* 40, no. 1 (2001): 70–73.

9. J. M. Jordan, C. G. Helmick, J. B. Renner, G. Luta, A. D. Dragomir, J. Woodard, F. Fang, T. A. Schwartz, L. M. Abbate, L. F. Callahan, M. D. Kalsbeek, and M. C. Hochberg, "Prevalence of Knee Symptoms and Radiographic and Symptomatic Knee Osteoarthritis in African Americans and Caucasians: The Johnston County Osteoarthritis Project," *Journal of Rheumatology* 34, no. 1 (2007): 172–80.

10. W. C. Shiel, "Osteoarthritis," MedicineNet, reviewed November 18, 2011, accessed May 24, 2012, www.medicinenet.com.

11. G. Slowik, ed., "What Are the Symptoms of Osteoarthritis?," ehealthMD, last modified April 23, 2012, accessed June 14, 2012, www.ehealthmd.com.

12. B. Rifkin, "How to Diagnose Osteoarthritis," Livestrong.com, last modified May 26, 2011, accessed June 23, 2012, www.livestrong.com.

13. K. D. Brandt, "Osteoarthritis Diagnosis: Avoiding Pitfalls," *Journal of Musculoskeletal Medicine* 27, no. 11 (2010): 445.

14. G. Rovetta, P. Monteforte, G. Molfetta, and V. Balestra, "A Two-Year Study of Chondroitin Sulfate in Erosive Osteoarthritis of the Hands: Behavior of Erosions, Osteophytes, Pain and Hand Dysfunction," *Drugs under Experimental and Clinical Research* 30, no. 1 (2004): 11–16; D. Uebelhart, E. J. Thonar, P. D. Delmas, A. Chantraine, and E. Vignon, "Effects of Oral Chondroitin Sulfate on the Progression of Knee Osteoarthritis: A Pilot Study," *Osteoarthritis Cartilage* 6 (suppl. A) (1998): 39–46.

15. Arthritis Today, "New Technology May Enable Early Diagnosis of Osteoarthritis," August 20, 2008, accessed May 24, 2012, www.arthritistoday.org.

11. PSORIATIC ARTHRITIS

1. Arthritis Research UK, "What Is Psoriatic Arthritis?," accessed May 24, 2012, www.arthritisresearchuk.org.

2. Mayo Clinic, "Psoriatic Arthritis: Causes," accessed May 24, 2012, www.mayoclinic.com.

3. Arthritis Foundation, "Psoriatic Arthritis," accessed May 24, 2012, www.arthritis.org.

4. M. J. Kaplan, "Cardiometabolic Risk in Psoriasis: Differential Effects of Biologic Agents," *Journal of Vascular Health and Risk Management* 4, no. 6 (2008): 1229–35.

5. Clinuvel Pharmaceuticals, "Psoriasis," accessed May 24, 2012, www.clinuvel.com.

6. WebMD, "Psoriatic Arthritis," accessed May 24, 2012, www.emedicinehealth.com.

7. WebMD, "Overview of Psoriatic Arthritis," updated June 21, 2012, accessed July 7, 2012, www.emedicine.medscape.com.

8. E. S. Tan, W. S. Chong, and H. L. Tey, "Nail Psoriasis: A Review," *American Journal of Clinical Dermatology* (2012): [published online ahead of print].

9. G. S. Kerr, J. S. Richards, H. Vahabzadeh-Monshie, C. Kindred, I. Sabahi, A. Treherne, and M. Alpert, "Psoriatic Arthritis in a Diverse Ethnic Cohort," *Arthritis and Rheumatism* 60 (suppl. 10) (2009): 528.

10. Mayo Clinic, "Psoriasis," accessed May 24, 2012, www.mayoclinic.com.

11. MedicineNet, "Psoriatic Arthritis," accessed May 24, 2012, www.medicinenet.com.

12. S. Kleinert, M. Feuchtenberger, C. Kneitz, and H. P. Tony, "Psoriatic Arthritis: Clinical Spectrum and Diagnostic Procedures," *Clinical Dermatology* 25, no. 6 (2007): 519–23.

13. R. Soltani-Arabshahi, R. Wong, B.-J. Feng, D. E. Goldgar, K. C. Duffin, and G. G. Krueger, "Obesity in Early Adulthood as a Risk Factor for Psoriatic Arthritis," *Archives of Dermatology* 146, no. 7 (2010): 721–26; A. Ogdie and J. M. Gelfand, "Identification of Risk Factors for Psoriatic Arthritis: Scientific Opportunity Meets Clinical Need," *Archives of Dermatology* 146, no. 7 (2010): 785–88.

14. National Psoriasis Foundation, "Research Priorities: Genetics," accessed May 24, 2012, www.psoriasis.org.

15. A. Albor, S. El Hizawi, E. J. Horn, M. Laederich, P. Frosk, K. Wrogemann, and Kulesz-Martin, "The Interaction of Piasy with Trim32, an E3-Ubiquitin Ligase Mutated in Limb-Girdle Muscular Dystrophy Type 2H, Promotes Piasy Degradation and Regulates UVB-Induced Keratinocyte Apoptosis through NFkappaB," *Journal of Biological Chemistry* 281, no. 35 (2006): 25850.

16. D. Mrabet, L. Laadhar, H. Sahli, B. Zouari, S. Haouet, S. Makni, and S. Sellami, "Synovial Fluid and Serum Levels of IL-17, IL-23, and CCL-20 in Rheumatoid Arthritis and Psoriatic Arthritis: A Tunisian Cross-sectional Study," *Rheumatology International* (2011): [published online ahead of print].

17. F. Cornelissen, A. Mus, P. S. Asmawidjaja, J. P. van Hamburg, J. Tocker, and E. Lubberts, "Interleukin-23 Is Critical for Full-blown Expression of a Non-autoimmune Destructive Arthritis and Regulates Interleukin-17A and RORγt in γδ T Cells," *Arthritis Research and Therapy* 11, no. 6 (2009): R194.

12. SEPTIC ARTHRITIS AND REACTIVE ARTHRITIS

1. Grolier, *The New Grolier Webster International Dictionary of the English Language* (New York: Grolier Incorporated, 1975), 2:879.

2. D. J. Wallace and M. Weisman, "Should a War Criminal Be Rewarded with Eponymous Distinction? The Double Life of Hans Reiter (1881–1969)," *Journal of Clinical Rheumatology* 6, no. 1 (2000): 49–54.

3. Wallace and Weisman, "Should a War Criminal Be Rewarded with Eponymous Distinction?," 49–54.

4. Merck and Co., "Septic Arthritis," Merck Source, accessed July 14, 2012, www.mercksource.com.

5. W. R. Fair, J. Couch, and N. Wehner, "Prostatic Antibacterial Factor: Identity and Significance," *Urology* 7, no. 2 (1976): 169–77.

6. M. P. Keith, "Gonorrheal Arthritis," Medscape, updated August 19, 2011, accessed July 14, 2012, www.emedicine.medscape.com.

7. Keith, "Gonorrheal Arthritis."

8. Mayo Clinic, "Reactive Arthritis (Reiter's Syndrome)," last modified March 5, 2011, accessed July 13, 2012, www.mayoclinic.com.

9. M. L. Cuéllar, L. H. Silveira, and L. R. Espinoza, "Fungal Arthritis," *Annals of Rheumatic Diseases* 51, no. 5 (1992): 690–97.

10. C. O'Callaghan and J. Axford, *Medicine*, 2nd ed. (Oxford: Blackwell Science, 2004).

11. O'Callaghan and Axford, *Medicine*.

12. S. G. Bowerman, N. E. Green, and G. A. Mencio, "Decline of Bone and Joint Infections Attributable to Haemophilus Influenzae Type B," *Clinical Orthopedics and Related Research* 341 (1997): 128–33.

13. R. Cotran, V. Kumar, N. Fausto, S. L. Robbins, and A. K. Abbas, *Pathologic Basis of Disease* (Philadelphia: Elsevier Saunders, 2005), 1310.

14. C. Kaandorp, H. Dinant, M. van de Laar, H. Moens, A. Prins, and B. Dijkmans, "Incidence and Sources of Native and Prosthetic Joint Infection: A Community-Based Prospective Survey," *Annals of Rheumatic Disease* 56, no. 8 (1997): 470–75.

15. J. S. Gaston and M. S. Lillicrap, "Arthritis Associated with Enteric Infection," *Best Practice and Research in Clinical Rheumatology* 17, no. 2 (2003): 219–39.

16. S. A. Paget, A. Gibofsky, J. F. Beary, and T. P. Sculco, *Manual of Rheumatology and Outpatient Orthopedic Disorders: Diagnosis and Therapy*, 4th ed. (New York: Lippincott, Williams, and Wilkins, 2000), ch. 36.

17. D. L. Goldenberg and D. J. Sexton, "Patient Information: Joint Infection," UpToDate, accessed July 13, 2012, www.uptodate.com.

18. P. D. Sampaio-Barros, A. B. Bortoluzzo, R. A. Conde, L. T. Costallat, A. M. Samara, and M. B. Bértolo, "Undifferentiated Spondyloarthritis: A Longterm Followup," *Journal of Rheumatology* 37, no. 6 (2010): 1195–99; A. J. Geirsson, H. Eyjolfsdottir, G. Bjornsdottir, K. Kristjansson, and B. Gudbjornsson, "Prevalence and Clinical Characteristics of Ankylosing Spondylitis in Iceland—a Nationwide Study," *Clinical and Experimental Rheumatology* 28, no. 3 (2010): 333–40.

19. L. M. Henrique da Mota, J. N. Carneiro, R. A. Lima, L. L. dos Santos Neto, and F. A. Lima, "[Reactive Arthritis in HIV-Infected Patients: Immunopathogenic Aspects]," *Acta Reumatológica Portuguesa* 33, no. 3 (2008): 279–87.

20. B. Alberts and A. Johnson, *Molecular Biology of the Cell*, 4th ed. (New York: Garland Science, 2002), ch. 24; National Center for Biotechnology Information and US National Library of Medicine, "Innate Immunity; Humoral Immunity; Cellular Immunity; Immunity; Inflammatory Response; Acquired (Adaptive) Immunity," last reviewed May 2, 2010, accessed June 4, 2012, www.ncbi.nlm.nih.gov/pubmedhealth.

21. Mayo Clinic, "Reactive Arthritis (Reiter's Syndrome)."

22. N. Sweiss, "Septic Arthritis Aspiration Techniques and Indications for Surgery," Medscape, updated February 7, 2012, accessed July 23, 2012, www.emedicine.medscape.com.

23. National Institute of Arthritis and Musculoskeletal and Skin Diseases (NIAMS), "Questions and Answers about Reactive Arthritis," updated September 2011, accessed June 9, 2012, www.niams.nih.gov.

24. S. L. Gorbach, "Lactic Acid Bacteria and Human Health," *Annals of Medicine* 22, no. 1 (1990): 37–41.

25. A. O. Malley, "Is a Negative Gram Stain in Suspected Septic Arthritis Sufficient to Rule Out Septic Arthritis?," BestBETs, accessed July 23, 2012, www.bestbets.org.

13. ENTEROPATHIC ARTHRITIS

1. C. Eustice, "What You Should Know about Enteropathic Arthritis," About.com, March 25, 2010, accessed July 13, 2012, www.arthritis.about.com.

2. R. Kitchen, C. Elizabeth, and T. Cowling, "Enteropathic Arthritis Overview and Facts," Health Guide Info, March 31, 2011, accessed July 16, 2012, www.healthguideinfo.com.

3. I. S. Alghafeeer and L. H. Sigal, "Rheumatic Manifestations of Gastrointestinal Diseases," July 17, 2012, www.arthritis-symptom.com.

4. Kitchen, Elizabeth, and Cowling, "Enteropathic Arthritis Overview and Facts."

5. M. Vann and N. Jones, "About Enteropathic Arthritis," Everyday Health, accessed July 17, 2012, www.everydayhealth.com.

6. Spondylitis Association of America, "Enteropathic Arthritis," accessed August 2, 2012, www.spondylitis.org.

7. Anemia.org, "Handouts: Anemia and Rheumatoid Arthritis," July 23, 2012, www.anemia.org.

8. American Association for Clinical Chemistry, "C-Reactive Protein," Lab Tests Online, accessed July 23, 2012, www.labtestsonline.org.

9. K. A. Solonen, "The Sacroiliac Joint in the Light of Anatomical, Roentgenological and Clinical Studies," *Acta Orthopedica Scandanavica* (suppl. 27) (1957): 1–127.

10. Solonen, "The Sacroiliac Joint in the Light of Anatomical, Roentgenological and Clinical Studies," 1–127.

11. D. Myers, "Colonoscopy," About.com, November 14, 2006, accessed June 23, 2012, www.coloncancer.about.com.

12. C. Galbreath, "Arthritis Foundation Announces Top 10 Arthritis Advances of 2008," Arthritis Foundation, accessed July 24, 2012, www.arthritis.org.

13. F. Van den Bosch, "Ankylosing Spondylitis and Extra-articular Manifestations," *European Musculoskeletal Review* 2 (2007): 25–26; V. Chandran and P. Rahman, "Update on the Genetics of Spondyloarthritis—Ankylosing Spondylitis and Psoriatic Arthritis," *Best Practice and Research in Clinical Rheumatology* 24, no. 5 (2010): 579–88; Unbound Medicine, "Enter-

opathic Arthritis," May 11, 2009, accessed July 20, 2012, www.harrisons.unboundmedicine. com.

14. Van den Bosch, "Ankylosing Spondylitis and Extra-articular Manifestations," 25–26.

15. Chandran and Rahman, "Update on the Genetics of Spondyloarthritis—Ankylosing Spondylitis and Psoriatic Arthritis," 579–88.

14. RELATED MANIFESTATIONS

1. R. P. Rapini, J. L. Bolognia, and J. L. Jorizzo, *Dermatology: 2-Volume Set* (St. Louis: Mosby, 2007), 602–3.

2. F. Franceschini and I. Cavazzana, "Anti-Ro/SSA and La/SSB Antibodies," *Autoimmunity* 38, no. 1 (2005): 55–63.

3. N. Delaleu, H. Immervoll, J. Cornelius, and R. Jonsson, "Biomarker Profiles in Serum and Saliva of Experimental Sjögren's Syndrome: Associations with Specific Autoimmune Manifestations," *Arthritis Research and Therapy* 10, no. 1 (2008): R22.

4. M. M. Ward, "Decreases in Rates of Hospitalizations for Manifestations of Severe Rheumatoid Arthritis, 1983–2001," *Arthritis and Rheumatism* 50, no. 4 (2004): 1122–23.

5. T. Saito, J. Sato, K. Kondo, M. Horikawa, K. Ohmori, and H. Fukuda, "Low Prevalence of Clinicopathologic and Sialographic Changes in Salivary Glands of Men with Sjögren's Syndrome," *Journal of Oral Pathology and Medicine* 28, no. 7 (1999): 312–16.

6. C. Eustice, "Sjogren's Syndrome Knocks Venus Williams Out of the Game," About.com, accessed June 23, 2012, www.arthritis.about.com.

7. G. P. Balint and P. V. Balint, "Felty's Syndrome," *Best Practice and Research in Clinical Rheumatology* 18, no. 5 (2004): 631–45.

8. K. A. Newman and M. Akhtari, "Management of Autoimmune Neutropenia in Felty's Syndrome and Systemic Lupus Erythematosus," Autoimmunity Reviews 10, no. 7 (2011): 432–37.

9. M. E. Suarez-Almazor, C. Spooner, and E. Belseck, "Penicillamine for Rheumatoid Arthritis," *Cochrane Database of Systematic Reviews* 2 (2000): CD001460.

10. Behcet's Disease Research Committee of Japan, "Behcet's Disease Guide to the Diagnosis of Behcet's disease (1972)," *Japanese Journal of Ophthalmology* 18 (1974): 291–94.

11. University of Washington Department of Orthopedics and Sports Medicine, "Behcet's Disease," accessed August 1, 2012, www.orthop.washington.edu.

12. National Health Service (UK), "Behcet's Disease," accessed August 1, 2012, www.nhs.uk.

13. M. Escudier, J. Bagan, and C. Scully, "Number VII Behçet's Disease (Adamantiades Syndrome)," *Oral Diseases* 12, no. 2 (2006): 78–84.

14. J. S. Pearce, "Neurological Symptoms of Adamantiades-Behçet's Syndrome," *Journal of Neurology, Neurosurgery and Psychiatry* 77, no. 8 (2006): 956–57.

15. H. O. Curth, "Recurrent Genito-oral Aphthosis with Hypopion (Behcet's Syndrome)," *Archives of Dermatology* 54 (1946): 179–96.

16. F. Davatchi, F. Shahram, and M. Akbarian, "Accuracy of Existing Diagnosis Criteria for Behcet's Disease," in *Behcet's Disease*, ed. B. Wechsler and P. Godeau, Excerpta Medica International Congress Series 1037 (Amsterdam: Excerpta Medica, 1993): 225–28.

17. C. G. Barnes, "Treatment of Behcet's Syndrome," *Rheumatology* 45, no. 3 (2006): 245–47.

18. J. H. Kim, V. Nam, H. S. Moon, J. O. Kim, and C. H. Sung, "The Effect of Thalidomide on Entero-Behcet's Disease," *Korean Journal of Pain* 22, no. 1 (2009): 104–6.

15. INITIAL APPROACHES TO RHEUMATIC AND JOINT PROBLEMS

1. Illinois Department of Public Health, "Factsheet—Facts about Arthritis," accessed April 29, 2012, www.idph.state.il.us.

2. J. Davis, "New Evidence Why RA Patients Should Quit Smoking," Arthritis Today, November 1, 2011, accessed June 5, 2012, www.arthritistoday.org.

3. D. Rodriguez, "The Emotional Side of Arthritis," Everyday Health, accessed May 2, 2012, www.everydayhealth.com.

4. Arthritis Foundation, "How to Care for Yourself," accessed May 2, 2012, www.arthritis. org.

5. S. Borland, "Arthritis Sufferers 40 Per Cent More Likely to Develop Fatal Heart Problems," *Daily Mail*, March 8, 2012, accessed June 14, 2012, www.dailymail.co.uk.

6. C. Eustice, "Rheumatologic Emergency—When You Should Go to the Emergency Room," About.com, last updated September 22, 2010, accessed July 6, 2012, www.arthritis. about.com.

7. W. C. Shiel, "Rheumatoid Arthritis—When Do I Call the Doctor," MedicineNet, accessed April 28, 2012, www.medicinenet.com.

8. B. McDonough, reviewer, "Joint Pain," Better Medicine, accessed April 28, 2012, www.localhealth.com.

16. PHARMACOLOGICAL TREATMENTS FOR ARTHRITIS

1. National Rheumatoid Arthritis Society, "Which Drugs Are Used," accessed May 5, 2012, www.nras.org.uk.

2. W. C. Shiel Jr., "First Line Rheumatoid Arthritis Medication and Second Line or Slow Acting Rheumatoid Arthritis Drugs," MedicineNet, accessed May 5, 2012, www.medicinenet. com.

3. S. Gottlieb, "Risk of Ulcer Soars with Combination of Arthritis Drugs," *British Medical Journal* 322, no. 7281 (2001): 258.

4. O. Ogbru, articles on arthritis drugs, MedicineNet, accessed May 6, 2012, www. medicinenet.com.

5. C. K. Zetterström, W. Jiang, H. Wähämaa, T. Ostberg, A. C. Aveberger, H. Schierbeck, M. T. Lotze, U. Andersson, D. S. Pisetsky, and H. H. Erlandsson, "Pivotal Advance: Inhibition of HMGB1 Nuclear Translocation as a Mechanism for the Anti-rheumatic Effects of Gold Sodium Thiomalate," *Journal of Leukocyte Biology* 83, no. 1 (2008): 31–38.

6. Arthritis Research UK, "Arthritis Information—Drugs," accessed May 6, 2012, www.arthritisresearchuk.org.

7. L. D. Settas, G. Tsimirikas, G. Vosvotekas, E. Triantafyllidou, and P. Nicolaides, "Reactivation of Pulmonary Tuberculosis in a Patient with Rheumatoid Arthritis during Treatment with IL-1 Receptor Antagonists (Anakinra)," *Journal of Clinical Rheumatology* 13, no. 4 (2007): 219–20.

8. O. Ogbru, articles on arthritis drugs, MedicineNet, accessed May 6, 2012, www.medicinenet.com.

9. K. Monson and A. Schoenstadt, section on drugs, eMedTV, accessed May 7, 2012, http://drugs.emedtv.com.

10. Drugs.com, "Drugs A–Z" section, accessed May 7, 2012, www.drugs.com.

11. O. Ogbru, "Valdecoxib—Bextra," MedicineNet, accessed May 7, 2012, www.medicinenet.com/valdecoxib/article.htm.

12. National Consumers League, "Medical Adherence," Script Your Future, accessed May 8, 2012, http://scriptyourfuture.org/medication-adherence.

17. NATURAL ARTHRITIS TREATMENTS AND SURGERY

1. C. Bailey-Lloyd, "Natural Alternatives vs. Prescription Drugs," IBringYouInfo.com, accessed May 15, 2012, www.alternative-medicine.ibringyouinfo.com.

2. Consumers Unified, "FDA Estimates Vioxx Caused 27,785 Deaths," Consumer Affairs, April 11 2004, accessed May 24, 2012, www.consumeraffairs.com/news04/vioxx_estimates. html.

3. T. Cohen, "The Hidden Risks of Top Herbal Remedies that Pharmacists Don't Tell Us About," *Daily Mail*, August 9, 2011, accessed June 12, 2012, www.dailymail.co.uk.

4. WebMD, "Hyaluronic Acid," accessed May 19, 2012, www.webmd.com.

5. E. Teeple, K. A. Elsaid, G. D. Jay, L. Zhang, G. J. Badger, M. Akelman, T. F. Bliss, and B. C. Fleming, "Effects of Supplemental Intra-articular Lubricin and Hyaluronic Acid on the Progression of Posttraumatic Arthritis in the Anterior Cruciate Ligament-Deficient Rat Knee," *American Journal of Sports Medicine* 39, no. 1 (2011): 164–72.

6. WebMD, "Heat and Cold Therapy for Arthritis Pain," accessed May 16, 2012, http:// arthritis.webmd.com.

7. N. Bagheri-Nesami, M. A. Mohseni-Bandpei, and M. Shayesteh-Azar, "The Effect of Benson Relaxation Technique on Rheumatoid Arthritis Patients," *International Journal of Nursing Practice* 12, no. 4 (2006): 214–19.

8. U. D. Krezel, "Relaxation Techniques for Arthritis Pain Relief," Outback Meditation, accessed May 18, 2012, http://outbackmeditations.com.

9. A. Dyson, "About Magnotherapy," The Alternative Guide, accessed May 17, 2012, www.altguide.com/therapydata/magnotherapy.html.

10. MedicineNet, "Massage Therapy," accessed May 18, 2012, www.medicinenet.com.

11. C. Bullen, "How to Travel with Arthritis," *USA Today*, accessed May 18, 2012, http:// traveltips.usatoday.com.

12. D. Zelman, reviewer, "Arthritis Supplements," WebMD, reviewed March 3, 2012, accessed May 18, 2012, www.webmd.com.

13. Arthritis Foundation, "Types of Surgery," accessed May 19, 2012, www.arthritis.org/ types-surgery.php.

18. ADDRESSING THE MENTAL ASPECTS

1. US Surgeon General, "Mental Health: A Report of the Surgeon General—Chapter 2, the Fundamentals of Mental Health and Mental Illness 1999," accessed April 11, 2012, www.surgeongeneral.gov/library/mentalhealth.

2. WHO International Consortium in Psychiatric Epidemiology, "Cross-national Comparisons of the Prevalence and Correlates of Mental Disorders," *Bulletin of the World Health Organization* 78, no. 4 (2000): 413–26.

3. National Institute of Mental Health, "Statistics," accessed June 5, 2012, www.apps.nimh.nih.gov.

4. J. M. Grohol, "Mental Health Statistics," PsychCentral, May 3, 2010, accessed July 12, 2012, http://psychcentral.com.

5. D. Lawrence, F. Mitrou, and S. R. Zubrick, "Smoking and Mental Illness: Results from Population Surveys in Australia and the United States," *BioMed Central Public Health* 9 (2009): 285.

6. Grohol, "Mental Health Statistics."

7. World Health Organization (WHO), *The World Health Report 2004: Changing History, Annex Table 3: Burden of Disease in DALYs by Cause, Sex, and Mortality Stratum in WHO Regions, Estimates for 2002* (Geneva: WHO, 2004).

8. Grohol, "Mental Health Statistics."

9. R. Nauert, "Happiness Enhances Health," PsychCentral, November 8, 2006, accessed July 12, 2012, http://psychcentral.com.

10. National Science Foundation (NSF), "Happiness Improves Health and Lengthens Life," *US News and World Report*, March 3, 2011, accessed July 12, 2012, www.usnews.com.

11. NSF, "Happiness Improves Health and Lengthens Life."

12. S. Rimer, "Happiness and Health," Harvard School of Public Health, accessed July 12, 2012, www.hsph.harvard.edu.

13. Rimer, "Happiness and Health."

14. P. Hagan, "The £1-a-Day 'Happy Pill' that Eases the Agony of Arthritis," *Daily Mail*, April 24, 2012, accessed July 12, 2012, www.dailymail.co.uk.

15. C. Eustice, "10 Ways to Improve Your Life with Arthritis," About.com, August 16, 2011, accessed July 12, 2012, www.arthritis.about.com.

16. L. B. Murphy, J. J. Sacks, T. J. Brady, J. M. Hootman, and D. P. Chapman, "Anxiety and Depression among US Adults with Arthritis: Prevalence and Correlates," *Arthritis Care and Research* 64, no. 7 (2012): 968–76.

17. T. Pederson, "Anxiety, Depression Affect One-Third of Arthritis Patients," PsychCentral, May 1, 2012, accessed July 12, 2012, http://psychcentral.com.

18. Pederson, "Anxiety, Depression Affect One-Third of Arthritis Patients."

19. Arthritis Ireland, "Coping with Emotions," accessed May 27, 2012, www.arthritisireland.ie.

20. C. Eustice, "When Does Sadness and Frustration Cross Over into Depression?," About.com, November 22, 2006, accessed July 12, 2012, www.arthritis.about.com.

21. Pederson, "Anxiety, Depression Affect One-Third of Arthritis Patients."

22. Pederson, "Anxiety, Depression Affect One-Third of Arthritis Patients."

23. EHealthMe.com, "Could Rheumatoid Arthritis Cause Agitation?," accessed July 12, 2012, www.ehealthme.com.

24. EHealthMe.com, "Could Rheumatoid Arthritis Cause Agitation?"

25. Arthritis Ireland, "Coping with Emotions."

19. EXERCISES FOR ARTHRITIS

1. Z. de Jong, M. Munneke, W. F. Lems, A. H. Zwinderman, H. M. Kroon, E. K. Pauwels, A. Jansen, K. H. Ronday, B. A. Dijkmans, F. C. Breedveld, T. P. Vliet Vlieland, and J. M. Hazes, "Slowing of Bone Loss in Patients with Rheumatoid Arthritis by Long-term High-Intensity Exercise: Results of a Randomized, Controlled Trial," *Arthritis and Rheumatism* 50 (2004): 1066–76.

2. H. Simon, reviewer, "Exercise In-depth Report," *New York Times*, accessed July 18, 2012, www.health.nytimes.com.

3. J. B. Bartholomew and D. E. Linder, "State Anxiety Following Resistance Exercise: The Role of Gender and Exercise Intensity," *Journal of Behavioral Medicine* 21 (1998): 205–19.

4. C. J. Pritzlaff-Roy, L. Widemen, J. Y. Weltman, R. Abbott, M. Gutgesell, M. L. Hartman, J. D. Veldhuis, and A. Weltman, "Gender Governs the Relationship between Exercise Intensity and Growth Hormone Release in Young Adults," *Journal of Applied Physiology* 92 (2002): 2053–60.

5. Harvard Medical School, "Does Exercise Contribute to Arthritis? Research Says No," November 10, 2009, accessed July 18, 2012, www.health.harvard.edu.

6. I. Mangani, M. Cesari, S. B. Kritchevsky, C. Maraldi, C. S. Carter, H. H. Atkinson, B. W. Penninx, N. Marchionni, and M. Pahor, "Physical Exercise and Comorbidity: Results from the Fitness and Arthritis in Seniors Trial (FAST)," *Aging Clinical and Experimental Research* 18 (2006): 374–80.

7. M. P. Tulppo, T. H. Mäkikallio, T. Seppänen, R. T. Laukkanen, and H. V. Huikuri, "Vagal Modulation of Heart Rate during Exercise: Effects of Age and Physical Fitness," *American Journal of Physiology* 274 (1998): H424–29.

8. Harvard Medical School, "Does Exercise Contribute to Arthritis?"

9. Harvard Medical School, "Does Exercise Contribute to Arthritis?"

10. S. Anitei, "Why Is Physical Exercise Important for Our Health?," Softpedia, August 22, 2007, accessed July 18, 2012, http://news.softpedia.com.

11. O. Johnston, J. Reilly, and J. Kremer, "Excessive Exercise: From Quantitative Categorisation to a Qualitative Continuum Approach," *European Eating Disorders Review* 19, no. 3 (2011): 237–48.

12. A. Lupu, "Too Much Physical Activity Brings about Serious Health Disorders," Softpedia, accessed July 18, 2012, http://news.softpedia.com.

20. APPROACHING ARTHRITIS AT HOME

1. K. E. Donahue, D. E. Jonas, R. A. Hansen, R. Roubey, B. Jonas, L. J. Lux, G. Gartlehner, F. Harden, T. Wilkins, V. Peravali, S. I. Bangdiwala, A. Yuen, P. Thieda, L C. Morgan, K. Crotty, R. Desai, and M. Van Noord, *Drug Therapy for Rheumatoid Arthritis in Adults: An Update*, No. 12-EHC025-EF (Rockville, MD: Agency for Healthcare Research and Quality, 2012).

2. L. S. Abramson, "Arthritis in Children," American College of Rheumatology, accessed April 22, 2012, www.rheumatology.org.

3. A. R. Kemper, R. Coeytaux, G. Sanders, H. Van Mater, J. W. Williams, R. N. Gray, R. J. Irvine, and A. Kendrick A. *Disease-Modifying Antirheumatic Drugs (DMARDs) in Children with Juvenile Idiopathic Arthritis (JIA)*, No. 11-EHC039-EF (Rockville, MD: Agency for Healthcare Research and Quality, 2011).

4. M. A. Rapoff, M. R. Purviance, and C. B. Lindsley, "Educational and Behavioral Strategies for Improving Medication Compliance in Juvenile Rheumatoid Arthritis," *Archives of Physical Medicine and Rehabilitation* 69 (1988): 439–41.

5. Donahue, Jonas, Hansen, Roubey, Jonas, Lux, Gartlehner, Harden, Wilkins, Peravali, Bangdiwala, Yuen, Thieda, Morgan, Crotty, Desai, and Van Noord, *Drug Therapy for Rheumatoid Arthritis in Adults.*

6. National Center for Biotechnology Information and US National Library of Medicine, "Arthritis," last reviewed February 2, 2012, accessed June 24, 2012, www.ncbi.nlm.nih.gov.

7. A. A. Stenger, M. A. van Leeuwen, and P. M. Houtman, "Early Effective Suppression of Inflammation in Rheumatoid Arthritis Reduces Radiologic Progression," *British Journal of Radiology* 37 (1998): 1157–63.

8. R. H. Wilkinson and B. N. Weissman, "Arthritis in Children," *Radiologic Clinics of North America* 26, no. 6 (1998): 1247–65.

9. Centers for Disease Control and Prevention (CDC), "Childhood Arthritis," accessed July 24, 2012, www.cdc.gov/arthritis/basics/childhood.htm.

10. Kemper, Coeytaux, Sanders, Van Mater, Williams, Gray, Irvine, and Kendrick, *Disease-Modifying Antirheumatic Drugs (DMARDs) in Children with Juvenile Idiopathic Arthritis (JIA).*

11. National Collaborating Centre for Women's and Children's Health (UK), *Feverish Illness in Children: Assessment and Initial Management in Children Younger Than 5 Years* (London, UK: RCOG Press, 2007).

21. FINDING MOTIVATION

1. "The Importance of Self-motivation," MotivationalWellBeing.com, last modified April 10, 2012, accessed June 21, 2012, www.motivationalwellbeing.com.

2. R. F. Booth, E. G. Webster, and M. S. McNally, "Schooling, Occupational Motivation, and Personality as Related to Success in Paramedical Training," *Public Health Reports* 91, no. 6 (1976): 533–37.

3. Natural News, "Most People with Arthritis Don't Get Enough Exercise," accessed July 3, 2012, www.naturalnews.com.

4. M. Shih, J. M. Hootman, J. Kruger, and C. G. Helmick, "Physical Activity in Men and Women with Arthritis: National Health Interview Survey, 2002," *American Journal of Preventive Medicine* 30, no. 5 (2006): 385–93.

5. C. Eustice, "How Do Arthritis Patients Perceive Exercise," About.com, accessed April 26, 2012, www.arthritis.about.com.

6. W. Thomas, M. W. Colligan, and M. Higgins, "Workplace Stress," *Journal of Workplace Behavioral Health* 21, no. 2 (2006): 89–97.

7. Centers for Disease Control and Prevention (CDC), "Prevalence of Doctor-Diagnosed Arthritis and Arthritis-Attributable Activity Limitation—United States, 2007–2009," *Morbidity and Mortality Weekly Report* 59, no. 39 (2010): 1261–65.

8. G. R. Kirkpatrick and G. N. Katsiaficas, *Introduction to Critical Sociology* (New York: Ardent Media, 1987), 261.

9. H. V. Long, "Discrimination against Elderly," LoveToKnow.com, last modified April 25, 2012, accessed May 12, 2012, www.seniors.lovetoknow.com.

10. A. Logsdon, "Ageism towards Senior Citizens—What Is Ageism Targeting Seniors?," About.com, last modified April 26, 2012, accessed May 23, 2012, www.learningdisabilities.about.com.

11. M. T. Compton, N. J. Thompson, and N. J. Kaslow, "Social Environment Factors Associated with Suicide Attempt among Low-Income African Americans: The Protective Role of Family Relationships and Social Support," *Social Psychiatry and Psychiatric Epidemiology* 40, no. 3 (2005): 175–85.

12. B. W. Penninx, J. M. Guralnik, M. Pahor, L. Ferrucci, J. R. Cerhan, R. B. Wallace, and R. J. Havlik, "Chronically Depressed Mood and Cancer Risk in Older Persons," *Journal of the National Cancer Institute* 90, no. 24 (1998): 1888–93.

13. W. W. Eaton, H. Armenian, J. Gallo, and D. E. Ford, "Depression Risk for Onset of Type II Diabetes: A Prospective Population-Based Study," *Diabetes Care* 19 (1996): 1097–102.

14. A. K. Ferketich, J. A. Schwartzbaum, D. J. Frid, and M. L. Moeschberger, "Depression as an Antecedent to Heart Disease among Women and Men in the NHANES I Study. *National Health and Nutrition Examination Survey*," *Archives of Internal Medicine* 160, no. 90 (2000): 1261–68.

15. B. S. Jonas and M. E. Mussolino, "Symptoms of Depression as a Prospective Risk Factor for Stroke," *Psychosomatic Medicine* 62 (2000): 463–71.

16. A. A. Ariyo, M. Haan, C. M. Tangen, J. C. Rutledge, M. Cushman, A. Dobs, and C. D. Furberg, "Depressive Symptoms and Risks of Coronary Heart Disease and Mortality in Elderly Americans," *Circulation* 102, no. 15 (2000): 1773–79.

17. J. T. Newsom, "Another Side to Caregiving: Negative Reactions to Being Helped," Portland State University, 1999, accessed April 27, 2012, www.upa.pdx.edu.

18. W. H. Ettinger, R. F. Loeser, S. P. Messier, G. D. Miller, T. Morgan, M. Pahor, J. Rejeski, M. A. Sevick, and J. D. Williamson, "Exercise and Dietary Weight Loss in Overweight and Obese Older Adults with Knee Osteoarthritis: The Arthritis, Diet, and Activity Promotion Trial," *Arthritis and Rheumatism* 50, no. 5 (2004): 1501–10.

19. S. Barlett, "Role of Exercise in Arthritis Management," Johns Hopkins Arthritis Center, accessed April 28, 2012, www.hopkinsarthritis.org.

20. C. E. Ross and D. Hayes, "Exercise and Psychologic Wellbeing in the Community," *American Journal of Epidemiology* 127, no. 4 (1988): 762–71, accessed April 28, 2012.

21. Department of Kinesiology and Health, Georgia State University, "The Benefits of Exercise," last modified November 6, 1997, accessed July 23, 2012, www2.gsu.edu/~wwwfit/benefits.html.

22. B. Thie, "The Benefits of a Healthy Lifestyle," BenefitsOfHealthyLifestyle.com, last modified April 28, 2012, accessed April 22, 2012, http://benefitsofhealthylifestyle.com.

23. A. H. Maslow, *Motivation and Personality*, 3rd ed. (New York: Harper and Row, 1987).

24. K. Perera, "The Importance of Self-esteem—Why It Matters," More-Selfesteem.com, accessed May 1, 2012, www.more-selfesteem.com.

25. J. Johnson, A. M. Wood, P. Gooding, P. J. Taylor, and N. Tarrier, "Resilience to Suicidality: The Buffering Hypothesis," *Clinical Psychology Review* 31, no. 4 (2011): 563–91.

26. C. Lawson, "The Connections between Emotions and Learning," Center for Development and Learning, accessed May 3, 2012, www.cdl.org.

27. J. B. Detweiler, A. J. Rothman, P. Salovey, and W. T. Steward, "Emotional States and Physical Health," *American Psychologist* 55, no. 1 (2000): 110–21.

28. R. Bacher, "Half of Americans Don't Get Second Opinion," MSNBC, accessed 4 May 2012, www.msnbc.msn.com.

22. COLLECTIVE EFFORTS

1. Centers for Disease Control and Prevention, "Arthritis Meeting the Challenge," accessed May 24, 2012, www.cdc.gov.

2. N. Shadick, "Patient Rheumatoid Arthritis Social Support Study (PARASS)," Clinical-Trials.gov, last modified February 2, 2012, accessed June 4, 2012, www.clinicaltrials.gov.

3. R. Suttle, "How to Set Up Health Care Focus Groups," eHow.com, accessed May 5, 2012, www.ehow.com.

4. D. E. Bender and D. Ewbank, "The Focus Group as a Tool for Health Research: Issues in Design and in Analysis," *Health Transition Review* 4, no. 1 (1994): 63–79.

5. J. Bahnson, P. Beal, M. Dignan, R. Michielutte, and P. Sharp, "The Role of Focus Groups in Health Education for Cervical Cancer among Minority Women," *Journal of Community Health* 15, no. 6 (1990): 369–75.

6. L. M. Butler, C. Dephelps, and R. Howell, "Focus Groups: A Tool for Understanding Community Perceptions and Experiences," Washington State University Extension, Computing and Web Resources, accessed May 24, 2012, http://cru.cahe.wsu.edu.

7. Region of Waterloo Public Health, "Focus Groups," accessed May 13, 2012, www.ahs.uwaterloo.ca.

8. M. A. Carey, "Comment: Concerns in the Analysis of Focus Group Data," *Qualitative Health Research* 5, no. 4 (1995): 487–95.

9. P. B. Works, "Issues Including Advantages and Disadvantages," PBworks, accessed May 15, 2012, http://focusgroups.pbworks.com.

10. S. Bernatsky, D. Feldman, M. De Civita, J. Haggerty, P. Tousignant, J. Legaré, M. Zummer, T. Meagher, C. Mill, M. Roper, and J. Lee, "Optimal Care for Rheumatoid Arthritis: A Focus Group Study," *Clinical Rheumatology* 29, no. 6 (2010): 645–57.

11. E. Amann, A. Cierza, M. Coenen, B. Kollerits, and G. Stucki, "Validation of the International Classification of Functioning, Disability and Health (ICF) Core Set for Rheumatoid Arthritis from the Patient Perspective Using Focus Groups," *Arthritis Research and Therapy*, accessed May 24, 2012, http://arthritis-research.com.

12. Arthritis Foundation, homepage, accessed May 24, 2012, www.arthritis.org.

13. Arthritis Foundation, "Events and Programs," accessed May 30, 2012, www.arthritis. org.

14. Arthritis Foundation, "Funding Opportunities," accessed May 25, 2012, www.arthritis.org.

15. Arthritis Foundation, "Research," accessed May 13, 2012, www.arthritis.org; Arthritis Foundation, "Advocacy," accessed May 24, 2012, www.arthritis.org.

16. Arthritis Foundation, "Why Join Congressional Arthritis Caucus," accessed May 14, 2012, www.arthritis.org.

17. D. Cooper, "Arthritis Support Groups: A Lot More Than What Meets the Eye," Canadian Arthritis Patient Alliance, accessed May 22, 2012, www.arthritispatient.ca.

18. Arthritis Foundation, "National Arthritis Action Plan," accessed May 13, 2012, www.arthritis.org.

19. Memorial Sloan-Kettering Cancer Center, "Patient-to-Patient Support Program," accessed May 23, 2012, www.mskcc.org.

20. M. Smith, R. Segal, and J. Segal, "Dealing with Depression: Self-help and Coping Tips," Helpguide, last modified May 2012, accessed June 11, 2012, www.helpguide.org.

23. CONCLUSION

1. Simmons, "Women Have Higher Food IQ's Than Men: National Study Makes It Official: Women Are More Health Conscious Than Men," PR Newswire, March 6, 2007, accessed April 17, 2012, www.prnewswire.com.
2. University of Queensland, "Hope Makes You Happier," April 23, 2012, accessed May 18, 2012, http://ns2.m1069.sgded.com; R. Gunatilaka and J. Knight, "Aspirations, Adaptations and Subjective Well-being of Rural Urban-Migrants of China," *Economics Series Working Papers* 381 (2008): 4–17; P. Frijters, G. Foster, and D. W. Johnston, "The Triumph of Hope over Regret: A Note on the Utility of Good Health Expectations," *Discussion Papers Series* 451 (2012): 2–23.
3. M. Bond, "Can Hope Heal?," Serendip Studio, Bryn Mawr, accessed May 18, 2012, www.serendip.brynmawr.edu.
4. J. Groopman, *The Anatomy of Hope* (New York: Random House, 2004).
5. M. Smith, R. Segal, and J. Segal, "Dealing with Depression: Self-help and Coping Tips," Helpguide, last modified May 2012, accessed June 11, 2012, www.helpguide.org.
6. J. D. Roth, "How to Build Confidence and Destroy Fear," Get Rich Slowly, last modified May 3, 2010, accessed May 23, 2012, www.getrichslowly.org.
7. S. Windholz, "Helpful Ways to Gain More Patience," Power Within, accessed May 22, 2012, www.being-inspired.com.
8. J. Lawson, "Developing Patience," Livestrong.com, accessed May 21, 2012, www.livestrong.com.
9. S. Williams, J. Weinman, and J. Dale, "Doctor-Patient Communication and Patient Satisfaction: A Review," *Family Practice* 15, no. 5 (1998): 480–92.
10. D. Roter and J. A. Hall, *Doctors Talking with Patients/Patients Talking with Doctors* (Westport, CT: Praeger Publishers, 2006).
11. A. Schattner, "The Silent Dimension: Expressing Humanism in Each Medical Encounter," *Archives of Internal Medicine* 169, no. 12 (2009): 1095–99; J. Tongue, H. Epps, and L. Forese, "Communication Skills for Patient-Centered Care; Research-Based, Easily Learned Techniques for Medical Interviews that Benefit Orthopaedic Surgeons and Their Patients," *Journal of Bone and Joint Surgery* 87 (2005): 652–58.
12. T. Bhattacharyya, H. Yeon, and M. B. Harris, "The Medical-Legal Aspects of Informed Consent in Orthopaedic Surgery," *Journal of Bone and Joint Surgery* 87 (2005): 652–58.
13. M. Morgan, "The Doctor-Patient Relationship," King Saud University Faculty, accessed May 23, 2012, http://faculty.ksu.edu.sa.
14. S. Daniel, "Why You Should See a Doctor Regularly," Professor's House, accessed May 24, 2012, www.professorshouse.com.

Bibliography

PREFACE

American Academy of Orthopedic Surgeons. "Arthritis: An Overview." Accessed July 4, 2012. www.orthoinfo.aaos.org.

BioMed Central. "Arthritis Research and Therapy." Accessed June 22, 2012. www.arthritis-research.com/content.

Centers for Disease Control and Prevention (CDC). "Arthritis in General." Accessed May 15, 2012. www.cdc.gov.

Eustice, C. "Arthritis: 10 Things You Should Know." About.com. Accessed July 13, 2012. www.arthritis.about.com.

CHAPTER 1

Amer, H., A. Swan, and P. Dieppe. "The Utilization of Synovial Fluid Analysis in the UK." *Rheumatology* 40, no. 9 (2001): 1060–63.

Copeman, W. *A Short History of the Gout and the Rheumatic Diseases*. Los Angeles: University of California Press, 1964.

Garrod, A. B. "Observations on Certain Pathological Conditions of the Blood and Urine in Gout, Rheumatism and Bright's Disease." Medico-Chirurgial Society of Edinburgh 31 (1848): 83–97.

———. *The Nature and Treatment of Gout and Rheumatic Gout*. London: Walton and Maberly, 1859.

Harrison, J., K. Kulkarni, M. Baguneid, and B. Prendergast. *Oxford Handbook of Key Clinical Evidence*. London: Oxford University Press, 2009.

Kersley, G. D., and J. H. Glyn. *A Concise International History of Rheumatology and Rehabilitation: Friends and Foes*. London: Royal Society of Medicine Services, 1991.

Low, G. "Thomas Sydenham: The English Hippocrates." *Australian and New Zealand Journal of Surgery* 69, no. 4 (1999): 258–62.

Lutz, P. *The Rise of Experimental Biology: An Illustrated History*. New York: Humana Press, 2002.

Marson, P. "*Gout and the Spider* by Jean de la Fontaine (1621–1695), or the Metamorphoses of a Rheumatologic Tale." *Reumatismo* 54, no. 4 (2002): 372–80.

McCarty, D. J., and J. L. Hollander. "Identification of Urate Crystals in Gouty Synovial Fluid." *Annals of Internal Medicine* 54 (1961): 452–60.

Nuki, G., and P. A. Simkin. "A Concise History of Gout and Hyperuricemia and Their Treatment." *Arthritis Research and Therapy* 8 (suppl. 1) (2006): 1–5. Accessed May 8, 2012.
Parker, G. *Philip II: Library of the World Biography.* London: Hutchinson, 1978.
Porter, R., and G. S. Rousseau. *Gout: The Patrician Malady.* New Haven, CT: Yale University Press, 2000.
Scholtens, M. "The Glorification of Gout in 16th- to 18th-Century Literature." *Canadian Medical Association Journal* 179, no. 8 (2008): 804–5.
Stein, M., and G. Taylor. *The Encyclopedia of Arthritis.* New York: Facts on File, 2004.
Syed, I. B. "Islamic Medicine: 1000 Years Ahead of Its Time." *Journal of the International Society for the History of Islamic Medicine* 2 (2002): 2–9.
Wright, L. F., R. P. Saylor, and F. A. Cecere. "Occult Lead Intoxication in Patients with Gout and Kidney Disease." *Journal of Rheumatology* 11, no. 4 (1984): 517–20.

CHAPTER 2

Atkinson, W., J. Hamborsky, and C. Wolfe, eds. "Diphtheria." In *Epidemiology and Prevention of Vaccine-Preventable Diseases*, 75–86. 12th ed. Washington DC: Public Health Foundation, 2011.
Choi, B. K., J. H. Verbeek, W. Wai-San Tam, and J. Y. Jiang. "Exercises for Prevention of Recurrences of Low-Back Pain." *Cochrane Database of Systematic Reviews* 1 (2010): CD006555.
Cleveland Clinic. "Diseases and Conditions." Accessed June 14, 2012. www.my.clevelandclinic.org.
Conner, M. G. "Understanding the Difference between Men and Women." Oregon Counseling. Accessed July 12, 2012. www.oregoncounseling.org.
Emson, H. E. "Health, Disease and Illness: Matters for Definition." *Canadian Medical Association Journal* 136, no. 8 (1987): 811–13.
Foster, S. "Structure and Function of Joints." Raw Food Explained. Accessed May 26, 2012. www.rawfoodexplained.com.
Gronowicz, A. *Béla Schick and the World of Children.* London: Abelard-Schuman, 1954.
Gunn, C. *Bones and Joints: A Guide for Students.* Atlanta, GA: Elsevier Health Sciences, 2002.
Katzenberg, A. M., and S. R. Saunders. *Biological Anthropology of the Human Skeleton.* Hoboken, NJ: John Wiley and Sons, 2011.
Lehman, T. J. *It's Not Just Growing Pains: A Guide to Childhood Muscle, Bone, and Joint Pain, Rheumatic Diseases, and the Latest Treatments.* New York: Oxford University Press, 2004.
Rosen, G. *A History of Public Health.* Baltimore: Johns Hopkins University Press, 1993.
Sayler, M. H. *The Encyclopedia of the Muscle and Skeletal Systems and Disorders.* New York: Infobase Publishing, 2005.
Schienberg, L. "More Than Skin Deep: The Scientific Search for Sexual Difference." In *The Mind Has No Sex*, 189–213. Cambridge, MA: Harvard University Press, 1991.
Schneider, M.-J. *Introduction to Public Health.* Burlington, MA: Jones and Bartlett Learning, 2010.
Schutkowski, H. "Sex Determination of Infant and Juvenile Skeletons: I. Morphognostic Features." *American Journal of Physical Anthropology* 90, no. 2 (1993): 199–205.
Smith, H. "Dinosaurs Suffered from Painful Arthritis, Say Scientists." Metro. May 15, 2012. Accessed May 16, 2012. www.metro.co.uk.
Steele, G. D., and C. A. Bramblett. *The Anatomy and Biology of the Human Skeleton.* College Station: Texas A&M University Press, 1988.
Thorpe, S. K., R. L. Holder, and R. H. Crompton. "Origin of Human Bipedalism as an Adaptation for Locomotion on Flexible Branches." *Science* 316, no. 5829 (2007): 1328–31.
Tulchinsky, T. H., and E. Varivikova. *The New Public Health.* Waltham, MA: Academic Press, 2009.
Turnock, B. J. *Public Health: What It Is and How It Works.* Burlington, MA: Jones and Bartlett Publishers, 2011.

Woolf, A. D., and B. Pfleger. "Burden of Major Musculoskeletal Conditions." *Bulletin of the World Health Organization* 81, no. 9 (2003): 646.

CHAPTER 3

Arthritis Foundation. "How to Care for Yourself." Accessed May 21, 2012. www.arthritis.org.
Coley, N. G. "Medical Chemists and the Origins of Clinical Chemistry in Britain (circa 1750–1850)." *Clinical Chemistry* 50, no. 5 (2004): 961–72.
Eustice, C. "How to Recognize the Signs and Symptoms of Arthritis." About.com. Updated January 15, 2012. Accessed June 16, 2012. www.arthritis.about.com.
Jupiter Infomedia. "History of Arthritis." 2008. India Netzone. Last updated March 10, 2009. Accessed June 28, 2012. www.indianetzone.com.
Shiel, W. C. "Ask the Experts: How Is Arthritis Diagnosed?." MedicineNet. Last editorial review November 29, 2006. Accessed May 17, 2012. www.medicinenet.com.
Soylent Communications. "Christiaan Barnard." Notable Names Database. Accessed July 14, 2012. www.nndb.com.

CHAPTER 4

Badeau, J. S., ed. *The Genius of Arab Civilization: Source of Renaissance.* 2nd ed. Cambridge, MA: MIT Press, 1983.
Bogduk, N., and L. Twomay. *Clinical Anatomy of the Lumbar Spine.* New York: Churchhill Livingstone, 1991.
Liebensen, C., ed. *Rehabilitation of the Spine: A Practitioner's Manual.* 2nd ed. Philadelphia: Lippincott, Williams, and Wilkins, 2007.
Nutton, V. "The Chronology of Galen's Early Career." *Classical Quarterly* 23, no. 1 (1973): 158–71.
Shealy, C. N., and P. Leroy. "New Concepts in Back Pain Management: Decompression, Reduction and Stabilization." In *Pain Management: A Practical Guide for Clinicians,* edited by R. Weiner, 239–57. Boca Raton, FL: St. Lucie Press, 1998.
Shiel, W. C. "Total Hip Replacement." MedicineNet. Accessed March 30, 2012. www.medicinenet.com.
Stevenson, D. C. "Works by Hippocrates." Massachusetts Institute of Technology Internet Classics Archive. Accessed June 26, 2012. www.classics.mit.edu.
Temkin, O. *Hippocrates in a World of Pagans and Christians.* Baltimore: Johns Hopkins University Press, 1991.

CHAPTER 5

Ahern, M., and M. Smith. "Rheumatoid Arthritis." *Medical Journal of Australia* 166 (1997): 88–161.
Gordon, M.-M., H. A. Capell, and R. Madhok. "Illiteracy in Rheumatoid Arthritis Patients as Determined by the Rapid Estimate of Literacy in Medicine (REALM) Score." *Rheumatology* 41 (2002): 750–54.
Harris, E., R. Budd, G. Firestein, M. Genovese, J. Sergent, S. Ruddy, and C. Sledge, eds. *Kelley's Textbook of Rheumatology.* Vol. 2. 8th ed. Philadelphia: Saunders Elsevier, 2004.
Koopman, W. J. *Arthritis and Allied Conditions: A Textbook of Rheumatology.* Philadelphia: Lippincott, Williams, and Wilkins, 1997.
Pincus, T. "Rheumatoid Arthritis: A Medical Emergency?." *Scandinavian Journal of Rheumatology* 100 (1994): 5–30.
Rodriguez, D. "Lifestyle Changes to Manage Arthritis Pain." Everyday Health. Accessed April 29, 2012. www.everydayhealth.com.

Silman, A. J., J. Newman, and A. J. MacGregor. "Cigarette Smoking Increases the Risk of Rheumatoid Arthritis: Results from a Nationwide Study of Disease-Discordant Twins." *Arthritis Rheumatology* 39 (1996): 732–35.

Warburton, D., C. W. Nicol, and S. S. Bredin. "Health Benefits of Physical Activity: The Evidence." *Canadian Medical Association Journal* 174, no. 6 (2006): 801–9.

CHAPTER 6

Harris, E., R. Budd, G. Firestein, M. Genovese, J. Sergent, S. Ruddy, and C. Sledge, eds. *Kelley's Textbook of Rheumatology.* Vol. 2. 8th ed. Philadelphia: Saunders Elsevier, 2004.

Koopman, W. J. *Arthritis and Allied Conditions: A Textbook of Rheumatology.* Philadelphia: Lippincott, Williams, and Wilkins, 1997.

Wolfe, F., and D. J. Hawley. "Remission in Rheumatoid Arthritis." *Journal of Rheumatology* 2 (1985): 245–52.

Wolfe, F., K. Ross, D. J. Hawley, F. K. Roberts, and M. A. Cathey. "The Prognosis of Rheumatoid Arthritis and Undifferentiated Polyarthritis Syndrome in the Clinic: A Study of 1141 patients." *Journal of Rheumatology* 12 (2005): 123–66.

CHAPTER 7

American Academy of Orthopedic Surgeons. "Questions to Ask Your Surgeon before Surgery." Accessed July 5, 2012. www.orthoinfo.aaos.org.

Cooper, N. J. "Economic Burden of Rheumatoid Arthritis: A Systematic Review." *Rheumatology* 39 (2000): 28–33.

Gold, S. *The Patient's Guide to Orthopedic Surgery.* Torrance, CA: Stuart M. Gold, 2010.

Harris, E., R. Budd, G. Firestein, M. Genovese, J. Sergent, S. Ruddy, and C. Sledge, eds. *Kelley's Textbook of Rheumatology.* Vol. 2. 8th ed. Philadelphia: Saunders Elsevier, 2004.

Hochberg, M. C., A. J. Silman, J. S. Smolen, M. E. Weinblatt, and M. H. Weisman, eds. *Rheumatology.* 3rd ed. New York: Mosby 2003.

Laskey, J. "Arthritis Questions to Ask Your Doctor." Everyday Health. Accessed June 27, 2012. www.everydayhealth.com.

National Institute of Arthritis and Musculoskeletal and Skin Diseases (NIAMS). "Questions and Answers about Arthritis and Rheumatic Diseases." Accessed April 30, 2012. www.niams.nih.gov.

Poznanski, A. K. "Radiological Approaches to Pediatric Joint Disease." *Journal of Rheumatology* 33 (1992): 78–93.

Quinn, C., and L. Greenbaum. *100 Questions and Answers about Arthritis.* Burlington, MA: Jones and Bartlett Publishers, 2007.

Siegfried, D., and D. Ray. "Calling All Rheumatologists." Arthritis Today. Accessed July 23, 2012. www.arthritistoday.org.

Wiesel, S. W., and J. N. Delahay. *Essentials of Orthopedic Surgery.* New York: Springer, 2010.

CHAPTER 8

Bizzaro, N., G. Mazzanti, E. Tonutti, R. Tozzoli, and D. Villalta. "Diagnostic Accuracy of the Anti-citrulline Antibody Assay for Rheumatoid Arthritis." *Clinical Chemistry* 47 (2001): 1089–93.

Gregersen, P. K., J. Silver, and R. J. Winchester. "The Shared Epitope Hypothesis: An Approach to Understanding the Molecular Genetics of Rheumatoid Arthritis Susceptibility." *Arthritis and Rheumatism* 30 (1987): 1205–13.

Thomas, T. F. *Conquering Rheumatoid Arthritis: The Latest Breakthroughs and Treatments.* New York: Prometheus Books, 2001.

CHAPTER 9

Arthritis Foundation. "Juvenile Rheumatoid Arthritis." Accessed May 24, 2012. www.arthritis.org.

Mayo Clinic. "Juvenile Rheumatoid Arthritis." Last modified October 20, 2011. Accessed May 14, 2012. www.mayoclinic.com.

Royal Australian College of General Practitioners, National Health and Medical Research Council (Australia). *Clinical Guideline for the Diagnosis and Management of Juvenile Idiopathic Arthritis.* Melbourne, Victoria: Royal Australian College of General Practitioners, 2009.

CHAPTER 10

Arthritis Foundation. "Osteoarthritis." Accessed May 24, 2012. www.arthritis.org.

Arthritis Today. "All about Osteoarthritis." Accessed May 24, 2012. www.arthritistoday.org.

Mayo Clinic. "Osteoarthritis." Last modified October 13, 2011. Accessed May 23, 2012. www.mayoclinic.com.

Srikulmontree, T. "Osteoarthritis." American College of Rheumatology. Last modified February 2012. Accessed May 13, 2012. www.rheumatology.org.

CHAPTER 11

American Academy of Dermatology. "What Is Psoriasis?." Last updated February 17, 2012. Accessed May 24, 2012. www.skincarephysicians.com.

Fitzgerald, O. "Psoriatic Arthritis." In *Kelley's Textbook of Rheumatology*, edited by E. Harris, R. Budd, G. Firestein, M. Genovese, J. Sergent, S. Ruddy, and C. Sledge. 8th ed. Philadelphia: W. B. Saunders Co., 2008.

Gladman, D. D. "Clinical Manifestations and Diagnosis of Psoriatic Arthritis." UpToDate. Accessed June 19, 2012. www.uptodate.com.

Mercier, L. R. "Arthritis, Psoriatic." In *Ferri's Clinical Advisor 2011*, edited by F. F. Ferri. Philadelphia: Mosby Elsevier, 2010.

National Psoriasis Foundation. "Psoriatic Arthritis." Accessed May 24, 2012. www.psoriasis.org.

CHAPTER 12

Keat, A. "Reiter's Syndrome and Reactive Arthritis in Perspective." *New England Journal of Medicine* 309 (1983): 1606–15.

Kvien, T. K., A. Glennås, K. Melby, K. Granfors, O. Andrup, B. Karstensen, and J. E. Thoen. "Reactive Arthritis: Incidence, Triggering Agents and Clinical Presentation." *Journal of Rheumatology* 21, no. 1 (1994): 115–22.

Reece, R. J., J. D. Canete, W. J. Parsons, P. Emery, and D. J. Veale. "Distinct Vascular Patterns of Early Synovitis in Psoriatic, Reactive, and Rheumatoid Arthritis." *Arthritis and Rheumatism* 42, no. 7 (1999): 1481–84.

CHAPTER 13

Bourikas, L. A., and K. A. Papadakis. "Musculoskeletal Manifestations of Inflammatory Bowel Disease." *Inflammatory Bowel Disease* 15, no. 12 (2009): 1915–24.

Chandran, V., and P. Rahman. "Update on the Genetics of Spondyloarthritis—Ankylosing Spondylitis and Psoriatic Arthritis." *Best Practice in Research and Clinical Rheumatology* 24, no. 5 (2010): 579–88.

Galbreath, C. "Arthritis Foundation Announces Top 10 Arthritis Advances of 2008." Arthritis Foundation. Accessed July 24, 2012. www.arthritis.org.

Kaufman, I., D. Caspi, D. Yeshurun, I. Dotan, M. Yaron, and O. Elkayam, "The Effect of Infliximab on Extraintestinal Manifestations of Crohn's Disease." Rheumatology International 25 (2005): 406–10.

Yüksel, I., H. Ataseven, O. Başar, S. Köklü, I. Ertuğrul, A. Ulker, U. Dağlı, and Saşmaz N. "Peripheral Arthritis in the Course of Inflammatory Bowel Diseases." *Digestive Diseases and Sciences* (2010) (published online ahead of print).

CHAPTER 14

Curth, H. O. "Recurrent Genito-oral Aphthosis with Hypopion (Behcet's Syndrome)." *Archives of Dermatology* 54 (1946): 179–96.

Franceschini, F., and I. Cavazzana. "Anti-Ro/SSA and La/SSB Antibodies." *Autoimmunity* 38, no. 1 (2005): 55–63.

Rapini, R. P., J. L. Bolognia, and J. L. Jorizzo. *Dermatology: 2-Volume Set.* St. Louis: Mosby, 2007.

CHAPTER 15

Arthritis Care. *Understanding Arthritis.* London: Arthritis Care, 2011.

Rizzo, T. H. "Ergonomic Workplace Tips." Arthritis Today. February 4, 2012. Accessed March 30, 2012. www.arthritistoday.org.

Rudd, R. E., E. K. Zobel, V. Gall, S. Ravven, and L. H. Daltroy. "Plain Talk about Arthritis and Key Words." Harvard School of Public Health. Accessed May 2, 2012. www.hsph.harvard.edu.

Shiel, W. C. "Arthritis." MedicineNet. Accessed April 28, 2012. www.medicinenet.com.

CHAPTER 16

American College of Rheumatology, section on "Medications." May 5, 2012. www.rheumatology.org.

National Health Service. "Rheumatoid Arthritis—Treatment." Last reviewed August 24, 2010. Accessed May 5, 2012. www.nhs.uk.

RxList. "The Internet Drug Index—A–Z Drug List." Accessed May 4, 2012. www.rxlist.com.

CHAPTER 17

Arthritis Foundation. "Benefits and Risks of Joint Replacement Surgery." Accessed May 19, 2012. www.arthritis.org.

Australian Rheumatology Association. *Patient Information on Hyaluronic Acid.* Melbourne: National Health and Medical Research Council, 2011.

WebMD. "Natural Treatments for Rheumatoid Arthritis." Accessed May 17, 2012. www.webmd.com.

———. "Vitamins & Supplements Center." Accessed May 18, 2012. www.webmd.com.

CHAPTER 18

Backman, C. L. "Arthritis and Pain: Psychological Aspects in the Management of Arthritis Pain." *Arthritis Research and Therapy* 8, no. 6 (2006): 221.

Delgado, J. L. *The Buena Salud Guide to Arthritis and Your Life.* New York: HarperCollins, 2012.

Sobel, D., and A. C. Klein. *Arthritis, What Exercises Work: Breakthrough Relief for the Rest of Your Life, Even After Drugs and Surgery Have Failed.* New York: St. Martin's Press, 1995.

CHAPTER 19

Goldberg, L. *The Healing Power of Exercise: Your Guide to Preventing and Treating Diabetes, Depression, Heart Disease, High Blood Pressure, Arthritis, and More.* New York: Wiley, 2000.

O'Driscoll, E. R. *Exercises for Arthritis: A Safe and Effective Way to Increase Strength, Improve Flexibility, Gain Energy, and Reduce Pain.* Southampton, NY: Hatherleigh Press, 2004.

Rama, S. *Exercises for Joints and Glands: Gentle Movements to Enhance Your Wellbeing.* Honesdale, PA: Himalayan Institute Press, 2007.

CHAPTER 20

Donahue, K. E., D. E. Jonas, R. A. Hansen, R. Roubey, B. Jonas, L. J. Lux, G. Gartlehner, E. Harden, T. Wilkins, V. Peravali, S. I. Bangdiwala, A. Yuen, P. Thieda, L. C. Morgan, K. Crotty, R. Desai, and M. Van Noord. *Drug Therapy for Rheumatoid Arthritis in Adults: An Update.* No. 12-EHC025-EF. Rockville, MD: Agency for Healthcare Research and Quality, 2012.

Meenan, R. F., P. M. Gertman, J. H. Mason, and R. Dunaif. "The Arthritis Impact Measurement Scales: Further Investigations of a Health Status Measure." *Arthritis and Rheumatism* 25 (1982): 1048–53.

Meenan, R. F., and T. Pincus. "The Status of Patient Status Measures." *Journal of Rheumatology* 14 (1987): 411–14.

CHAPTER 21

Centaur Communications. "Workplace Stress: Show Your Commitment." *Employee Benefits* (2008): S13.

Knittle, K. P., V. De Gucht, E. J. Hurkmans, T. P. Vlieland, A. J. Peeters, H. K. Ronday, and S. Maes. "Effect of Self-efficacy and Physical Activity Goal Achievement on Arthritis Pain and Quality of Life in Patients with Rheumatoid Arthritis." *Arthritis Care and Research* 63 (2011): 1613–19.

Schumann, I. "Motivation's Effect on Mental and Physical Health." Earthling Communication. Last modified April 25, 2012. Accessed July 23, 2012. www.earthlingcommunication.com.

CHAPTER 22

National Arthritis and Musculoskeletal Conditions Advisory Group (NAMSCAG). "Evidence to Support the National Action Plan for Osteoarthritis, Rheumatoid Arthritis and Osteoporosis: Opportunities to Improve Health-Related Quality of Life and Reduce the Burden of Disease and Disability." Accessed May 24, 2012. www.health.gov.au.

Patient Rheumatoid Arthritis Social Support Initiative. "Why Have a Peer Support Partner?." Accessed May 24, 2012. www.parassstudy.org.

Rao, J. K., R. Arick, K. Mihaliak, and M. Weinberger. "Using Focus Groups to Understand Arthritis Patients' Perceptions about Unconventional Therapy." *Arthritis Care and Research* 11, no. 4 (1998): 253–60.

CHAPTER 23: CONCLUSION

Martin, E., D. Russell, S. Goodwin, R. Chapman, and P. Sheridan. "Why Patients Consult and What Happens When They Do." *British Medical Journal* 303, no. 6797 (1991): 289–92.

Sullivan, K. "What to Do When Someone You Love Is Chronically Ill." Jigsaw Health. Accessed May 20, 2012. www.jigsawhealth.com.

Van de Kar, A., A. Knottnerus, R. Meertens, V. Dubois, and G. Kok. "Why Do Patients Consult the General Practitioner? Determinants of Their Decision." *British Journal of General Practice* 42, no. 361: 313–16.

Index

AAOS. *See* American Academy of Orthopedic Surgeons

acupuncture: as a technique, 150; at home, 249

Adamantiades-Behçet's disease, 327n14

adipocytes, 28

aerobic exercise: in a study, 330n6; in other water exercises, 243

AIDS, 187

alternative methods, 249

alternative treatment: as natural method of healing, 219; for relief of pain, 205; Methods, 249–250; option, 119

American Academy of Orthopedic Surgeons, 120

analgesics, 208; commonly prescribed, 207; help in inflammation, 177; quick relief, 208

anemia, 146, 149, 151; screening for, 182; in blood tests, 182; in Felty's syndrome, 192; Ankylosing spondylitis, 63, 136, 185, 317n18

anti-TNF. *See* anti-tumor necrosis factor agents

anti-tumor necrosis factor agents, 140

arthritis: acute, 11; anatomy and pathology, 57; benefits of treatment, 208; causes and symptoms, 75; chronic, 311n50; gouty, 11; history, 53; in infants, 251; infectious, 39; introduction, 3; juvenile rheumatoid, 143; pathology, 64;

psoriatic, 163; heumatoid, 10, 131, 311n36; role of nutrition, 224; signs and symptoms, 83, 84; swelling and inflammation in arthritis, 89; treatments, 207, 328n1

arthritis at home, 247–256; adolescents, 253; early detection in children, 247; mobility of joints for transfers, 247; schoolchildren, 252; significance, 247; toddlers, 251

arthritis mutilans, 165

arthritis pain, 107, 135, 209; deeper look on, 86; diminished fever in, 203; relief from corticosteroids, 207; types of, 87

arthrodesis surgical option, 228

arthrology: arthron, 11; history of, 4; medical knowledge, 5; not the science, 11; seek to raise awareness, 93

arthroplasty: demographics of procedures in, 123–124; on shoulders, 117; surgical options, 229; when medications do not work, 51

arthroscopy: degree of specialization, 122; demographics, 124; screening procedure, 100; surgical options, 228

australopithecus fossils, 24

autoimmune deficiency syndrome, 164

autoimmune disease: causes, 81; in relation with interleukin, 67; in rheumatoid arthritis, 163; may intervene with HLA, 65; on JRA, 145, 150; on psoriatic

About the Author

Naheed Ali, MD, began writing professionally in 2005 and later trained at the Harvard Medical School Continuing Medical Education program. He has taught at colleges in the United States and written several books on medical topics. Additional information is available at NaheedAli.com.